Alphabet
KIDS

of related interest

Kids in the Syndrome Mix of ADHD, LD, Asperger's, Tourette's, Bipolar and More!
The one stop guide for parents, teachers and other professionals
Martin L. Kutscher MD
With a contribution from Tony Attwood
With a contribution from Robert R Wolff MD
ISBN 978 1 84310 810 8 (hardback)
ISBN 978 1 84310 811 5 (paperback)

The Complete Guide to Asperger's Syndrome
Tony Attwood
ISBN 978 1 84310 495 7 (hardback)
ISBN 978 1 84310 669 2 (paperback)

Dietary Interventions in Autism Spectrum Disorders
Why They Work When They Do, Why They Don't When They Don't
Kenneth J. Aitken
ISBN 978 1 84310 939 6

ADHD – Living Without Brakes
Martin L. Kutscher MD
Illustrated by Douglas Puder, M.D.
ISBN 978 1 84310 873 3 (hardback)
ISBN 978 1 84310 816 2 (paperback)

"What a valuable resource to help parents find their way through the bewildering vocabulary of psychiatric labels. An easy-to-read, quick way in to what is known and how to get help. Books like *Alphabet Kids* are essential if we are to bridge the gap between professionals and families."

—*Professor Simon Baron-Cohen, Director, Autism Research Centre, Cambridge University*

"I wish I'd had Robbie Woliver's book to guide me in the early days of my journey with my daughter ...it provides valuable practical information and advice from a wide array of impressive experts that can very well make the difference in the quality of your child's life. *Alphabet Kids* should be in every household; it is an essential guide for all parents and should be required reading for all teachers."

—*Cathy Moriarty-Gentile, Academy award-nominated actress, child's health advocate, and parent of a daughter with special needs*

"Medical diagnosis and treatment is complex and overwhelming for many families... *Alphabet Kids*, does an excellent job of translating complex medical conditions and terminology into language that parents can understand. Filled with helpful and accessible information about numerous disabilities, it also provides a wealth of useful information on signs and symptoms for parents to watch for, the diagnostic process, treatment options, and prognoses and links to other resources. This is a tremendous resource for families and others that work with kids with disabilities."

—*Matthew Cohen, Adjunct Professor of Mental Health Law at Loyola University of Chicago School of Law, and author of* A Guide to Special Education Advocacy

"A necessity for every household! An invaluable reference tool for every pediatric specialist and educator. As our contemporary culture strives to increase knowledge, elevate awareness, and decreases the stigma of developmental, neurobiological, and psychological disorders, Robbie Woliver presents an incredibly comprehensive guide. *Alphabet Kids* impressively offers a range of relatable vignettes, relevant symptoms, and a wealth of helpful resources, providing clarity and answers...all in one, easy to read, positive and encouraging book!"

—*Dr. Kimberly Williams, Psy.D., Neuropsychologist, Assistant Research Scientist, NYU Child Study Center*

"I wish *Alphabet Kids* were available 18 years ago when those nagging questions were keeping my wife and I up nights. It would have led us in the right direction and resulted in needed early interventions. Insightful, informative and understandable. A must read for any parents losing sleep."

—Jeffrey Cohen, father of two children living with Fragile X Syndrome
and Chair Public Policy, National Fragile X Foundation

"When a child is struggling, parents worry. What's wrong? Whom do we see? Where do I find help? Thanks to Robbie Woliver, parents now have a comprehensive resource, *Alphabet Kids*, to help them help their child."

—Larry B. Silver, M.D., Clinical Professor of Psychiatry,
Georgetown University Medical Center, former acting director and deputy director of the National
Institute of Mental Health (NIMH), and author of The Misunderstood Child:
A Guide For Parents of Children With Learning Disabilities

"Robbie Woliver provides us with an encyclopedic overview of children's developmental and mental conditions. Weaving extensive research with personal empathy, he provides parents and practitioners with an extremely useful resource, as we work to identify and improve the life of children with special needs."

—Martin L. Kutscher, M.D., pediatric neurologist and author of Kids in the Syndrome
Mix of ADHD, LD, Asperger's, Tourette's, Bipolar and More!,
ADHD: Living without Brakes, *and* Children with Seizures

"*Alphabet Kids* will be very important because it describes a panoply of disorders ranging from physical to emotional, and hereditary, which have often been perceived as conduct disorders or conditions so unresolvable there is no help. This book will encourage both parents and professionals to use available tools and to make contributions that will further enhance the prognosis for so many."

—Vivian Hanson Meehan, president and founder of ANAD
(National Association of Anorexia Nervosa and Associated Disorders)

Alphabet KIDS

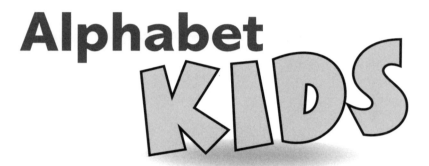

From ADD to Zellweger Syndrome

A Guide to Developmental, Neurobiological
and Psychological Disorders
for Parents and Professionals

Robbie Woliver

Jessica Kingsley Publishers
London and Philadelphia

First published in hardback in 2009
Paperback edition first published in 2010
by Jessica Kingsley Publishers
116 Pentonville Road
London N1 9JB, UK
and
400 Market Street, Suite 400
Philadelphia, PA 19106, USA

www.jkp.com

Disclaimer: The information in this book does not constitute medical advice, nor is it a substitute for discussion between patients and their doctors. Medical information and recommendations are often subject to debate and are likely to change over time. This material is not intended to be all-inclusive. Full discussion of the approved indications, usefulness, side effects, risks, monitoring, drug interactions, etc., of medications is beyond the scope of this book. Not all of the medications discussed in this text have U.S. Food and Drug Administration approval for use in children, or for some of the indications that they are commonly used for. Current detailed medication information can be found from many sources, including your doctor, the manufacturer's package insert and Web site, and the U.S. Food and Drug Administration Web site at www.FDA.gov.

Library of Congress Cataloging in Publication Data
Woliver, Robbie.
Alphabet kids : from ADD to Zellweger syndrome : a guide to developmental, neurobiological and psychological disorders for parents and professionals / Robbie Woliver.
  p. cm.
Includes bibliographical references and index.
  ISBN 978-1-84905-822-3 (pbk. : alk. paper) 1. Behavior disorders in children--Encyclopedias. 2. Neurobehavioral disorders--Encyclopedias. 3. Child development deviations--Encyclopedias. 4. Syndromes--Encyclopedias. 5. Diseases--Acronyms--Encyclopedias. I. Title.
RJ506.B44W65 2010
618.92'89003--dc22

                           2009048268

British Library Cataloguing in Publication Data
A CIP catalogue record for this book is available from the British Library

ISBN 978 1 84905 822 3

Printed and bound in the United States by
Thomson-Shore, 7300 Joy Road, Dexter, MI 48130

To Marilyn
and
our wonderfully fascinating children,
Cory and Emma, who inspired this book.

Contents

M

N

O

P

R

S

Acknowledgments

First and foremost, I want to thank Jessica Kingsley for creating, with Jessica Kingsley Publishers, an oasis for parents who are searching for answers. The books she publishes are ones that helped me in my own personal search, and I knew from the start that this was the right publishing company for *Alphabet Kids*. Jessica has been enthusiastic about this project from the moment it was brought to her and I'm appreciative of her knowledge, support, and mission.

Thanks to Jed Morey and the *Long Island Press* for giving me a platform to create the award-winning newspaper series "Our Children's Brains," which has become my obsession. Three of those stories (on APD, ASD, and OCD) are revised and included in this book, and two chapters of this book were revised and adapted for the series (ADHD and Asperger).

Thank you to April Jimenez for assistance on several of the "Brains" stories that ran in the *Press*; Mo Ibrahim for assistance on the APD "Brains" story; Annie Blachley, Michael Patrick Nelson, and Josh Stewart for their editing skills on the "Brains" series; and extra thanks to Annie and Michael for their editing assistance on additional chapters of this book. Michael Martino Jr. and Tim Bolger, two *Press* colleagues, have provided much support as well. I also appreciate the support of Autism United founder and *Spectrum* Magazine publisher Evelyn Ain, who is always able to get answers to any questions; Robert Rooney at Jessica Kingsley Publishers for being the first to support this project; Mary Lou Bertucci for her superb editing work; and Lisa Clark for overseeing the project so well.

And my dear friend Andree Abecassis of the Ann Elmo Literary Agency.

Many, many people provided information for this book:

Of great help to me in understanding the global picture of Alphabet Disorders was Temple Grandin, Ph.D., who provided me with insight into what it's like to live with autism; Larry B. Silver, M.D., expert in the field of attention-deficit/hyperactivity disorder and learning disabilities, for his professional and personal assistance, for his time both in person and on the phone, and for his indispensable book *The Misunderstood Child*; Ravi Sockalingam, Ph.D., senior lecturer at the University of Canterbury, New Zealand, for his overview of auditory processing disorders—it was inspiring to learn about his life's work with indigenous people around the world; Aina-Nelago iimbili, a Namibian psychologist and neurotherapist, who provided extraordinary insight into childhood disabilities in Africa, as she currently struggles to gain funding to open a clinic for these children; and Sabine Naessén, M.D., Ph.D., an expert on eating disorders, who provided a very thorough global view of eating disorders.

For more inspiration, it's hard to beat the daily battles of Guillermo Tyberg and his daughter Daniela, who has Tourette syndrome among numerous other disorders, and Guillermo's global perspective living in various countries such as Israel and Argentina; Sean Partington, who lives near Toronto with his wife and their three children, who all have Alphabet Disorders; Vicki Hodgson-Brown, manager of Aboriginal Services Unit Disability Services SA, Department for Families and Communities, an aboriginal woman from Australia whose children are afflicted with many Alphabet Disorders from autism to panic disorder. She needed permission from the aboriginal elders before she could discuss her story with me, and I thank them for letting her share her moving and cautionary story; Rekha Ramachandran, Ph.D., president of the Down Syndrome Federation of India, where one in 750 live births results in Down, a syndrome her 21-year-old daughter Babli has lived with and persevered through. Rekha is a specialist in depression and Down syndrome. Unfortunately, I couldn't tell all their stories, but the information imparted was invaluable to the book and inspiring. The list just goes on and on.

The following people provided immeasurable help, whether it was through interviews, permission to use previously published quotes, excerpts from their books, or results of their studies. Most importantly, I want to thank the parents from around the world who graciously shared their stories about their own unique Alphabet Kids.

Thank you, all of the following: Oddvar Aamdal, Norway; Evelyn Ain, Autism United and Spectrum Publications; Carrie Allison, Autism Research Centre, Department of Psychiatry, University of Cambridge, Douglas House, U.K.; American Psychiatric Association (APA); American Speech-Language-Hearing Association (ASHA); Angelman Syndrome Foundation; Anxiety Disorders Association of America; The Arc of the United States; Attention Deficit Disorder Association (ADDA); Dr. Joseph Attias, Schneider Children's Hospital, Israel; Tony Attwood, M.Sc., Ph.D., AFBPsS, MAPS, MCCP, associate professor, Griffith University, Queensland, Australia; Anna Baldursdóttir, communication officer, UNICEF Iceland; Warren Barlowe, Long Island OCD Support Network (LIOCDSN); Patty Romanowski Bashe, MS.Ed.; Fred Baughman, M.D., neurologist; Associate Professor Annette Beautrais, Ph.D., principal investigator, Canterbury Suicide Project, Christchurch School of Medicine, Christchurch, New Zealand; Cindy Beles, triage advocate, Prader-Willi Association; Teri James Bellis, Ph.D., chairperson, Department of Communication Disorders, University of South Dakota, and chairperson, ASHA Working Group on APD; Oded Ben-Arush, Psy.D., clinical director, Israeli Center for the Treatment of Obsessive-Compulsive Disorders, Moshav Mesilat Zion, Israel; Will Beswick, www.DoYouPanic.co.uk; Sigrún Birgisdottir, manager, Icelandic Autistic Society, and her daughter Eydís; Eric Bixel, French Association for Cockayne Patients, and his son Baptiste; Robert Bock, National Institutes of Health; Dr. Jeff Bradstreet, founder, International Child Development Resource Center, Florida; *British Journal of Psychiatry*; Robert Budd, chief administrative officer, Family Residences and Essential Enterprises, Inc. (FREE), Long Island, New York; Richard Budnyj, secretary, FOLKS–Friends of Landau-Kleffner

Syndrome, U.K.; Elizabeth Burns, vice president, Tourette Syndrome Association of Australia; Dr. Ioav Cabantchik, professor, head, Life Sciences Institute, Hebrew University of Jerusalem, Israel; Haylee and Tim Carroll and their children Ian, Eden, and Gage; Centers for Disease Control and Prevention (CDC); Childhood Apraxia of Speech Association of North America (CASANA); Children's Hospital Boston; Vanessa Christian; Margarette Christie, director, Cri du Chat Support Group of Australia (CDCSA), and her daughter Mindy; Jackie Clark, president and executive director, Share and Care Cockayne Syndrome Network; Monica Coenraads, Rett Syndrome Research Foundation; Coffin-Lowry Syndrome Foundation (CLSF); Arlene Cohen, Fragile X Foundation, and her children Joshua and Allison Cohen; Melissa Cohen; Tracy Colletti-Flynn, Tourette Syndrome Association; Barrie and Alastair Cooper, National Autistic Society, Scotland; Robert Cooper, founder, AD/HD Foundation of Canada; Cornelia de Lange Syndrome Foundation/USA; Jean Cottraux, M.D., Ph.D., Anxiety Disorder Unit, Hospital Neurologique, Lyon, France; Hilary Craig, B.A., B.Ed., M.Ed., Davis Dyslexia Facilitator, HILS Services, Kuala Lumpur, Malaysia; Andrew Cuddy, Esq., author of *The Special Education Battlefield*; Dr. Christopher Cunniff, Arizona CDC Autism Study; Professor Alfred Cuschieri, Department of Anatomy, University of Malta; Tony Daranyi and his daughter Ali; Michelle Darwin, director, Ehlers-Danlos National Foundation (EDNF), and her daughter Nikki; Omaida De Frias, Policentro de Salud de Juan Díaz, Miniserio de Salud, Panamá, República de Panamá; Gary S. Dell, Ph.D., professor, Psychology, University of Illinois at Urbana-Champaign; Pamela de Witt, Hearing Service executive, Cork, Ireland; Petra Dillman, Autism Namibia; Richard Downing; Sharon Downs, Cloud 9 Children's Foundation (Asperger), New Zealand; Pat Dreibelbis, director, Program Services, Charcot-Marie-Tooth Association (CMTA); Maureen Durkin, Ph.D., epidemiologist, University of Wisconsin; V. Eapen, Ph.D., FRCPsych, professor of Child Psychiatry, Faculty of Medicine and Health Sciences, Al Ain, United Arab Emirates; Dr. Carlo Faravelli, professor of Psychiatry, Department of Neurology and Psychiatry, Florence University, Italy; Heather Flaharty and her son Caleb; Michele Foster, National Eating Disorder Information Centre (NEDIC), Toronto, Ontario, Canada; Dr. Roger D. Freeman, clinical head, Neuropsychiatry Clinic, British Columbia, Children's Hospital, Vancouver, BC; French Cockayne Association; Ellayne S. Ganzfried, M.S., CCC-SLP, executive director, National Aphasia Association; Dr. Miriam Gatt, principal medical officer, Department of Health Information, Malta; Dr. Ellen Giarelli, co-investigator, Pennsylvania CDC Autism Study; Charles Giglio, president, Learning Disabilities Association of America (LDA); Cynthia Gold, president, Smith-Lemli-Opitz/RSH Foundation; Temple Grandin, Ph.D., professor, Animal Science, Colorado State University; Arwa El Amin Halawi, president, Lebanese Autism Society; Karen Hamman and her daughter Nika Louise, Namibia; Cynthia Harding, Autistic Unit, Browns' School; Steven Harulow, communications manager, Royal College of Speech and Language Therapists (RCSLT), U.K.; Maha Helali, Advance, Egypt, and her son Mostafa; Melanie Herzfeld, Au.D., audiologist, Woodbury, NY; Dr. Paul Hubert, national director, Autism Netherlands; Kathy Hunter, parent, founder, president, and director of Family Support, International Rett Syndrome Foundation; Hala T. Ibrahim, special education educator, Jordan; Marie Insulander, psychologist, Kognitivt Forum, Gothenburg, Sweden; International Dyslexia Association (IDA); Dr. Sujatha Jagadeesh, consultant geneticist and paediatric dysmorphologist, Fetal Care Research Foundation, Chennai, India; Hema Jairam and Gita, We Can Trust Autism Resource Center, Chennai, India; Dr. Michael Johnson, University of Illinois Medical Center; Jack Katz, Ph.D., audiologist and Advisory Board member, National Association of Future Doctors of Audiology (NAFDA); Alan Kazdin, Ph.D., Yale Parenting Center and Child Conduct Clinic; Roy Keenan, *Bamford Review of Mental Health and Learning Disabilities*, N. Ireland; Andrea S. Kelly, Ph.D., lecturer, University of Auckland, Faculty of Medical and Health Sciences, Section of Audiology; Colleta G. Kibassa, M.D., UNICEF, Zimbabwe; Barbara Kirby, OASIS; Susan Koniak, Esq.; Pirjo Korpilahti, professor of Logopedics, University of Turku, Finland; Robert J. Krakow, Esq., A-CHAMP; Marianne Kuzemtshenko, Autism, Estonia; Dr. Siu-Man LAM, senior medical officer, Child and Adolescent Psychiatric Team, Castle Peak Hospital, Hong Kong; Cindy Lauren, Ehlers-Danlos National Foundation (EDNF); Learning Disabilities Association of America; Lesch-Nyhan Disease Registry (LNDR), New York University School of Medicine; Dr. Florence Levy, University of New South Wales, Australia; Pina LoGiudice, N.D., naturopath, Syosset, New York; Deborah Lott; Jay Lucker, Ed.D., director and founder, National Coalition on Auditory Processing Disorders (NCAPD), Inc.; Brendan A. Maher, Ph.D.; Marie Concklin Malloy, Cornelia de Lange Syndrome Foundation; Riddhima Manek, behavior therapist, Ummeed Child Development Centre, Mubai, India; Courtney E. Martin, Ehlers-Danlos National Foundation (EDNF); The Mayo Clinic, Rochester, Minnesota; Patricia McDowell and Gary Maxwell, Northern Ireland Statistics and Research Agency (NISRA), Community Information Branch, Department of Health, Social Service and Public Safety; Alex Melrose, New Zealand ADHD Organization; Liisa Miettinen, speech-language therapist, Riihimäki Health Center, Finland; Anisa Missaghi, UNICEF, Finland; Michelle Mitchell; Marthese Mugliette, chairperson, Down Syndrome Association, Malta; Muscular Dystrophy Association; Brenda Smith Myles, Ph.D., associate professor, University of Kansas; Sabine Naessén, M.D., Ph.D., senior consulting doctor in Obstetrics and Gynecology, Karolinska University Hospital, Stockholm, Sweden; Michiko Nagashima, UNICEF Tokyo, Japan; Abigail Natenshon, MA, LCSW, GCFP, psychotherapist; National Alliance on Mental Illness (NAMI); National Association for Down Syndrome (NADS); National Attention Deficit Disorder Information and Support Service (ADDISS); National Autistic Society (NAS); National Center for Learning Disabilities (NCLD); National Dissemination Center for Children with Disabilities (NICHCY); National Down Syndrome Society (NDSS); National Eating Disorders Association (NEDA); National Institute of Mental Health (NIMH); National Institute of Neurological Disorders and Stroke (NINDS); National Institute on Deafness and Other Communication Disorders

(NIDOCD); National Institutes of Health (NIH); National Joint Committee on Learning Disabilities (NJCLD); Nemours Foundation; Fugen Neziroglu, Ph.D., clinical director, Bio-Behavioral Institute, Great Neck, New York; Shana Nichols, Ph.D., Fay J. Lindner Center for Autism and Developmental Disorders, Bethpage, New York; Eva Naputuni Nyoike, director, Acorn Special Tutorials, National Autistic Center, Kenya; Christopher Jon Olesch; Roberto Olivardia, Ph.D., clinical instructor, Harvard Medical School; Dr. John M. Opitz; Ian Osborn, M.D., psychiatrist, Penn State University; Elizabeth Ouellette and her son Yohan; Kathleen Page, M.A., pediatric audiologist, Hearing Education, Assessment and Related Services (H.E.A.R.S.), Smithtown, New York; Siobhan Parker, St. John of God Hospitaller Services, Dublin, Ireland; Sean Partington, Canada; Judith W. Paton, M.A., audiologist, San Mateo, California; Penn State Children's Hospital; Fred Penzel, Ph.D.; Professor Alan K. Percy, M.D., scientific director, International Rett Syndrome Association; Patricia Perkins, co-founder, executive director, Obsessive-Compulsive Foundation (OCF); Sydney Pettygrove, Ph.D., epidemiologist, co-investigator, Arizona CDC Autism Study; Peter Pierri, executive director, Developmental Disabilities Institute (DDI), Smithtown, New York; Anita Pilika, psychiatrist, National Center for Growth, Development and Rehabilitation of Children (NCGDRCH), Tirana, Albania; Donna Pincus, Ph.D., director, Child and Adolescent Fear and Anxiety Treatment Program at Boston University; Dr. Theresa Pitt, Aud.D., F.S.H.A.A., Audiology Services, Wexford, Ireland; Craig Polhemus, executive director, Prader-Willi Foundation; Prader-Willi Alliance; PRISMS (Parents and Researchers Interested in Smith-Magenis Syndrome); *Psychiatric Times*; *Psychology Today*; Patricia Quinn, M.D., director, National Center for Gender Issues and ADHD; Dr. See King Emilio Quinto, psychiatrist, associate professor of Psychiatry, San Carlos and Francisco Marroquín Universities, associate professor of Cognitive Psychotherapy, Galileo University of Guatemala, School of Family Therapy and Counseling, clinical director of Centro de Terapia Cognitiva-SIAD, Guatemala; Don Ralbovsky, Office of Communications, NIH; Rekha Ramachandran, Ph.D., president, Down Syndrome Federation of India, and her daughter Babli; Ronald M. Rapee, Ph.D., professor, Department of Psychology, director, Centre for Emotional Health, Macquarie University, Sydney, Australia; Veronika Raudsalu, president of Estonian Logopedists Union, Estonia; Rett Syndrome Research Foundation; Rotary Club of Santa Monica/ Center for Healthy Aging; Byron P. Rourke, Ph.D., FRSC, Department of Psychology, University of Windsor, Canada; Katya Rubia, Ph.D., child psychiatrist, Institute of Psychiatry, Denmark Hill, affiliated with King's College in London, U.K.; Sheila Daly Russo, M.Ed./CCC-SLP, and David W. Bailey, M.D., Early Intervention Program, University of Florida Health Science Center; Dr. Yoichi Sakakihara, Department of Child Care and Education, Research Center for Child and Adolescent Development and Education, Ochanomizu University, Tokyo, Japan; Kerrylea Sampson, group facilitator and peer support coordinator, Social Phobia Support Group, Joint Anxiety Disorders Group, Christchurch, N.Z.; Ayadil Saparbekov, Health and Nutrition Officer, UNICEF,

Ashkhabad, Turkmenistan; Dr. Kurtis Sauder and Zachary Sauder; Pia Savage; Richard Schloss, M.D.; Caryl Schonbrun; *The Scientist*; Sensory Processing Disorder Foundation; Sensory Processing Disorder Resource Center; Larry B. Silver, M.D., child and adolescent psychiatrist, clinical professor, psychiatry, Georgetown Medical Center, Washington, D.C., and former acting director and deputy director, NIMH; Nidhal Singhal, Action For Autism/India; Jari Sinkkonen, Finland; Jennifer L. Smart, Ph.D., postdoctoral research fellow, University of Auckland, Department of Psychology, Discipline of Speech Science and Faculty of Medical and Health Sciences, Section of Audiology; Dr. John So, psychiatrist, Hong Kong; Rita Serpa Soares, psychologist, APPDA-Lisbon, Associação Portuguesa para as erturbações do Desenvolvimento e Autismo (Portuguese Association for the Development and Disorders of Autism); Bodil Solberg, child and youth psychiatrist, cognitive therapist, and supervisor, Region Centre, Oslo, Norway; Marie Soskova-Campion, Marino Therapy Centre, Dublin, Ireland; Jill Stacey, Autism South Africa; John Stack, Marino Therapy Centre, Dublin, Ireland; Debbie Staveley, Indigenous Psychological Services, East Victoria Park, Western Australia; Dr. Robert D. Steiner, professor, Pediatrics and Molecular and Medical Genetics, vice chair, Research, Department of Pediatrics, Deputy Director, Oregon Clinical and Translational Research Institute, Doernbecher Children's Hospital, Oregon Health and Science University; Dr. Anne Stewart, Oxfordshire and Buckinghamshire Mental Health Partnership NHS, U.K.; Andrea Stolz; Sheila and John Hudson Symons; Dr. Ariel Tenenbaum, director, Down Syndrome Medical Center, Hadassah Mt. Scopus University Medical Center, Jerusalem, Israel; Ellenmorris Tiegerman, Ph.D., director, founder, School for Language and Communication Development, Glen Cove, New York; Jana, Dave, and Kaitlyn Tovey; Dr. Nikki Turner, director, Immunisation Advisory Centre Senior Lecturer, University of Auckland, New Zealand; Guillermo Tyberg and his daughter Daniela, Argentina; UNICEF; UNICEF Malaysia; Dr. Jim Vacca, department chair of Special Education and Literacy, C.W. Post College, Greenvale, New York; Priscilla L. Vail, M.A.T., educator; Professor Dr. Rutger Jan van der Gaag, Radboud University Nijmegen Medical Center, Karakter University Center, Child and Adolescent Psychiatry, the Netherlands; Dr. David Veale, president of the British Association for Behavioural and Cognitive Psychotherapies, U.K.; Melissa Barnes Walker and her son Jacob; Huei-Shyong Wang, M.D., Division of Pediatric Neurology, Chang Gung Children's Hospital, Taiwan, president, Taiwan Tourette Family Association; Rosie Wartecker, executive director, Tourette Syndrome Foundation of Canada; We Move; Diane Whiteoak, hospital manager, The Huntercombe Hospital, Edinburgh, Scotland; Professor Ingvard Wilhelmsen, Institute of Medicine, University of Bergen Haraldsplass Deaconal Hospital, Bergen, Germany; Sheri Woliver-Jones, Esq.; Shirley Woliver, Doug and Patti Wood, Grassroots Environmental Education; World Health Organization; Yvonne Wren, research speech and language therapist, Speech and Language Therapy Research Unit, Frenchay Hospital, Bristol, U.K.; The Yale Developmental Disabilities Clinic; Dr. Yushiro Yamashita, professor of Pediatrics, Kurume University; Marshalyn Yeargin-Allsopp, M.D., neurobiologist, chief, CDC Autism Program; William Yule, Ph.D., emeritus professor, Applied Child Psychology, King's College London Institute of Psychiatry, U.K.; Dr. Kathryn Zerbe, Menninger Clinic; Jon-Kar Zubieta, M.D., Ph.D., Mental Health Research Institute, University of Michigan; and Jen and Jane Zwilling, and hundreds of others around the world who answered a question or two or took the time to refer me to someone else. This has been an amazing adventure.

Introduction

One in six.

That's how many children are estimated to have special needs due to what I refer to as Alphabet Disorders: those interconnected neurobiological, developmental, and genetic illnesses that are rising in prevalence. With language-based disabilities alone, it has been estimated that up to 20 percent of the population is affected. In some studies, the rate for autism is as high as one in ninety-four. Anxiety, eating, and mood disorders are growing at alarming rates.

That is an extraordinary number—one in six—and many in the know believe that statistic is too low. Experts such as Patti Wood, executive director of Grassroots Environmental Education, think that startlingly high statistic does not accurately reflect the actual frequency of these disorders in children. "I truly believe that is a conservative number," Wood says, "especially because there are so many undiagnosed cases, and it's an old [Centers for Disease Control] statistic." She believes it is closer to one in four.

Think about it: one out of every four—or even six, for that matter—children have some sort of physical, developmental, or mental-health disorder. Add to that the new kind of spelling bee that has become an unfortunate international phenomenon—one that has stung a whole generation of children. You know the kind of child affected by this affliction; he or she is the kid who has multiple alphabetic diagnoses: ADHD, OCD, ODD, ASD, APD, SAD, COS, PDD, SID … There are millions of these Alphabet Kids plagued by clusters of these disorders.

While more and more children are being diagnosed—along with millions of adults who have suffered quietly for their entire lives with these same, often inherited, disorders—many others go undiagnosed or misdiagnosed. Sometimes one diagnosis is treated and another one that was not attended to reveals itself. These disorders are often genetic, so, for some adults, it is not until their own children are diagnosed that they themselves receive a too-little, too-late diagnosis. Many of these are spectrum disorders, and as the spectrum stretches, so does the prevalence number. Of course, statistics rise because of growing awareness, ongoing strides in research, and improved diagnosis techniques. It is also believed that, because so many Alphabet Kids have not yet even been incorporated into published studies or are just beginning to be included, the rates will rise even more dramatically.

Alphabet Disorders are usually not singular, autonomous ailments; they are often concurrent with each other. They are *comorbid*—existing together simultaneously—and the mix makes for significant trouble. It is becoming more and more common for a child to be diagnosed with any combination of these disorders.

Many parents are desperately trying to get a handle on what exactly is wrong with their child, whether it is a life-threatening genetic disease, a complex and considerable disability, or just "quirky" behavior that negatively impacts some aspect of the child's wellbeing. The situation is not black and white for those parents with children who are Alphabet Kids. The symptoms often blend into each other, or one might mimic another. These parents often have only rigid official criteria to follow, yet what might seem like autism to a parent might not be officially diagnosed as such because one of the main ASD (autism spectrum disorder) criteria isn't apparent or might be overshadowed by another symptom of a secondary disorder. A child's condition might seem like TS (Tourette syndrome) to the parent, but the cough he has might not be recognized as a vocal tic by the doctor, so a crucial element of the TS diagnosis would be lost. The child might not seem to be paying attention—but is it APD (auditory processing disorder) or ADHD (attention-deficit/hyperactivity disorder)? Or both? A child just might seem a bit "off," exhibiting symptoms from various disorders—pragmatic speech problems, repetitive behavior, clumsiness, anxiety, noise and tactile sensitivity, always asking "What?," exhibiting a slight tic, not being able to follow directions, exhibiting obsessions and compulsions, inability to maintain proper friendships—how many of you are shaking your heads now thinking, "That's my kid"?

Often the parents' gut feelings are correct—they know something is wrong—but they are intimidated into submission by medical professionals until, unfortunately, the condition exacerbates into something more serious. That's bad news because, for almost all Alphabet Kids, early intervention is the key to success.

The purpose of this book is to serve as a resource and guide for parents as they journey through the muddle of symptoms and possible diagnoses when they suspect something is wrong with their child. In easy-to-understand language, *Alphabet Kids* is a comprehensive, go-to guide that will provide a helpful set of signposts for parents to follow as they attempt to understand their child and fight for the proper diagnosis and treatment. One particular element that I hope proves useful for anyone searching for answers regarding Alphabet Kids is the extensive symptoms list in each chapter. This is the exact type of guide that would have proved so valuable to me when I began my personal journey with my own Alphabet Kids, which started twenty years ago. In effect, this book has been in research mode for the past two decades.

Alphabet Kids is *not* a medical text. Anything parents read here that might spark a light of recognition in them should be taken up with medical experts. This book will not provide parents with an official diagnosis for their child, but it can serve as a roadmap, providing parents with possible destinations that can be further researched so that the parent can become as well-informed as possible when visiting the medical specialists.

Alphabet Kids is not only geared to help parents and their young child, it will aid those older children who missed out on early intervention, those teenagers who are first being diagnosed, and even adults who struggle with undetected disorders in silence. And then there are those who are outgrowing their initial diagnoses and growing into new ones.

This book will also indicate where these Alphabet Disorders intersect. The reason doctors, educators, and parents are having so much trouble with accurate diagnoses is that Alphabet Kids' disorders cluster, blend, or, as is too often the case, have only one of the many concurrent problems attended to. With some disorders mimicking or being overshadowed by others, the child is still impacted by hidden or unnoticed disorders, and therein rests many unaddressed problems.

But what about overdiagnosing? Does every symptom have to lead to a disorder? It seems as if every child is suddenly being labeled and, in some cases, people complain and fear that these children are being unnecessarily overdiagnosed. There seems to be an Alphabet Disorder for almost every behavior, from those caused by serious, rare genetic diseases to more common LDs (learning disabilities) that hinder our children's academic and social progress, and even to what seems like normal, everyday behaviors. There are the colorfully named disorders such as CCS (clumsy child syndrome), HPS (happy puppet syndrome, listed in this book as AS, Angelman syndrome), and CDC (cri du chat [cry of the cat] syndrome), along with more-to-the-point ODD (oppositional defiant disorder) and SAD (separation anxiety disorder).

Sometimes it feels as if every type of behavior has a disorder attached to it. Years ago, when I first announced my intentions about writing a book about Alphabet Kids, my young daughter, Emma, joked that she would contribute a disorder for her then-annoying teenaged brother Cory: TNT, or explosive personality disorder. "Great joke," I told her.

Then, as I began researching this project, what behavioral disorder do I come across in medical literature? EPD—explosive personality disorder.

Inattention, defiant behavior, feeling blue, clumsiness—they all sound like common behaviors. The key, however, to these conditions and all Alphabet Disorders is that, when a behavior starts to have a negative impact on the child's functioning and wellbeing in different areas of daily life (home, school, and social interaction), it becomes a serious problem—a clinical disorder, one with strict diagnostic criteria—and not just a troublesome personality trait or a superficial label.

When diagnoses are done properly, those labels are important. The key is getting the right diagnosis from the start. If being labeled with Alphabet Disorders from A–Z helps a child obtain needed intervention and services, it is worth it. But with more and more children being diagnosed with so many concurrent disorders, obtaining that correct label might be very difficult. Perhaps there will be a slew of new umbrella diagnoses created, older ones such as MSDD (multisystem developmental disorder) revitalized, or existing ones such as PDD–NOS (pervasive developmental disorder–not otherwise specified) broadened in order to accommodate these children.

One of the most pressing questions of our day is how parents, children, family members, friends, employers, doctors, educators, researchers, and advocates can manage through all these physical, neurobiological, social, and psychological problems from which our children seem to be suffering in greater numbers. And the ultimate question is how to help these tens of millions of Alphabet Kids.

One way to achieve that goal is to start connecting the dots between these often-interrelated disorders. As you read through these chapters, especially the extensive "Signs and symptoms" sections of each chapter, you will find that many disorders have similar symptoms, some are even interchangeable, and most interconnect.

As comorbid disorders, they are already connected in the child, but not always in the minds of diagnosticians. Some doctors "ghettoize" their diagnosis, closing off disciplines that are not their own. That does a great disservice to the child. To repeat a main point in this book: millions of these Alphabet Kids either go undiagnosed or are misdiagnosed. Some who have OCD (obsessive-compulsive disorder) are treated for that condition, but then their ADHD goes unchecked. Some who had dramatic ASD symptoms have outgrown them, but still have lingering SID (sensory integration disorder) issues. Children might be on medication for their ADHD, but their APD deficits are still present and ignored. Many children who have ODD (oppositional defiant disorder) might have a combination of ADHD and APD. And too often when LDs should be the diagnosis the child goes undiagnosed for years. Many Alphabet Kids fit the requirements for PDD or MSDD, but their diagnoses never move beyond their dyspraxic, hyperlexic, OCD, or sensory symptoms.

Alphabet Kids are like snowflakes: It seems like no two are alike. They have a little bit of one disorder, a touch of another, a dash of a third. Pick one from column A and two from column B.

We need a holistic approach to treating Alphabet Kids.

How many stunned parents have left a diagnostician's office with their child, holding a list of six or seven of the above disorders as diagnoses? They entered with a bunch of concerns about their child, and left with an Alphabet Kid. Now what?

Finding the cause is imperative, but it is a challenge. These disorders are often genetic or inherited, but some are caused by environmental factors or trauma. There is a large school of thought that many are caused, or at least exacerbated, by vaccines, antibiotics, toxins in our environment, food allergies, and additives. No sides are taken in this book, and most theories are laid out for the reader to consider. The one thing that is agreed upon is that there needs to be some sort of predisposition in the child for factors like toxins or vaccines to have their ill effects. We need to continue supporting research studies that determine why these disorders are so prevalent and growing exponentially, how they are related, and how to cure or treat them.

Depending on the severity of the disorder, children are affected and compensate in myriad ways. Whether they are severely impaired or slightly brushed by a disorder (the milder form can be worse in a way because then misdiagnoses might occur or the diagnosis might be missed altogether), and as is repeated throughout this book, these children need early detection and early intervention. Besides not addressing the symptoms, which is critical, lack of early intervention wastes the child's time, energy, and brain power as he or she develops compensatory skills instead of the real ones.

Proper diagnosis and early intervention cannot be stressed too much. The remarkable statistics listed below indicate that our children and our society are experiencing a crisis:

According to the 2002 annual report to Congress by the U.S. Department of Education, one out of every five people in the United States has a learning disability, including almost three million children ages 6 through 21. These children require immediate diagnoses and special education or special modifications in school.

The Centers for Disease Control (CDC) estimates that at least 4.4 million American children are diagnosed with ADHD and many advocates believe that the true number is much higher.

In the National Institute of Mental Health-funded National Comorbidity Replication Survey, published in 2005, it was reported that half of all serious adult psychiatric illnesses start by 14 years of age. Intervention is needed as soon as possible, so these children have their mental disorders in check by the time they become adults.

Take the disturbing statistics surrounding ASDs, one of the most talked-about examples of the rapid rise in prevalence of any neurobiological disorder. The increase, while no surprise to parents of children on the spectrum, is downright frightening. It is now believed that autism affects one in 150 children. That figure is dramatically up from five years ago when it affected one in five hundred children. According to Austim Speaks, the new statistic means that almost three children are diagnosed each hour, sixty-seven children are diagnosed a day, and two thousand children diagnosed each month. In New Jersey, where diagnosis is better than some of the other states involved in the CDC study from which the one-in-150 statistic was determined, the number was closer to one in ninety-four. The Vaccine Autoimmune Project for Research and Education reports that it is as high as one in sixty-seven if you extrapolate ages in prevalence studies. Whatever the rate, this disorder's increase is startling. And early detection and intervention can make a world of difference.

While autism seems to be on everyone's mind, it is the Alphabet Kids who have made that one-in-150 statistic so dramatic. This staggering statistic covers the *entire* autism spectrum, adding the millions of children who are high-functioning; have been diagnosed with AS (Asperger syndrome); fall under the autism spectrum catch-all (PDD–NOS); or those who are even mildly touched by the spectrum. Also add to this mix the many children who are misdiagnosed as autistic, and those autistic children misdiagnosed as something else.

Even rare genetic disorders that you would think would be cut-and-dry are misdiagnosed or undiagnosed. As has been mentioned previously, the actual prevalence numbers are considered much higher than officially stated (that's the reason so many "rare" disorders are included in this book). The criteria for these disorders are evolving every day, and, as they do, millions of previously uncounted Alphabet Kids will eventually make our current statistics for all disorders even more extreme.

According to studies, almost every family is somehow impacted by a child with an Alphabet Disorder. If it is not your own child, it is your sibling, niece or nephew, grandchild, friend, neighbor, student, or child of a coworker. And if the research is true and many of these disorders are genetic in nature, then multiply that number by the adults in their lives who also suffer from these comorbid disorders.

In my hundreds of interviews for this book, and in my own experience, one thing stands out: *parents have to act as advocates for their children*. They have to learn everything there is about their child's symptoms and diagnoses, and they have to become informed in all aspects of their child's care, from diagnosis to treatment to prognosis. Parents of Alphabet Kids have become better informed than their doctors in many cases, and in doing so they have helped make their child's life better.

A number of parents I interviewed have become experts in their field. Some have returned to school and have become doctors themselves. Some have become special-education teachers, advocacy lawyers, and even genetic researchers. I have spoken with parents who have started foundations and advocacy organizations for their child's disorder. But there are also many parents who are lost. They might be just starting their journey, or they just don't have the time to immerse themselves in the disorder because they are so busy with their day-to-day struggle keeping their child on track, or even alive, whether inserting and cleaning feeding tubes throughout the day or working six hours a night studying with a child who can't memorize or comprehend.

Many of the chapters in this book begin with a brief profile of a child who suffers from the disorder covered in that chapter. You will see a commonality: co-occurring conditions, years of misdiagnoses, and parents at odds with their doctors and educators. There are many mothers and fathers represented in this book who were patronized by their child's pediatrician because they kept returning time after time, saying, "But I know there's something wrong," and the doctor brushed them off as a hysteric first-time mother or a clueless, overbearing father. And time after time, the parent was proved right. Of course, it's not always a battle. Other parents talked about that special doctor or therapist or teacher who noticed one slight symptom that enabled them to find the answer to what was wrong with their child.

Unfortunately there is no "Gotcha!" here; no reason for the parent to gloat when proven right, because it is often too late then to take advantage of what is the key treatment for almost all Alphabet Kids: early intervention.

Some of the profiles of Alphabet Kids, brief as they might be, are profound. You will never forget now-37-year-old Philip Baker, imprisoned in a twisted LNS (Lesch-Nyman syndrome) body, believed to be mentally retarded in his youth, but actually far from it. You will be inspired by the Tovey family, who have an RS (Rett's syndrome) daughter, and are hoping to bring two more RS girls into their home as foster children. Richard Downing, a 21-year-old who has OCD, will stun you with his fight against forty-eight different demons. Haylee Carroll, who was only 18 when she had her first of two children with the fatal disorder CS (Cockayne syndrome), will break your heart with the story of her young children's valiant struggle. You will cheer on Dr. Kurtis Sauder, who learned a valuable lesson after his son was diagnosed with PKU (phenylketonuria) and he found himself lost and confused. He now realizes the value of sitting with his own patients and giving them all the time they need to have all their questions answered.

They all have something to teach us.

I have spoken to hundreds of parents and specialists around the world in more than thirty countries. Whether it is the U.S. or the U.K., South Africa or Turkmenistan, Finland or Panama, Japan or Israel, the prevalence of Alphabet Kids is on the rise. The disorders are found everywhere, and they exhibit themselves similarly, if not identically, worldwide, although I have found some circumstances where culture or geography might influence the manifestation of the disorder (for example, some autistic children in the Netherlands have been observed with windmill obsessions, while, in Kenya, the obsession is wild animals). But for the most part, even with obsessions, it is the same around the world—trains, mechanical operations, dates, popular cartoon characters, etc. What varies most dramatically worldwide about Alphabet Disorders is how the specific condition is perceived, diagnosed, and treated. Awareness of the disorders and acceptance of the children are growing around the world, but not fast enough. In rural India, some parents feel that their autistic child doesn't deserve services, while in parts of Namibia a disabled child is regarded as "cursed."

I wish you the best of luck in your search. I hope the information you find in this book helps lead you to the right kind of specialist, early detection, the correct diagnosis, timely intervention, effective treatment, and a good prognosis for your child. It will be daunting, but you cannot give up. You are your child's best and most important advocate. Don't forget the interconnectivity of these disorders—and remember your ABCs.

What You Need to Know

Throughout this book, certain terms are repeatedly used. While some may be familiar, they are used in a special way in this volume:

Children

The generic terms *children* and *child* are used throughout the book in reference to both children *and* adolescents, from birth through age 19.

Comorbidity

Throughout this book, you will see that the disorders listed within often occur concurrently, or comorbidly, with each other. It is important to be aware of the comorbidity of these disorders. Why? The associations and connections between them might better enable diagnosticians to reach more accurate diagnoses and allow researchers to find better diagnostic tools, cures, and treatments.

As mentioned in the introduction, neurobiologically based Alphabet Disorders are often comorbid in a child; in fact, it is rare when they are seen on their own. The perfect example is ADHD. Epidemiologic studies have revealed comorbidity rates of between 50 percent and 90 percent for ADHD. Since the symptoms of ADHD are the same as seen in many comorbid psychiatric conditions, some experts have suggested that they are not comorbid at all, but rather "symptom clusters." It has been suggested that, if one primary disorder can account for all the symptoms, those symptoms should not be relegated to a comorbid disorder. On the other hand, if both disorders contribute to the child's disabilities or impairments, both should be considered, say experts.

So you need to be careful. When the disorders are truly comorbid, one might overshadow another, diverting the diagnostician's attention, or they can mimic each other. A Tourette child's tic can imitate the driven behavior of OCD or the perseverative or repetitive behaviors associated with autism. Or, for that matter, the child could, and very well likely might, have all three disorders. And it makes sense, doesn't it, that, if a child has several of these disorders, which is often the case, he or she would also develop stress-related anxiety and mood and behavioral disorders? Comorbid disorders also tend to intensify one another. Even a mild manifestation of a condition, when added to the mix of disorders, syndromes, and symptoms often found in a single Alphabet Kid, can create havoc for that child and ramp up concurrent disorders to disabling levels.

It is important to have all the disorders your child has properly diagnosed because there are different treatments for the same types of symptoms, depending on the disorder.

And as stated throughout this book, if your doctor tells you that your child only has one singular condition, don't stop there—look further into it.

That's what *Alphabet Kids* is all about—the interconnectivity of these disorders and how to sort them out properly.

DSM and *ICD*

The *DSM* (*Diagnostic and Statistical Manual of Mental Disorders*) is the manual published by the American Psychiatric Association that lists mental disorders and the diagnostic criteria for those disorders. The *ICD* (*International Statistical Classification of Diseases and Related Health Problems*) is a similar guide used mostly outside of North America and compiled by the World Health Organization, part of the United Nations. The most recent version of the *ICD* is the *ICD-10*, second edition.

The *DSM* and *ICD* are referred to throughout *Alphabet Kids*, but their criteria are not always identical.

Doctors, researchers, insurance companies, and lay people use these guides in different ways—some use them as be-all definitive bibles, while others use them as flexible guides to help direct the professional toward a diagnosis that makes sense. These guides have caused their share of controversy (e.g., up until 1974's *DSM-II*, homosexuality was listed as a disorder, and childhood autism wasn't recognized until 1994's *DSM-IV*), with those who discount their criteria and disorder classifications—or lack of classifications—as a too-conservative approach. But many other professionals do use these guides for a wide variety of purposes.

The *DSM* has been revised five times since its debut in 1952, the last time being the fourth edition (*DSM-IV*), listing 297 disorders. The next edition is expected in 2012 (*DSM-V*). The latest version referred to in *Alphabet Kids* is the *DSM-IV-TR* (fourth edition, text revised), the interim revision between the *DSM-IV and DSM-V* published in 2000. It is the most up-to-date revision of this essential reference. Unless otherwise indicated, the general term *DSM* will refer to that revised edition. The *ICD* is in its tenth revision. The *DSM* and *ICD* both have similar criteria and classifications, but, when they differ, the *DSM* classification will be used (e.g., *DSM*'s *selective mutism* is used instead of the *ICD*'s *elective mutism*). In many cases, the commonly used names for some of these disorders are used instead of either guide's terminology, such as with the condition hyperlexia.

IEP (individualized education program)

In the U.S., the IEP is an individualized education program, while, in the U.K. and Canada, it is an individualized education plan. In the U.S., it is mandated by the Individuals with Disabilities Education Act (IDEA), which requires that public schools provide an IEP, detailing modifications and services for every child with a disability if that child meets the requirements.

NIH (National Institutes of Health); NIMH (National Institute of Mental Health)

The NIH, a division of the U.S. Department of Health and Human Services, is the main federal agency for conducting and supporting medical research and is composed of twenty-seven institutes and centers, including the NIMH, which is the world's largest scientific organization "dedicated to research focused on the understanding, treatment, and prevention of mental disorders and the promotion of mental health."

Signs and symptoms

One of my favorite parts of this book is the extensive list of "Signs and symptoms" in each chapter. What makes these lists different from those you've already seen is that they not only include officially acknowledged symptoms, but they also incorporate anecdotal ones culled from hundreds of interviews with parents of *Alphabet Kids*, specialists who deal with them, and those who have the disorder. These additional symptoms are often less discussed or rarer than the established ones suggested by the *DSM* or *ICD*, but, for that very reason, they might turn out to be the one missing key needed for a diagnosis.

Be careful with these symptoms; sometimes they are also signs of other disorders, but often they are signs that are present in normal, typical children. For example, *fatigue* might mean nothing on its own, but when it is tied to other symptoms, it could complete the puzzle for a disorder such as CMT (Charcot-Marie-Tooth disease). Also remember that this is an exhaustive list and that your child will most likely *not* have everything on it—sometimes it might take one or two symptoms to make a diagnosis. Also you will notice that some symptoms contradict themselves: "no eye contact" and "intense eye contact." Keep in mind that many of the conditions covered within are syndrome and spectrum disorders with a wide range of symptoms, some conflicting with others. And, finally, don't be alarmed if your child's symptoms match fifteen of twenty signs on the list. Some are minor, benign, or purely descriptive, all there to help you complete a picture. A child with two symptoms on a more severe level can be more highly impacted than a child with fifteen mild symptoms.

Sources and resources

At the end of each chapter, you will find a section titled "Sources and resources." This contains information on the first places to look for information on a particular disability or disorder. The contacts list provides an organization's name, often a telephone number, and a Web site address when available. It would be impossible to list all the organizations, centers, hospitals, and government agencies that can be of help, but these references are a starting point for parents looking for information.

In addition, this section also contains the primary sources for that chapter, unless the information was taken largely from personal interviews that I conducted. In particular, when a quotation is used in a chapter, you will find the source information for that quotation. There are hundreds of professionals, parents, educators, and advocates around the world who provided information to me for the book, and, due to the interconnected nature of Alphabet Disorders, the information gathered from each individual or organization often helped me with research for multiple chapters. The names of those individuals and organizations can be found in the "Acknowledgments" section of the book.

The organizations cited in this section are listed alphabetically, and the order does not indicate a preference or primary source for the chapter.

SSRIs

Selective Serotonin Reuptake Inhibitors (SSRIs) are mentioned in many chapters. SSRIs are antidepressants that slow the removal or reabsorption of essential neurotransmitters in the brain. Neurotransmitters are chemicals that move signals between the brain's neurons. The most popular antidepressants that are currently used for a variety of disorders are SSRIs, which help restore the neurotransmitter serotonin in the brain. Serotonin is a neurotransmitter involved especially in mood regulation, fear, and energy.

These drugs have fewer side effects than other antidepressants, but they can take a month or two to take effect. For depression, the National Institute of Mental Health reports that the medication must be taken for at least four-to-nine months to prevent recurrence, warning that some medications such as SSRIs must be stopped gradually, through a doctor's guidance, to give the body time to adjust. SSRIs are not addictive, but they can cause symptoms of addiction withdrawal if stopped abruptly.

SSRIs are available in both extended (XR) and controlled (CR) release forms, and sometimes lower doses are more effective than higher ones. When first begun, sometimes SSRIs can exaggerate depression or even suicidal feelings; in such cases, a doctor should be consulted immediately. SSRIs often contain a "black box warning," a label that cautions of potential feelings of suicide as an adverse reaction. There is a great debate about the efficacy of these drugs, with many experts pointing to research showing evidence for a significant increase in suicide in children and teens who use these drugs, especially Strattera (atomoxetine). Because of this controversy, some doctors have begun pulling back on the routine use of these drugs. Other doctors, however, swear by them. Parents considering these drugs for their child should seek out several opinions and make sure that, if medications are taken (and ended), it should be under strict guidance of a doctor.

SSRIs include sertraline (Zoloft, Lustral, Serlain), citalopram (Celexa, Cipramil, Seropram, Talam, Emocal, Sepram), fluoxetine (Prozac Fontex, Seronil, Sarafem, Fluctin), fluvoxamine (Luvox, Faverin), paroxetine (Paxil, Seromex, Seroxat, Aropax, Deroxat, Rexetin, Xetanor, Paroxat), and escitalopram (Lexapro, Cipralex, Esertia).

Some foods are high in serotonin: simple carbohydrates such as candy, soft drinks, sugar, honey, teas, and sweets boost the serotonin level but are short-lasting, for only an hour or two; complex carbohydrates such as bread, pasta, cereal, starchy vegetables, potatoes, and rice increase serotonin, but they can inhibit it as well. Foods rich in the amino acid tryptophan such as turkey, meat proteins, fruits, and mushrooms help raise the level.

Supplements such as St. John's Wort and SAMe (S-Adenosylmethionine) also raise serotonin levels. However, it is important to discuss the use of any supplement with your child's doctor. Some supplements are not compatible with some drugs, and the child may suffer a reaction if a supplement and a drug interact.

While low serotonin can cause a myriad of mental problems, too much serotonin in the brain can be bad, too. Serotonin syndrome can occur when serotonin is mixed with drugs called monoamine oxidase inhibitors (MAOIs) or even supplements like St. John's Wort. Some SSRIs can cause serious birth defects and childhood health problems.

"Terms used in this chapter"

At the beginning of each section, you will see the heading "Terms used in this chapter." These are the acronyms and initialisms that are most prevalent in the following section, a special "alphabet," as it were, for that one chapter. If a term is not used more than once in a chapter, I have provided its full name and not used an abbreviation. However, given the importance of some acronyms, such as ED (eating disorder), IEP (individualized education program), LD (learning disability), and NIH (National Institutes of Health), I have added these to the "Terms" heading, even if they are used only once. I did this because it is important that parents of Alphabet Kids become familiar with such acronyms, which will often figure in some way in their child's care.

◊ **Warning** ◊

◊ Do not give children medication, vitamins, or supplements without first consulting a doctor.

◊ Any medication mentioned in this book is for informational purposes only and should be discussed with a specialist.

◊ Never take a child off medication without guidance from a doctor. If you don't like what a doctor prescribes, or are unsure, go for a second or third opinion.

ADD/ADHD (Attention-Deficit Disorder; Attention-Deficit/Hyperactivity Disorder)

AN (Anorexia Nervosa)

APD (Auditory Processing Disorder)

AS (Aarskog Syndrome)

AS (Angelman Syndrome)

AS (Asperger Syndrome)

ASD (Autism Spectrum Disorder)

ADD/ADHD

Attention-Deficit Disorder; Attention-Deficit/Hyperactivity Disorder

Terms used in this chapter: ADHD will be the generic term used for the ADD–ADHD spectrum of attention deficits. ADD (attention-deficit disorder); ADHD (attention-deficit/hyperactivity disorder); ADHD–NOS (attention-deficit/hyperactivity disorder–not otherwise specified); APD (auditory processing disorder); ASD (autism spectrum disorder); CBD (childhood bipolar disorder); CDC (Center for Disease Control); *DSM* (*Diagnostic and Statistical Manual of Mental Disorders*); *ICD* (*International Classification of Diseases*); LD (learning disability); NIH (National Institutes of Health); NIMH (National Institute of Mental Health); OCD (obsessive-compulsive disorder); SID (sensory integration disorder); TS (Tourette syndrome); WHO (World Health Organization); WPA (World Psychiatric Association)

Sound familiar?

Don: "OK, Lauren, pay attention. The War of 1812 was fought by the United States against the United Kingdom and its colonies when President James Madison sent his war message to Congress. When was the war?"

Lauren: "1932?"

"No, Lauren, it was 1812. What was the name of the war?"

"The 1812 Act."

"No. It was the War of 1812. Who sent the war message to Congress?"

"Benjamin Franklin."

And on it goes.

Lauren, 13, is a smart girl, but it isn't easy for her to study. She has been on and off the honor roll for several years, one quarter barely passing, the next attaining As and Bs. But from this actual dialogue, recalled by Don, her father, it's difficult to imagine the Lauren who struggled with studying the War of 1812 as the girl who can sometimes do so well academically.

Let's look more closely at that study session. Don says it's all about Lauren's attention deficit and lack of interest in the subject at hand. During the brief discourse, Lauren would stare off into space, interrupting with unrelated statements and questions, interject an American slave spiritual she had learned in her school's chorus, sustain a prolonged faux-coughing fit, play with her father's hair, entangle her hand in a nearby curtain, contort her body into moves a Gold Medal gymnast would be proud of, doze off, and execute a well-planned burping attack.

Don notes that immediately after the study session, which took approximately an hour for just one War of 1812 section, he overheard his daughter singing along to the hit novelty pop song

"Fergilicious." She matched every nuance, every abstract syllable—all memorized down to the most subtle nonsense word. Why she could memorize that, but not remember what year the War of 1812 began, was beyond him.

In school, it's a bit of a different story. Lauren, who is generally well-behaved, doesn't interrupt class with songs or burping, but she does daydream, tap her pencil, shake her leg, stare out the window, and sing "Fergilicious" in her head.

But another aspect of Lauren and her attention problems confused her parents, and that was a misperception that caused them not to initially consider a diagnosis of ADHD. Lauren can sit for hours, immersed in something that interests her, like a video game or a TV show. Nothing can distract her—no tangential thought or conversation, no motor restlessness, no shaking the leg, or tapping a pencil. Total concentration.

On the other hand, typical of Lauren's behavior when overwhelmed by something—whether it is studying or the pressure of a social situation—is that she starts losing control. She becomes hyper and silly, often acts inappropriately; and although she knows it is happening and that it is not acceptable behavior and might even be turning off her peers, she cannot control her actions.

When she is with friends, for example, Lauren will act in a way that even she refers to as "annoying." She calls it that because that's what her peer group calls it, and this behavior has had long-lasting social repercussions.

In 2005, Lauren's attention-deficit disorder was diagnosed as the "inattentive" type. This does not seem as outwardly dramatic as the type her friend Caroline has, the "hyperactive" type, but it is equally debilitating. When she is with Caroline, who was diagnosed with ADHD when she was 8, all is complete chaos. Caroline's more manic behavior takes over, with loud, boisterous, overly energetic actions, causing Lauren to retreat, despite Caroline's being an engaging and sweet young girl. The two types of attention-deficit disorders—inattentive and hyperactive—make for a volatile mixture between the young friends. And although Lauren is very aware of Caroline's inappropriate behavior, she cannot stop it in herself.

Lauren has ADHD—attention-deficit/hyperactivity disorder.

Did you know?

The modern concept of the ADHD was introduced by the English pediatrician Sir George F. Still in 1902 when he explained children's significant behavioral problems as neurologically based, as opposed to attributing the problems to the children's being poorly raised, which had been conventional thinking at the time. Now, those who had previously been explained away as "fidgety" were discussed in a more serious light—as children having neurological disabilities.

Since then, tens of thousands of specialists and countless studies have examined the disorder, named "minimal brain dysfunction" by doctors in the 1950s. The theory was that children with the disorder had been suffering from externally acquired brain damage. Through the years the disorder has had several names, including hyperkinetic disorder—which is how it is classified in the *ICD*—but it wasn't until the 1980s, when it was determined that the disorder was more complex than previously thought, that it was named attention-deficit disorder in the *DSM-III*. In 1994, the *DSM-IV* described attention-deficit/hyperactivity disorder.

Considered mostly genetic in nature, ADHD is a neurobehavioral syndrome in which the patient displays impulsive, uncontrollable behaviors and has difficulty maintaining attention, as well as possibly exhibiting motor restlessness. It is estimated that as many as 15 percent of American children might have this lifetime disorder. Sixty-five percent of children with ADHD may continue to experience symptoms into adolescence and into adulthood.

The following are the specific subtypes of ADHD and the *DSM-IV-TR* criteria for diagnosis:

Inattention

- often fails to give close attention to details or makes careless mistakes in schoolwork, work, or other activities
- often has difficulty sustaining attention in tasks or play areas
- often does not seem to listen when spoken to directly
- often does not follow through on instructions and fails to finish schoolwork, chores, or duties in the workplace (not due to oppositional behavior or failure to understand instructions)
- often has difficulty organizing tasks and activities
- often avoids, dislikes, or is reluctant to engage in tasks that require sustained mental effort (such as schoolwork or homework)
- often loses things necessary for tasks or activities (toys, school assignments, pencils, books, tools)
- often is distracted by extraneous stimuli
- often is forgetful in daily activities

Hyperactivity-Impulsivity

Hyperactivity:

- often fidgets with hands and feet and squirms in seat
- often leaves seat in classroom or in other situations when staying seated is required
- often runs about or climbs excessively in situations when it is inappropriate (in adolescents, this might be subjective feeling of restlessness)
- often has difficulty playing or engaging in leisure activities quietly
- often is on the go or often acts as if driven by a motor
- often talks excessively

Impulsivity:

- often blurts out answers before questions have been completed
- often has difficulty awaiting turn
- often interrupts or intrudes on others—butts into conversations, games

Combined type

The child exhibits six or more symptoms of inattention and six or more hyper-impulsive symptoms for at least six months. This type is referred to as ADHD, also used for the generic disorder.

Inattentive type

The child exhibits six or more symptoms of inattention and six or fewer symptoms of hyper-impulsive behavior for at least six months. Don't be confused—a child can have inattentive type and still have hyperactive tendencies. This type is often referred to as ADD.

Hyperactive type

The child exhibits six or more symptoms of hyperactive-impulsive behavior and fewer than six behaviors of inattention for at least six months. Again, although the child has the hyperactive type, he or she might still exhibit areas of inattention. This type is referred to as ADHD.

How it is manifested

While they have difficulty concentrating, children with the inattentive type of ADHD do have the ability to focus on things of interest to them. That causes great difficulty in school because schoolwork is not usually one of those interests, so the children are often faced with academic underachievement. Their inability to stay organized affects them in many ways at home and school, showing up as the inability to complete homework, chores, or simple tasks. These children are often viewed as "lazy," but that is not the case.

These inattentive children also have problems in the social realm because they seem disinterested and are unable to keep up with their peers. They sometimes lack the social skills appropriate to their age group. The need for stimulation can manifest itself in inappropriate behaviors and lead to further social ostracism and even discipline problems. It can also result in physical harm because the ADHD child might attempt to show off by being inappropriately hyper, or even reckless, and, when he or she is older, the child might experiment with actual stimulants such as alcohol or drugs. These children can easily become outcasts and are often considered oddballs by schoolmates.

Melissa Cohen, at 36 years old, still bears the scars of her childhood inattentive-type ADHD. A customer-service representative from Medford, New York, Cohen says she spent most of her youth feeling isolated because of the disorder; and, since an ADHD diagnosis was virtually unheard of in the 1970s and 1980s, she was often mislabeled.

"Try being a teenager and not being able to fit into that tiny, little, perfect circle that girls are supposed to fit into," remembers Cohen, who says she was labeled as "dumb" by students and teachers alike. Cohen was finally diagnosed when she was 19. By then, she had missed out on crucial early intervention, says Ellenmorris Tiegerman, Ph.D., director and founder of the School for Language and Communication Development in Glen Cove, New York.

"Most of these kids were either diagnosed as having conduct disorders, or [were considered] just as bad kids. It was believed that there is this voluntary component—that the kid had control issues, not a spectrum disorder, and unfortunately they were dealt with [like kids with behavioral issues]," says Dr. Tiegerman.

"The teachers told my parents that I was unreachable, that I just couldn't learn and that was it," says Cohen, who would often daydream in class or forget what she learned minutes after she wrote it down.

Larry B. Silver, M.D., author of *The Misunderstood Child*, says children like Lauren and Melissa with inattentive ADHD often appear uninterested or detached, and have taken on the monikers of "airhead" and "space case."

Although it is difficult for inattentive-type children to make friends because of their sometimes odd behaviors and difficulty in maintaining conversations, it is believed that they still make deeper friendships than the more hyper, social ADHD children, when they do finally make friends.

Most of us are familiar with the seemingly wild, out-of-control, hyper child, but those with inattentive ADHD can fall through the cracks because of their introverted behaviors. These inattentive children often like solitary activities and can become completely immersed in a video game or TV show. However, they have difficulty reading, sometimes because of an additional LD, and can sit with a book in front of them for an hour and never get past the first paragraph.

Hyperactive children are a whole different story. They are often regarded as the "annoying kids"—the ones who don't stop talking, excessively babbling on, or who are excitable and in constant motion. Full of energy, they frequently attract friends either because they are outgoing or because they behave badly—young children are often attracted to the troublemaker in class. But once they have made friends, it's not easy for these children to maintain friendships due to their bouncing-off-the-wall nature. ADHD kids, with their minds constantly racing, often miss conversation's subtleties and details.

One of the most common questions brought up in ADHD discussions is, "When is it ADHD and not just typical childhood behavior?"

Impairment is the answer: if the behaviors negatively affect the child's daily academic, family, and social functioning, the child is said to have a disorder. And there is a strict list of criteria for a diagnosis.

Although it seems as if every other child is labeled ADHD nowadays, there is a real difference between rambunctious or dreamy children and those with true ADHD. It is important to remember that disorders are viewed as beyond the norm when the symptoms' frequency is more prevalent or more severe than in other children at the same level of development. All disorders are judged by that standard, and it is no different for ADHD.

Again, certain criteria are followed to determine the ADHD diagnosis, and although some might argue with various aspects of the criteria, the basics are still the foundation of current diagnosis.

Aside from the specific attention problems caused by the disorder, there is another potential concern. These ADHD kids, with all their academic and social problems, trying to keep up with their schoolwork and social pressures, are at a much higher risk for anxiety, behavioral and mood disorders, substance abuse, and delinquency. Studies and anecdotal information have shown that children with ADHD are less likely to play with other children or participate in after-school activities. Only half of the parents of ADHD kids report that their children have "many good friends." In fact, according to the 2001 I.M.P.A.C.T. Survey (Investigating the Mindset of Parents about ADHD & Children Today), by the New York University Child Study Center, ADHD children are twice as likely to be picked on at school and have three times as much difficulty getting along with their peers.

ADHD is often comorbid, or concurrent, with mood, behavioral, anxiety, conduct, and sleep disorders, OCD, TS, bed-wetting, substance abuse, and more. Conduct disorder is highly common in about 60 percent of ADHD kids and can be secondary to ADHD problems. One in eight ADHD children also has emotional disorders. Autism can occur with ADHD. Sometimes the two conditions are mistaken for each other or ADHD is ignored and considered as part of the autism manifestation when in fact it is separate and can be treated as such.

One disorder in particular has a unique connection to ADHD—APD, especially if the child has the inattentive type of ADD. The two, which can be comorbid, have similar symptoms and are often mistaken for one another. The inability to process what is heard in one disorder can easily be misread as inattention in the other.

ADHD can also easily be mistaken for CBD. The symptoms in the manic phase of CBD are very similar to hyperactive ADHD: impetuosity, hyper-talkativeness, impatience, attention problems, overactivity, etc. Many children diagnosed with CBD have ADHD.

Poor academic achievement due to attention deficits can be mistaken for LDs, or vice versa. ADHD children can also exhibit visual and sensory integration disturbances. Parents should be careful when their child is tested, especially with most LDs and other Alphabet Disorders. Since ADHD kids do not normally have lower IQs, a low test score may be a result of their poor attention span or LDs rather than an accurate assessment of the IQ itself.

"I'd say that half of the children diagnosed with ADHD also have a learning disability—they overlap often," says Dr. Tiegerman, and Dr. Silver strongly agrees. It is one of the main themes of his book, which states that up to 50 percent of children with ADHD also have LDs.

In 2006, the NIH spent $115 million on ADHD research; the 2007 amount was $107 million and it is expected to be the same for 2008. There are global studies galore on this disruptive and oft-misunderstood disorder. The numbers will likely continue to rise worldwide as more nations begin to understand and track the disorder. Parents need to use the same directive with the medical, scientific, and educational establishment as they use with their children: "Pay attention."

By the numbers

ADHD, no matter what study you read, affects many children. The *DSM* reports that as many as 7 percent of school children suffer from the disorder. The 2005 National Health Interview Survey, conducted by the CDC and National Center for Health Statistics, reported that 4.4 million American children between 3 and 17 years old—6.5 percent—have ADHD, and that boys, at 9.2 percent, were more than twice as likely as girls, at 3.8 percent, to have ADHD. It is now commonly believed that ADHD affects boys and girls at the same rate but that boys are simply referred to services more often than girls are.

Katya Rubia, Ph.D., a child psychiatrist at the Institute of Psychiatry in Denmark Hill, affiliated with King's College in London, who specializes in ADHD, says that the U.K.'s statistics are similar to those from NIMH, citing a rate of between 3 and 5 percent of children having ADHD. She adds, however, that studies suggest that the U.S. statistic could be as high as 15 percent.

"This is a bit controversial," Dr. Rubia says, "as some studies suggest the prevalence rate is not higher in the U.S., but the disorder is more known and therefore more often diagnosed."

But, as the British advocacy group National Attention Deficit Disorder Information and Support Service (ADDISS) reports, and the 2000 study "Guidance on the Use of Methylphenidate (Ritalin, Equasym) for Attention Deficit/Hyperactivity Disorder (ADHD) in Childhood" by the National Institute of Health and Clinical Excellence (NICE) states, "Not all children who might meet the diagnostic criteria for ADHD are diagnosed." That is a widely held, global view.

In the U.S.—which is often behind the U.K.'s statistical curve for reported prevalence rates for such disorders as autism—ADHD's rate seems to be higher. The highest rate, reported in a 2005 National Institute of Health Science study, titled "Summary Health Statistics for U.S. Children: National Health Interview Survey, 2003," was for multiple-race boys at 23.1 percent and multiple-race girls at 11.5 percent, for children between 10 and 17. The CDC estimates that, out of the 4.4 million youth diagnosed with ADHD by a healthcare professional nationwide, as of 2003, 2.5 million were receiving medication for the disorder. In 2003, 7.8 percent of school-aged children were reported by their parent to have an ADHD diagnosis.

Genetics is a big factor with ADHD, as with many other Alphabet Disorders. The Attention Deficit Disorder Association (ADDA) reports that, if a parent or close relative has ADHD, there is a 30 percent chance that a child will have it as well. Dr. Silver, the former acting director of NIMH, says it's more like 50 percent.

Florence Levy, M.D., of the University of New South Wales, Australia, conducted a study on heritability for ADHD. The results indicated that there was a 91 percent chance that if one twin had ADHD, the other one would also. Compared to other behavioral disorders, that statistic is very high. In contrast, at 13 percent, there was a much lower effect on the heritability of ADHD between non-twin siblings growing up in the same environment.

The worldwide view of ADHD is difficult to coalesce into one unified perception because of inconsistent studies and diverse diagnostic criteria. For example, the WHO utilizes different criteria than the *DSM*. WHO's criteria is the *ICD*. There are also different names for the disorder: in Scandinavia, it is DAMP (deficits in attention, motor control, and perception), while HKD (hyperkinetic disorder) is still used in other European nations.

The 2003 study, "The Worldwide Prevalence of ADHD: Is It an American Condition?," conducted by the WPA, found that the ADHD diagnosis in one in twenty American children was pretty much universal:

> *Analysis ... suggests that the prevalence of ADHD is at least as high in many non-U.S. children as in U.S. children, with the highest prevalence rates being seen when using DSM-IV diagnoses. Recognition that ADHD is not purely an American disorder and that the prevalence of this behavioral disorder in many countries is in the same range as that in the U.S.A. will have important implications for the psychiatric care of children.*

Throughout the world, some countries such as Iceland, Australia, Italy, India, and Sweden report a lower prevalence of ADHD symptoms. That could stem from many factors, including the predominance of American research, conflicting criteria, unfamiliarity with diagnoses, cultural differences or lifestyle, and environmental impact. The WPA study reported a high prevalence of ADHD symptoms of 19.8 percent for children in the Ukraine, location of the 1986 Chernobyl nuclear disaster, compared with 9.7 percent for the U.S. sample. While the study doesn't say that the higher Ukrainian numbers are due to environmental and psychosocial effects of Chernobyl (it explains that there was no "appropriate Ukrainian control group"), they appear to be strong factors.

Alex Melrose of New Zealand's ADHD Association, Inc., based in Auckland, believes that different social and cultural contexts and environments are important ADHD factors.

"While we are convinced ADHD is a neurobiological condition, we are not convinced that, in every individual or family, it is an undesirable, damaging, or limiting condition," he says. "Also, although the main numbers of our membership are made up of folk who are European/Caucasian in origin and thus share a common—more or less—attitude to notions of individuality and family, there exists in New Zealand a significant population of Maori and Polynesian people who do not necessarily share these notions of individuality and who do not see certain behaviors as problematic, but which in other societies would be classified as ADHD."

Yoichi Sakakihara, M.D., of the Department of Child Care and Education at the Research Center for Child and Adolescent Development and Education in Tokyo, does not believe in cultural differences between children around the world regarding most Alphabet Disorders. But he does think there are differences, when it comes to ADHD: "There are some differences in ADHD and learning disabilities. The incidence of conduct disorder among children with ADHD seems less in Japan."

Yushiro Yamashita, M.D., professor of pediatrics at Japan's Kurume University and a member of the committee to develop Japan's new ADHD guidelines, has strong thoughts about the disorder. He says that, in Japan, the diagnosis of ADHD has increased over the past decade, but the number of psychiatrists, psychologists, and pediatric neurologists trained to treat ADHD has remained stagnant.

"There is growing awareness of ADHD in Japan, not only in the field of medicine, but [also] in the field of education," Dr. Yamashita says. "More and more children are being diagnosed, but there are only two hundred child psychiatrists and about three hundred pediatric neurologists who see children with developmental disorders in Japan."

Dr. Yamashita says that not only are there few services for children with ADHD in Japan, but there isn't even official approval for ADHD medication for them even if they are able to find a doctor who will properly diagnose them. According to Dr. Yamashita, methylphenidate, the stimulant used in popular ADHD drugs Concerta and Ritalin, is under strict-use regulations and behavior-modification therapies are not covered by national insurance. Clinical trials of Concerta, however, recently were completed and approval for the drug from the Japanese government came in December 2007.

Dr. Yamashita says that ADHD is one of Japan's biggest health concerns. "There has been a long-held theory that certain disorders like ADHD and learning disabilities such as dyslexia were higher in the U.S. either because the prevalence was actually higher or because the U.S. was spearheading most of the original research. The most prevalent developmental disorder [in Japan] may be ADHD. I do not think that ADHD is not as prevalent [in Japan] as it is in the U.S.," he says. "We had a survey in our city ... for elementary school teachers, based on *DSM-IV* criteria, and the prevalence was 3–5 percent among elementary school children. The recognition is increasing in Japan, but ADHD is still underdiagnosed in Japan."

In Namibia, Aina-Nelago iimbili, M.D., has more culturally based concerns about ADHD: "ADHD is very common in Namibia and the children with ADHD are definitely not that well accepted. The different cultures we have, except Afrikaans and Colored, were very strict and expect people to just behave as everyone else, which makes it a problem with ADHD. Nowadays societies are more flexible than before, and ADHD is better accepted than before, but it still depends on which part of the country. For example, the central part, the capital city, is more accepting than rural areas where kids will be beaten for being ADHD."

Nikki Turner, M.D., a specialist in immunization and preventative child-health issues in New Zealand, has another view on prevalence rates: "The rise in rates of ADD could be due to diagnostic approaches, that is, the more you look the more you find, and also the modern need to categorize something that is probably a normal variant of human behavior, because the current framework of families and schools are not well equipped to deal with this sort of child."

Signs and symptoms

- being meddlesome
- carelessness
- daydreaming
- decreased physical activity of the body, slow motion (hypoactivity)
- disorganization
- fidgeting
- forgetfulness
- hasty decision-making
- hyperactivity
- inattention
- interrupting
- lack of concentration
- lethargy
- listlessness
- memory problems
- negative conduct behaviors
- passivity
- poor planning skills
- sloppiness

Cause

There are a number of theories as to what causes ADHD. They are good to know, because some might be appropriate to your child—but it is important to keep in mind that some won't be.

It all starts in the brain—a miswired brain.

According to the NIH, researchers are concentrating on the cerebrum's frontal lobes. This area assists with activities such as planning ahead; problem solving; motor function; spontaneity; understanding other people's behavior; judgment; and coordinating, controlling, and executing one's behavior, especially controlling impulses. The right and left lobes communicate with each other through the corpus callosum, the nerve fibers connecting the lobes.

The body's motor coordination is controlled by the basal ganglia, serving as the connection between the cerebrum and cerebellum. Studies show that specific areas of the brain exhibit diminished blood flow and less activity in people with ADHD. The studies also indicate that certain structures in the ADHD brain are somewhat smaller. The basal ganglia and the cerebral vermis have become popular research targets in investigating ADHD and other Alphabet Disorders, especially autism.

ADHD results from deficiencies in the brain's dopamine neurotransmitter systems, which help brain cells communicate. Specifically being studied, the NIH reports, is an abnormality in the dopamine D4 receptor gene, which is associated with abnormal risk-taking behavior, hyperactivity, movement, cognition, motivation, and pleasure.

NIMH scientists have also discovered a link between the ability to pay attention for a prolonged time and brain-activity levels. Through positron emission tomography (PET) scans, scientists can observe the working brain. NIMH scientists measuring glucose levels (glucose supplies the brain with energy) in the areas that control attention and inhibit impulsive behavior discovered that ADHD brains used less glucose, indicating that low brain activity might cause inattention.

The brain works harder when it isn't receiving enough neurochemicals, neurotransmitters, and other brain chemicals produced by neurons, searching for ways to increase the chemicals. Children with ADHD have to find some movement, some activity to stimulate their brain—either a physical activity like running or spinning around or other stimulation such as yelling or incessant talking, TV watching, or video game playing. They crave any kind of stimulation.

It's easy to see how closely related so many neurobiological disorders are, and how easily they mimic each other: ADHD impulsivity could easily be mistaken for OCD, the impassivity of inattentive ADHD could easily be confused with APD and the children with ADHD who need self-stimulation, making it difficult to differentiate between the actions of a Tourette sufferer or "stimming" (self-stimulating) activities such as the rocking or hand-flapping prevalent in ASDs.

Other conditions may cause ADHD and ADHD-like behaviors, such as FAS (fetal alcohol syndrome), thyroid disorders, or acquired trauma such as severe head injuries. If a parent suspects ADHD, a psychiatrist's diagnosis alone might not suffice. A medical doctor should see the child to rule out the above conditions.

It seems as if more and more children are being diagnosed with ADHD. Does this mean that there is an epidemic?

Some experts such as Dr. Rubia contend that there are many reasons a child develops ADHD, which get even more complex through the development of the disorder. Environmental factors related to ADHD, experts say, can include birth complications, lead poisoning, adverse living circumstances, and one that almost all experts agree on—genetic factors (having an ADHD mother or father is common). Rubia lists single motherhood, diet and food additives, and the TV and video-game culture as factors in the rising rate.

Some doctors, such as Syosset, New York-based naturopath Pina LoGiudice, N.D., agree that food additives are a big problem for those susceptible to ADHD. "What's in the food is a disaster. What we're feeding children in the schools is a travesty—colors, dyes, hydrogenated oils—kids can't detoxify themselves until they are about 12," says LoGiudice, who says that lead paints in toys as well as plastics are also at fault. She adds that, when TVs and video games are added "to the overload of a chemical burden, it all becomes too much stimulation for a young brain to handle."

Environmental factors also cause ADHD, as is suggested by the high Chernobyl rates. The organization Grassroots Environmental Education thinks our children are little Chernobyls with all the environmental toxins they're subjected to from synthetic turf in the school yard to bottled water they drink.

And there are always new theories. On November 16, 2007, the latest research reported in *Proceedings of the National Academy of Sciences* ties the brain disorder to a developmental delay. The outer layer of gray matter, or cortex, develops by thickening from back to front during childhood and thins out during adolescence after setting loose unused neurons. Observing the brain during its height of maturation at its ultimate thickness has revealed that, in ADHD children, this thickness is reached three-to-five years later than in their nonaffected peers. The worst delays are in the section of the brain that determines attention and planning skills. These new data explain the observation that some children outgrow ADHD, as their brains slowly become similar to those of their peers' brains.

Diagnosis

Your child should first be given a full physical exam by his or her pediatrician to rule out other disorders. If ADHD is suspected, the child should be referred to a neurologist or mental-health expert such as a pediatric psychiatrist or psychologist.

Consistency in behavior is an important diagnostic tool. If a child displays rowdy behavior during recess but behaves in the classroom and at home, the child might not have ADHD. If a child displays some ADHD symptoms but is not impaired in schoolwork, friendships, or peer relationships, he or she also would not necessarily be diagnosed with ADHD. The NIH says that, to obtain an ADHD diagnosis, a child must exhibit "long-term, excessive and pervasive behaviors which occur more than the child's peers." It must be determined whether the behavior is continuous or the child is acting out because of a temporary event or traumatic incident. The *DSM* requires that there be clear evidence of clinically significant impairment in social, academic, or (in teens) occupational performance, which is a key to a good diagnosis and a strong argument that ADHD is indeed a disorder and not just a label for a group of misbehaviors of bad or lazy kids. But be careful with this one, a child might exhibit different symptoms in different settings.

In *The Misunderstood Child*, Dr. Silver addresses, head-on, the spate of misdiagnoses and lack of diagnoses so often associated with these children. He says that, out of all the disorders responsible for hyperactive, impulsive, or inattentive behavior, ADHD is the least common—anxiety is the first, depression is the second, neurologically based Alphabet Disorders such as OCD, LDs, SID, and tactile sensitivity are third. The *least* common cause is ADHD. This is the main reason for the huge numbers of misdiagnoses.

The point of the *DSM* is to help rule out disorders—it sets guidelines. It cannot always be taken literally. Labeling our children is a problematic venture because these disorders constantly evolve, and chances are that, if your child has only one label, it just might not be the whole picture. Not all children with ADHD have only ADHD; they may also have comorbid anxiety disorders as well. Autistic children are not solely autistic; they might also have ADHD, APD, OCD, and SID—take your pick. They are not always regarded as autonomous disorders when manifested in a disease like autism, but they could be and they might need to be addressed as such. So, when a doctor gives a child a one-label diagnosis of ADHD, the parents' first question should be "And what else does my child have?" because something else is probably hidden behind the obvious diagnosis, and it needs to be treated with the main diagnosis.

And then there is ADHD–NOS, one of many NOS (not otherwise specified) disorders in the Alphabet Disorder spectrum. ADHD–NOS includes prominent symptoms of inattention or hyperactivity-impulsivity that do not meet the criteria and are, according to the *DSM*, "not better accounted for by another mental disorder"—or, as many parents describe it, "What the doctor can't figure out." That's where the spectrum and interconnectivity aspects come in—at these NOS points in the diagnosis of ADHD and other Alphabet Disorders, boundaries dissolve and guessing begins.

You, as the parent, might just know the best diagnosis. You see your child in his or her natural habitat—if you feel your child has ADHD, but he or she does not fit all of the official criteria, go through all the NOS possibilities—even ones the most revised *DSM* have not yet made official—keep pursuing it. Perhaps a child has only four, not six, of the *DSM*'s required symptoms. Insist on a full-spectrum, holistic view of your child. A child with two required symptoms might actually have a more debilitating problem than a child with six symptoms, but he or she will not receive a diagnosis. How ADHD manifests itself can change dramatically with each child.

The *DSM* offers some assuring words on ADHD: the symptoms of some ADHD children start weakening in early adolescence, stabilizing the disorder's most extreme aspects. As mentioned earlier, a recent study indicated that ADHD may be more a result of delayed maturation of the brain than a defect in the brain.

It is easy to misinterpret a child's condition if he or she has impassive symptoms and also be aware that gender stereotyping can lead to missed, misdiagnosed, or disregarded symptoms. Rowdy, lively boys and quiet, shy girls can easily be incorrectly diagnosed by a doctor who doesn't regard the whole picture, and only views them in their expected gender roles. Parents should not be fooled by stereotypical behaviors. As with other neurobiological and psychological Alphabet Disorders, the difference between boys and girls is becoming less and less divergent with each new study.

Patricia Quinn, M.D., director of the National Center for Gender Issues and ADHD, says, "Girls often remain undiagnosed until mid-life when they seek treatment for themselves or their children. Often they are diagnosed as anxious in elementary school or depressed in high school and beyond."

Falling through the cracks happens more than it should.

There are generally fewer studies on girls, and the disorder is much less well understood in girls. According to ADHD expert Dr. Rubia, behaviorally, girls are generally more inattentive and do not suffer much from overactivity symptoms—therefore, not that obviously recognized—so girls' ADHD symptoms are often missed. Girls cause fewer classroom disturbances and disruptions than boys but can have the same attention deficits. Brain imaging shows no differences between sexes in brain abnormalities; boys and girls with ADHD both have certain abnormalities, particularly in the frontal lobes and cerebellum.

In the U.K.'s last child mental-health survey of 2005, 86 percent of ADHD children were boys. This factor also contributes to girls being under- or misdiagnosed—and the belief that it is a predominantly male disorder. In the U.S., about four boys to every girl are diagnosed with ADHD, but the number rises to more than twelve boys to one girl when the statistics deal with children referred to counseling. In other words, disruptive boys are referred for counseling much more than inattentive or even disruptive girls.

Many children who suffer with the more misunderstood inattentive type of ADHD are often diagnosed later, in middle school or even high school, as Dr. Quinn suggests, because of their more passive nature, but the damage is often already done by then.

It is important to remember that inattentive children's problems are more internal—they are unable to organize work, concentrate, or pay attention, and they are often labeled as underachievers. They are smart and capable, but seemingly unmotivated, disorganized, and disinterested. The fact is, they *cannot* concentrate, stay organized, or focus their attention. As they move up in school and have more complicated schedules (academically and logistically) and as organization and paying attention become more important to their success, their day becomes more problematic and the disability more obvious. The ADHD kids, especially boys, with their more obvious outward behavior, are recognizable from the get-go.

Treatment

Even though symptoms may be different, treatment is much the same for all types of attention disorders: medication (stimulants and antidepressants), psychological counseling, special-education support, and behavior modification—mostly cognitive behavioral therapy (CBT), which helps change bad behavior patterns and replaces them with more positive, effective ones.

Medicating the ADHD child is one of the most provocative topics regarding all of the Alphabet Disorders. Some parents report that their ADHD children's lives improved dramatically with drugs, while others say their children became listless and severely depressed. Some suicides have been attributed to ADHD drugs.

How many children taking drugs like Ritalin say they feel as if a veil has been lifted from their eyes; that the world seems clearer; that they can finally concentrate; that they feel renewed and, in turn, have become more successful in school, at home, and with their peers, boosting their performance and self-esteem? Might that not alleviate the need for drugs like Zoloft, because the anxiety disorders would then subside?

On the other hand, there are many medicated ADHD children who become robotic or overly tired, or even worse, mentally unstable. There is never an easy answer for the parents of Alphabet Kids.

Dr. Silver feels strongly that, if the child has true ADHD, medication is the answer. He says that if a drug is not working it means, (a) it's the wrong drug, (b) it is the wrong dosage, or (c) the child does not have ADHD.

Many ADHD drugs such as Cylert, Concerta, and the long-popular and perhaps grossly overprescribed Ritalin have the same classification as such powerful drugs as cocaine and morphine and can, in some cases, affect children in a harmful way. Cylert, for example, has such serious side effects that it is rarely the first course of action.

Let's get into pharmacy mode: Amphetamines and dextroamphetamines such as Adderall, Dexedrine, Dextrostat, and Focalin are recommended for young ADHD sufferers, ages 3 and older. Concerta and Ritalin LA are long-acting stimulants called methylphenidates. Metadate ER, Metadate CD, and Ritalin SR are extended-release drugs prescribed for ages 6 and older.

The newest drug finding favor among parents and doctors is Strattera. This nonstimulant, atomoxetine, works on the brain chemical norepinephrine, whereas stimulants concentrate on dopamine; both neurotransmitters are believed to play a role in ADHD. Studies show that Strattera has had marked improvement in symptoms.

But drugs can also have negative results, affecting the child's mood, appetite, physical development, social interaction, sleep patterns, and more. Side effects include irritability, tics, insomnia, impatience, agitation, lethargy, depression, and physical ailments such as appetite problems, digestive disturbances, and headaches. Drugs that help so many children can turn other children, who had only focus and behavior difficulties, into more of a physical and emotional mess.

Many parents who are unhappy with the results of prescription drugs turn to natural remedies such as Omega-3 and essential fatty acids, calcium, magnesium (calming minerals), iron, zinc, GABA (gamma-aminobutyric acid, which calms the body as tranquilizers do without the negative side effects), trimethylglycine, vitamin B complex (needed for brain function and digestion), extra B3 (niacin), B5, and B6, zinc, selenium, brewer's yeast (a natural source of B vitamins), vitamin C (antistress vitamin), and probiotics. Also popular is valerian root, a calming herb. Your child's psychiatrist will probably scoff at alternative methods. Naturopaths might be more likely to suggest alternatives than your traditional medical provider. As with medications, no vitamin, herb, or supplement should be given to children without consulting a health professional first.

Some experts believe that allergies play a great part in this disorder. The supplement quercetin, a powerful antioxidant, has been shown to be effective for allergies and for some children with hyperactivity.

Parents should always keep in mind the comorbid nature of these interconnected Alphabet Disorders. Remember to address the coexisting disorders such as anxiety that are often associated with ADHD. Many of these children might already be on allergy medicine, antidepressants, and antianxiety drugs for mood or anxiety disorders, or a variety of other medications. It might be wise to consider the interactions for a child taking an ADHD medication like Ritalin, while they are also on allergy medication, antibiotics for ear infections, and antidepressants and drugs for anxiety or mood disorders such as OCD, panic attacks, or depression.

Stimulant drugs come in long- and short-term forms, making it easier to manage the child's therapy. For example, sustained-release drugs can be taken before leaving for school, lasting so long that the child does not have to disrupt the day by going to the nurse for a new dose. And maybe the child doesn't need the drug as much in school as he or she does at home. There are many alternatives. Again, check with your doctor, and don't be ashamed to ask for a second or even third opinion.

Frequently, if the child doesn't respond to the drug in a week, the doctor adjusts the dosage. If there is still no desired response, the doctor should change the drug. It is believed that one in ten children do not respond to these medications.

The NIMH, in its "Multimodal Treatment Study of Children with Attention Deficit Hyperactivity Disorder," an intensive study that first published its findings in 1999, indicated that combination treatments (drugs and therapy) were the most effective treatment for ADHD.

Help doesn't always come in a little bottle with a twist-off cap. Behavior modification techniques and various therapies are effectively utilized to target specific needs and symptoms that cause impairment in an ADHD child.

Occupational therapy can also help an ADHD child with sensory issues—heightening ability to better command their physical actions, as in controlling body movements, along with developing control over their senses. Vision therapy is becoming popular, not only for ADHD children but for other Alphabet Disorders, especially autism. This improves the visual skills enough, in numerous ways, to allow the child to pay attention and understand what he sees, whether it is written language, a specific item, or a physical action. Training helps children to track, fixate, and focus and to learn how to sustain their attention. And it is not just about visual conditions; therapy also helps with auditory skills.

One other aspect of your child's behavior that should immediately be addressed by an occupational therapist or psychologist is social skills. The CDC strongly suggests that parents help their ADHD child build and strengthen peer relationships.

Under the federally legislated Rehabilitation Act of 1973, Americans with Disabilities Act, and Individuals with Disabilities Education Act (IDEA), ADHD is recognized as a disability, and special-education accommodations should be available in your school district. Numerous modifications can be made for your ADHD child through an IEP, from seating in front of the class to focus on the teacher to quiet testing rooms with extended testing time.

Prognosis

There is no cure for ADHD. Symptoms can be controlled, but ADHD is a chronic condition. Many children outgrow some of the symptoms, but it usually carries through to adulthood. Most ADHD children and adults learn compensatory ways to handle the attending problems, and they live full, productive lives. Without treatment, however, studies have shown a large percentage of ADHD adults turn to substance abuse and promiscuous sex and experience academic failure and problems with the law. And while there are torturous years for an ADHD child trying to study, make friends, play sports, or just behave, when they get older, they just might find the hyperactivity of ADHD to be a benefit in activities like multitasking at work.

Whatever the case, the ADHD child needs to be attended to. He or she should not be written off as lazy, stupid, or badly behaved. With the proper intervention, the ADHD child can be helped.

Sources and resources

When you check out these organizations, you might want to check out which might be funded or run by pharmaceutical companies.
4adhd.com (www.4-adhd.com)
Adders.org (www.adders.org)
ADDitude Magazine (www.additudemag.com)
Addvance.com (www.addvance.com)
A.D.D. Warehouse (www.addwarehouse.com)
ADHDAwareness.org (www.adhdawareness.org)
AD/HD Foundation of Canada (www.adhdfoundation.ca)

ADHD.net (www.adhd.net)

ADHD News.com (www.adhdnews.com)

Attention Deficit Disorder Association (www.add.org)

Attention Deficit Information Network (www.addinfonetwork.com)

Attention Deficit Resource Network, Canada (www.adrn.org)

Centers for Disease Control 2005 National Health Interview Survey (www.cdc.gov/nchs/nhis.htm).

Children and Adults with Attention Deficit (www.CHADD.org)

Learning Disabilities Association of America (www.ldaamerica.org)

The National Attention Deficit Disorder Information and Support Service (www.addiss.co.uk)

National Institute of Health and Clinical Excellence (www.nice.org.uk)

National Institute of Health Science (www.nihspro.com)

National Resource Center on ADHD (www.help4adhd.org)

New York University Child Study Center (www.AboutOurKids.org)

Oneaddplace.com (www.oneaddplace.com)

Proceedings of the National Academy of Sciences (www.pnas.org)

Shire: ADHDsupport.com (www.adhdsupport.com). This website is connected to the pharmaceutical industry

Larry B. Silver, M.D., *The Misunderstood Child: Understanding and Coping with Your Child's Learning Disabilities*, 4th ed. (New York: Three Rivers Press, 2006).

World Psychiatric Association (www.wpanet.org)

See the mental-health contacts under "General Resources" in the appendix for more sources used in this chapter.

AN

Anorexia Nervosa

Terms used in this chapter: AN (anorexia nervosa); ANAD (National Association of Anorexia Nervosa and Associated Disorders); *DSM* (*Diagnostic and Statistical Manual of Mental Disorders*); ED (eating disorder); NAMI (National Alliance on Mental Illness); NEDA (National Eating Disorders Association); NIMH (National Institute of Mental Health); OCD (obsessive-compulsive disorder)

Sound familiar?

John Stack grew up in County Kerry, Ireland, in a small town called Castleisland, so it was a big adjustment for him to move to Dublin to attend Trinity College at age 17.

Having suddenly to take responsibility for his life was hard for John. He shared a room with another student who barely studied, wasn't academically inclined, and was very athletic—all opposite characteristics of John's. His roommate began physically abusing him, and John failed his first year's exams.

"I felt so humiliated and that I had let my parents down," John recalls. "I remember distinctly changing in an instant." He started a routine of strict study and exercise. "I passed the exams," he says, "but lost a whole part of my personality."

When he returned to college, he vowed that he would not fail anything "ever again." And so an obsession was hatched. He studied, exercised, and read all he could on exercising. "I guess I read the wrong stuff because the sources I read were all about weight loss," he now says.

"In my clouded wisdom, I felt that dieting would be good for me. I started by just cleaning up my diet, not eating junk food. Then I started limiting other food and generally restricting my calorie intake. And, then I started to exercise more—a thirty-mile cycle every morning before college."

He also began to lose weight very quickly, and he developed a distorted body image.

"I hated what I saw in the mirror and pushed myself harder and ate less, all the while trying to cope with college, everyday life, and my other commitments."

Within a couple of months, John was emaciated. "I suffered in silence," he says.

Eventually he asked his family for help and saw a doctor who bluntly told him he had an eating disorder.

"I was relieved actually, because someone had finally told me what was wrong with me. I suspected but couldn't accept that I, a man, could have a female problem."

The following week, John started seeing a therapist.

John got his weight up again but never got to deal with the issues behind the condition. After graduating from college, he began working for the Dublin City Council as an engineer. And his problems got worse.

"I started to lose any sense of self-worth and self-esteem that I had managed to acquire working with the therapist. Very quickly, I started to lose weight again, this time dropping to a dangerously low 112 lbs [John is 6 feet tall]."

Unable to concentrate on work, John took a leave of absence and signed himself into a hospital-based in-patient treatment program, which was a disaster.

"Everything was procedural and focused merely on restoring and maintaining a healthy body weight," John recalls. The wrong body weight.

After twelve weeks, he was discharged at a heavier weight. "I was even further from recovery now," he says.

It took about three months for John to lose all the weight again.

"My family was terrified for me and they were shocked by my appearance," John recalls. "I was getting worse and worse."

He returned to Dublin and called the Marino Therapy Centre to make an appointment.

"I made the appointment, and, when I'd finished the call, I promised myself that if it didn't work, I would kill myself," John states. "I couldn't go on any longer."

But Marino was different from his hospital stay because he felt, at Marino, the staff understood him.

"In Marino, I got the opportunity to talk, and they listened. I was never judged, and I was not

told what to do at the start. Rather, I was encouraged to analyze my thoughts and see that they were irrational and bad for me. I was encouraged to think about the negative thoughts I had about myself and to replace them with positive affirmations. Naturally, there were sessions that dealt with my health and nutrition, too."

Progress, John says, was "excruciatingly slow." The more he became aware about the condition, the worse he seemed to get. But when he was informed he had very severe osteoporosis (57 percent bone density), it was a wake-up call. At first, he was annoyed because the news, he felt, "would interfere with my (self-destructive) lifestyle."

That evening he says he went to church and "cried my eyes out." This was six years into his struggle with anorexia.

"It got me thinking," he says. "I had to beat this. I studied everything I could find about treating osteoporosis naturally. I started going to the gym and lifting weights and forced myself to eat more food. I must have been stronger and more determined because usually someone in the early stages of recovery from an ED will not have the strength to eat more food."

John credits the biggest boost to his recovery to the results of his second osteoporosis scan, which indicated that his bone density was normal again. He had reversed his osteoporosis in only a year and a half.

"Now, I knew I could beat the condition," he says. "I also realized that I wanted to help people. So I started to study for a personal training certificate. Now, I knew I was almost recovered."

He was soon featured in Muscle and Fitness *magazine.*

"I never found why I suffered from this condition," John says. "I do not believe that there is any one cause. I was predisposed to having the condition from the time I was born. My childhood was a mixture of emotions. I was unhappy with myself. From a very young age, I have memories of wanting to die. I felt worthless. However, anybody would have thought that I was the happiest child alive. Dad runs a theatre as a hobby, but I was the better actor because I lived a lie.

"For years, I refused to accept that I could possibly have a girl's disease. In Ireland, we don't talk about our problems either, especially men, but I suppose that might be universal. If you showed any sign of weakness, it would be like letting your father down. So, I tried to deal with my problems on my own. Furthermore, there is a complete lack of awareness about the condition, both in general and that it can happen to males. Also, there is very little support available for people suffering from it. Inpatient programs are all attached to psychiatric institutions; if you're admitted to an [emergency room], as soon as your vital signs pick up, you are discharged. There is little or no financial support for treatment unless you are admitted to an inpatient hospital program. And treatment is expensive, primarily because you cannot put a time limit on how long it will take to recover."

At present, John is still working as an environmental engineer with Dublin City Council, and he runs a personal training and sport-conditioning business. He is also a model with a Dublin modeling agency and a careworker with the Marino Therapy Centre.

Most experts in the field of EDs believe that these disorders such as AN are like alcoholism, and that they are incurable. Those who have AN learn to live with it. The position at Marino is different. They believe that you can be completely recovered from it.

"I have recovered," John states proudly, "and I am very happy with my life now."

John had AN—anorexia nervosa.

Did you know?

"Between 5 and 20 percent of individuals struggling with anorexia nervosa will die. The probabilities of death increases within that range depending on the length of the condition," reports Kathryn Zerbe, M.D., of the Menninger Clinic in Houston, Texas.

How's that for a wake-up call?

AN, often described as the relentless pursuit of thinness, is a serious, often chronic, and life-threatening eating disorder. Research indicates that about 10 percent of female adolescents have anorexia, and the rate for men is growing as well.

While anorexia literally means "loss of appetite," it is somewhat misleading because those suffering with AN don't lose their appetite: they fight it, controlling their hunger.

When a person's regard for food or weight does not fit the norm, it is considered an ED, and AN is one of the most dangerous. While food disorders are easy to define, they are difficult to detect and treat. Because of this, the conventional wisdom is that the rates are much, much higher than statistics indicate.

Although Dr. Hilda Bruch, a leading authority on eating disorders since the 1930s and the author of the breakthrough book *The Golden Cage: The Enigma of Anorexia Nervosa*, first published in 1978, brought the disorder public, "anorexia" was not officially declared a disorder until its first entry in the 1980 edition of the *DSM-III*.

The *DSM-IV-TR*, compiled in 2000, defines AN as a refusal to maintain minimal body weight within 15 percent of an individual's normal weight. In 2000, Michael Johnson, M.D., wrote for the University of Illinois Medical Center Web site section on AN that "The individual with anorexia nervosa typically loses 25 percent or more of his or her original body weight."

Symptoms of AN include an intense fear of gaining weight, a distorted body image, and, in women, amenorrhea (absence of at least three consecutive menstrual cycles when they are otherwise expected to occur).

However, in 2005, in its report on AN, the Mayo Clinic warned that the *DSM* criteria "are not without some controversy": "Some medical professionals believe these criteria are too strict. Some people may not meet all of these criteria but still have an eating disorder and need professional help. Indeed, as more is learned about anorexia, the diagnostic criteria may evolve."

The NAMI, along with countless other professional organizations and medical experts, warns about the seriousness of starvation—which is basically what AN is—and weight loss and cautions that medical complications related to AN are life-threatening.

NEDA pulls no punches when describing AN: "Anorexia nervosa is a serious, potentially life-threatening eating disorder characterized by self-starvation and excessive weight loss."

NAMI describes those with AN as people who usually lose weight by reducing their total food intake and exercising excessively. Many persons with this disorder, they say, restrict their intake to fewer than 1,000 calories per day and most avoid fattening, high-calorie foods and eliminate meats. An anorexic will exist on a low-calorie vegetable diet or just live on lettuce, carrots, popcorn, and diet soda. Vivian Hanson Meehan, D.Sc., president of ANAD, warns, "families need to be aware that starving child who suddenly begins eating and gaining weight may have switched to bulimia, much is equally dengerous."

While AN revolves around food, it is a more complicated disease than just wanting to be skinny. Anorexia is a coping mechanism for young girls and boys who have emotional problems. Their idea of self-worth is skewed: the skinnier they are, the better they think they are. And they are always struggling for that belief in themselves.

All EDs are most likely to have their onset in pre- or postpuberty, but they can occur at any time.

According to NEDA and the American Psychiatric Association, AN is one of the most common psychiatric diagnoses in young women, in whom they say it typically appears in early to mid-adolescence.

By the numbers

Although AN predominately affects adolescent girls and young adult women, it also occurs in younger girls and boys and in adolescent boys, as well as in older men and women. The Mayo Clinic reports that it could be as high as 10 percent of adolescent girls who have AN.

NAMI reports that more than 90 percent of all those who are diagnosed (as opposed to the population who remain undiagnosed) with AN are female—the disorder has been known as a girl's illness. However, the number of males with AN is now estimated at 10 percent of those suffering with the disease and many experts expect that number to grow. And it is not only a disorder for adolescents: according to NAMI, children as young as 7 have been diagnosed.

The problem is worldwide. According to a March 2007 report in *The Scotsman*, around one in every one hundred young people aged between 12 and 25 in Great Britain has AN. And the age profile of AN sufferers is falling, with the youngest recorded case in Britain just 8 years old.

Signs and symptoms

The major warning signs of AN are obvious: preoccupation with food and a refusal to maintain normal body weight. AN sufferers have an irrational body image, always believing they are fat when they can actually be emaciated.

There are two types of anorexia categories—classic anorexia (restrictive eating) and binge eating/purging—but as with almost all disorders, there is a lot of overlapping and interconnecting and nothing is really black and white. No matter how the anorexic gets there, the outcome is their still being dangerously underweight.

The food restrictors

By limiting their food intake, weight is lost. They also try to lose weight by exercising excessively.

The bingers and purgers

By binging and purging, weight is lost by eliminating food and calories by vomiting after eating or by misusing laxatives, diuretics, or enemas. Some may binge, eating excessive amounts of food, and then purge. Others may purge after eating only a small amount, such as a single piece of candy.

Combination

The Mayo Clinic reports that people with AN frequently move back and forth between these two categories, or they may adopt a combination of these behaviors.

The following are the physical and psychological trouble signs as the child's nutritional health becomes decimated.

Physical

- abnormal blood counts (indicating, e.g., anemia)
- abnormally slow heart rate
- brittle nails
- constipation
- decreased production of acid by the stomach
- dehydration
- developing fine, downy hair all over the body, including the face, to help keep the body warm (lanugo)
- disappearance of fat under the skin
- dizziness
- dry, yellow, and inelastic skin
- fainting
- fatigue
- feeling cold because the body temperature is dropping (hypothermia)
- fluid accumulation in the arms, legs, and abdomen
- frequent, sometimes fatal diarrhea
- impaired ability to fight infections and repair wounds
- irregular heart beat
- lack of balance, unsteady gait
- lack of menstruation in females (amenorrhea)
- lowered blood pressure
- lowered testosterone level in males
- osteoporosis

- reduced heart size
- reduced size of interior of the digestive tract
- reduced size of ovaries in females
- reduced size of testes in males
- respiratory failure
- slow breathing and reduced lung capacity
- starvation
- thinning or brittle hair
- tingling in hands and feet
- weight loss and thin appearance (the most obvious signs)

Psychological and behavioral

- body dysmorphia (unhappiness with body shape and size)
- denial—believes others are overreacting to his/her low weight or eating habits
- denial of hunger
- depression
- development of food rituals (eating foods in certain orders, excessive chewing, rearranging food on a plate)
- difficulty eating with others
- difficulty expressing feelings
- emotionless or unfluctuating mood
- feels fat even though others say he/she is already very thin
- focus on certain body parts (e.g., arms, buttocks, thighs, stomach)
- insomnia
- irritability
- lack of concentration or clear thinking
- low self-esteem—uses weight as a measure of worth
- lying about eating habits
- need to be in control
- obsessive and excessive exercising
- obsessive-compulsive behaviors
- perfectionism—strives to be the neatest, thinnest, smartest, etc.
- possible conflict over gender identity or sexual orientation
- preoccupation with body building, weight lifting, or muscle toning
- preoccupation with food, calories, fat grams, and diet
- preoccupation with weight, constantly weighing self
- refusal to eat certain foods, and then moving on to not eating certain categories of food (high fat, carbohydrates)
- rigid, inflexible thinking, "all or nothing"
- social isolation

Eating habits

- avoiding fattening, high-calorie food
- cutting food into very small pieces
- denial of hunger
- diet of low-calorie vegetables, foods like lettuce, carrots, or popcorn
- elimination of meats
- reduction of food intake (fewer than 1,000 calories a day)
- refusal to eat
- refusing to eat in front of others

Cause

There is a lot of focus on the etiology of anorexia. The common belief is that, as with many diseases, it is a combination of biological, psychological, and sociocultural causes. The Mayo Clinic has broken it up into ten causes.

(1) *Biological*

Eating disorders tend to run in families, with female relatives being the most-often affected. According to NAMI, a girl has a ten-to-twenty times higher risk of developing AN if she has a sibling with the disease, and other organizations point to the connection between mother and daughter, all indicating a genetic link. Studies of twins also support the theory of genetics.

The Mayo Clinic suggests that three traits associated with AN—perfectionism, sensitivity, and perseverance (focus on a particular interest)—could have genetics as a contributor. Specialists agree that EDs tend to run in families. The lifetime risk of developing an ED for a first-degree relative of an individual with an eating disorder is 6 percent compared to only 1 percent among relatives of controls, as reported in the *Psychiatric Times*, by Deborah Lott in "Eating Disorders and the Family: Controversies and Questions."

The NIMH reports that "eating disorders are not due to a failure of will or behavior; rather, they are real, treatable medical illnesses in which certain maladaptive patterns of eating take on a life of their own."

As with other Alphabet Disorders, predisposition also seems to be a key. NAMI asserts that brain chemistry plays a big role: studies have shown that anorexics have impacted biochemistry—they have decreased neurotransmitters serotonin and norepinephrine, just as do other psychiatric patients who suffer from mood and behavioral disorders like depression and OCD. NAMI also reports that anorexics tend to have elevated cortisol (a brain hormone released in response to stress) and vasopressin (a brain chemical found to be abnormal in patients with OCD).

Once again we see the interconnectivity of the Alphabet Disorders.

(2) *Psychological*

Anorexia may have psychological or emotional components. Common traits include the need to be perfect (academically, socially, athletically, etc.) and low self-esteem or self-worth. There has also been a connection drawn between sexually abused girls and EDs. Then there's the extreme need to be perfect, which leads to the never-thin-enough aspect of the disorder. OCD tendencies are believed to enable anorexics to battle hunger and maintain their odd, strict diets.

As Deborah Lott reported in the *Psychiatric Times*, "For some young women, having total mastery over one's eating and one's body is a very concrete way of achieving a tangible, measurable success. 'If you can achieve a certain weight, you can convince yourself that you've succeeded,' [Dr. Kathryn] Zerbe said."

(3) *Sociocultural*

Thin. Thin. Thin. It's all children and young adults see on TV, read in magazines, and observe in schoolmates. Thin equals popularity, success, and happiness, or so it is thought. Peer pressure to be thin is always there for girls. On television, they see sickly, rail-thin waif celebrities become famous for being, well ... sickly and rail-thin. Multiply that message by hundreds of similar ones that are thrown at young girls throughout the day, every day.

Recently, on the *Teen People* magazine Web site, under the "favorite celebrities" list, out of the sixty-eight female celebrities included, all but three were thin, ranging from the young emaciated Olsen twins to the then-44-year-old skinny actress Demi Moore.

(4) *Dieting*

When everyone starts telling a child that he or she is looking good as the child is dieting and losing weight, that positive reinforcement is going to stick, along with looking in the mirror and seeing the changes the child was hoping for. The problem is when dieting becomes excessive.

(5) *Unintentional weight loss*

Sometimes children or adolescents will lose weight unintentionally, because of illness or being too busy to eat, and, as can occur during a diet, when the compliments come pouring in, they might have such an effect on the child that he or she will want, and need, more of what the child perceives to be positive reinforcement. So he or she then begins to lose weight intentionally.

(6) *Weight gain*

Gaining weight happens to almost everyone. As opposed to the unintentional weight loss, weight gain will often garner some negative comments. Also, the child's self-esteem might be lowered, on its own, without outside help, because he or she is unhappy with the gain. If the resulting attempt to lose that weight gets out of control, that's where the trouble lies.

(7) *Puberty*

When children go through prepuberty and puberty, they might gain weight. They also see the changes that are happening to their friends. During this time, when they are more sensitive than usual, criticism (even casual comments) and doubts about their bodies can become a very volatile combination.

(8) *Transitions*

Who doesn't crave a piece of cake when he or she is depressed? What teenager doesn't want to eat a box of donuts after breaking up with a first love? Nervous about starting a new school? Eat. You were bullied in school today? Eat. Chatting on the phone in the kitchen with your best friend? Eat? Waiting for your report card to arrive in the mail? Eat. Speaking of the mail, is your college acceptance letter arriving today? Eat. Eat. Eat.

All life changes cause stress, and one of the easiest ways to calm that stress, many people find, is to eat. Some dishes are even called "comfort foods." When the world is spinning out of control, it's easy to think, "Well, I have control of what I put in my stomach," and the sad irony is how out of control that becomes.

(9) *Sports, work, and artistic activities*

For children and adolescents, there are certain activities that require them to be fit, but it is important to keep them on track and know when too much is too much. Specific disorders are associated with trimming down, overexercising, and bulking up. Parents should not count on coaches to intervene. While many coaches have a child's best interest at heart, some just want to win—at any expense. Parents should check into any sport or activity such as theater or dance with which their child gets involved because some of them require certain weight levels, and sometimes the ways to achieve that are dangerous.

(10) *Media and society*

While it's difficult to censor everything a child watches and reads, it's important to talk to them to sort out what is healthy and what is not in what they see and hear. Remember when you were a child, and think about how difficult it might be for your kids to resist the images of the celebrities who are so omnipresent in their world.

When 21-year-old model Ana Carolina Reston died from AN in November 2006, it was the beginning of a series of deaths from AN of young women from the prosperous area of São Paulo, the fashion center of Brazil. Reston lived on a diet of apples and tomatoes. Following Reston's death after collapsing at a photo shoot in Japan, Brazilian supermodel Gisele Bündchen told the newspaper *Folha de São Paulo*, "Unfortunately, with the competition that exists in our milieu, a lot of girls attach more importance to work and certain notions of beauty than to their health. To go hungry in order to copy a certain standard is a big mistake and is not going to guarantee anyone's success."

Shocked by Reston's death, following the lead of Spain in banning underweight models and canceling the Madrid Fashion Week, the annual São Paulo Fashion Week now requires models to be at least 16 years old and provide a health certificate.

The Spanish ban of their Fashion Week was further inspired by the death of 22-year-old Luisel Ramos during a fashion show in her home of Uruguay. Ramos, who was skeletal and whose weight was considered "starvation" level by World Health Organization guidelines, died of a heart attack soon after she exited a Montevideo catwalk. It was reported that, for three months, all she consumed was lettuce and Diet Coke. Six months later, in February 2007, her 18-year-old sister, Eliana, died, also of a heart attack attributed to malnutrition.

London's Mayor Ken Livingstone stopped funding for London Fashion Week, he said, unless "stick-thin" models were banned. Around the world, from Israel to Italy to New York City, banning underweight models became the order of business. And even in France, which did not support the Madrid ban, the fashion designer Jean Paul Gaultier made his statement by hiring his first plus-size model.

Body image is the one reason younger girls are so vulnerable to EDs. Their need to fit in and look like their skinny peers, along with the role models they see in magazines and on TV, are cited as reasons for the slide into AN. They start dieting, which soon turns addictive and obsessive. Young girls are overwhelmed with images of skinny rock stars, skinny actresses, and dangerously skinny models. They see the skinny athletes at school and often wallow in the shadow of rail-thin popular girls at school. The same goes for boys. In a way, it's worse for them because, as prevalent as public awareness is becoming for girls with AN, there is little knowledge or acceptance of AN in boys.

There is also a large psychological component. For young teens who are fighting a myriad world of changes and confusion, having "control" over one aspect of life—in this case, eating—gives them a sense of power.

Diagnosis

There are simple ways to diagnose AN from a simple physical exam (checking for weight and height, blood-pressure changes, and skin dryness). The child will need a complete blood count, as well as tests for kidney, thyroid, and liver functions. A check of electrolytes is crucial, as is a urinalysis. Bones might be broken, so an X-ray should be suggested (which could also check lungs). The heart will be checked out through an electrocardiogram, as well as X-rays.

A psychological exam is also required.

Treatment

There are several ways to try to nip AN in the bud.

One important direction is to expand public awareness. Many advocacy groups are fighting the image of skinny-as-good that is so heavily portrayed in the media. And it is having an effect.

Parents, teachers, medical doctors, and psychiatrists are now becoming more aware of the risk factors and danger signs: low self-esteem, body obsession and dissatisfaction, and dieting.

Remember that anorexics are out of control. It is almost impossible for them to help themselves and pull themselves out of the quicksand. They don't want treatment. They want to be thin. But they have to get to a doctor and get help.

Why must anorexics get help, even if it's against their wishes?

Anorexics are at risk for death. The disease does damage to all major organs and body systems. Anorexics slowly starve themselves, and starvation damages the whole body—from the brain to the heart. Anorexics suffer everything from heart and kidney failure to stroke and broken bones. Blood pressure drops, bones get brittle, kidneys stop filtering, and the brain misfires—in other words, the body shuts down. NAMI, in its "Fact Sheet on Anorexia Nervosa," reports that AN is among the psychiatric conditions having the highest mortality rates, *killing up to 6 percent of its victims!*

Death can happen suddenly, without warning. And it could happen to an anorexic who is not necessarily skeletal or even terribly underweight. Electrolyte imbalances cause great cardiac disturbances and often result in irregular heartbeats and, eventually, to the breakdown of the entire body.

Another concern is the co-occurrence of other disorders that can make the disease even more difficult to treat.

If a person with anorexia becomes severely malnourished, every organ in the body can sustain damage. This damage may not be fully reversible, even when the AN is under control.

The NIMH reports the following, in the section "The Numbers Count: Mental Disorders in America":

> *The course and outcome of anorexia nervosa vary across individuals: some fully recover after a single episode; some have a fluctuating pattern of weight gain and relapse; and others experience a chronically deteriorating course of illness over many years. The mortality rate among people with anorexia … is about 12 times higher than the annual death rate due to all causes of death among females ages 15–24 in the general population. The most common causes of death are complications of the disorder, such as cardiac arrest or electrolyte imbalance, and suicide.*

Once the AN child is stable physically, treatment usually involves individual psychotherapy; family therapy, during which parents help their child learn to eat again and maintain healthy eating habits on his or her own; and group therapy, so the child learns he or she is not alone, that they do have a problem, and that the problem is treatable.

Behavioral therapy such as cognitive behavioral therapy (CBT), which helps replace the child's negative behavioral patterns with positive ones, has been proven effective for helping anorexics return to healthy eating habits.

The AN child needs and can find support from a variety of sources (pediatrician, nutritionist, dietician, mental health counseling, hospitalization, family support, advocacy support groups) and many therapies (psychotherapy, cognitive-behavioral, group and family therapy).

Prognosis

There is good news. AN can be treated if caught in time, and when the weight is restored, many patients can reverse their ill effects.

As with most disorders, AN benefits from early intervention, and depending on the severity of the complications it can be helped through out-patient therapy, self-help, or hospitalization. NAMI reports on its Web site that a weekly one- to three-pound weight gain, with a total weight gain of 10 percent of normal, is the desired goal.

It is important to know that, as with alcoholism or other illnesses that cannot be cured but can be successfully treated, AN is a lifelong struggle. Anorexics can rid themselves of their symptoms and feel and become healthier, but the "thinness" lure can return and the anorexic remains vulnerable, especially in times of stress. It is of utmost importance to complete treatment. Ending too soon will negate all the hard work put into it.

Warning

Believe it or not, there are pro-anorexia Web sites on the Internet, and your number one priority as a parent is to keep your child away from them. The AN child or the one who is prone to become anorexic is completely vulnerable to the dangerous camaraderie engendered on these sites, with incorrect information being disseminated and a propaganda-like positive image of thinness portrayed on the site.

Sources and resources

Hilda Bruch, *The Golden Cage: The Enigma of Anorexia Nervosa*, with a new introduction by Catherine Steiner-Adair, Ed.D. (Cambridge, MA: Harvard University Press, 2001).

Deborah Lott, "Eating Disorders and the Family: Controversies and Questions," *Psychiatric Times* XV, no. 9 (1998): 952–80.

Mayo Clinic (www.mayoclinic.com)

National Alliance on Mental Illness (www.nami.org). See especially "Fact Sheet on Anorexia Nervosa."

National Eating Disorders Association (www.nationaleatingdisorders.org)

The National Institute of Mental Health (www.nimh.nih.gov)

The Scotsman (http://thescotsman.scotsman.com)

University of Illinois Medical Center (www.uimc.discoveryhospital.com)

See the "ED: Eating Disorder" chapter for more sources and resources for this chapter.

APD

Auditory Processing Disorder

Terms used in this chapter: ADD (attention-deficit disorder); ADHD (attention-deficit/hyperactivity disorder); APD (auditory processing disorder); ASHA (American Speech-Language-Hearing Association); IEP (individualized education program); LD (learning disability); NAFDA (National Association of Future Doctors of Audiology); NCAPD (National Coalition on Auditory Processing Disorders); OCD (obsessive-compulsive disorder); PDD–NOS (pervasive developmental disorder–not otherwise specified)

Did you know?

"What?"

One word.

Just one word your child repeats could indicate big trouble—perhaps years of future struggle.

You probably know a child who often asks, "What?" But if you notice that he or she asks it consistently or in what you might think are inappropriate situations (like close one-on-one discussion), that child needs to be checked by a specialist. The child may have a disorder that is suddenly gaining a lot of attention—CAPD (central auditory processing disorder), more popularly known as APD. If the condition is caught in time, the child can be helped. If not, he or she could have a world of problems ahead—academic, social, emotional, and physical.

APD is a condition in which children have difficulty cognitively processing sounds, language, and/or phonemes (the smallest unit of speech sound). Judith W. Paton, M.A., an audiologist from San Mateo, California, describes APD as "a physical hearing impairment, but one that does not show up as a hearing loss on routine screenings or an audiogram. Instead, it affects the hearing system 'beyond the ear,' whose job it is to separate a meaningful message."

An APD child can have any combination of problems. While some APD children develop compensatory skills enabling them to succeed in school, it is still not easy for them. Compensatory skills take up working memory (think of RAM—random-access memory—in a computer), and working memory then suffers. The disorder is a hindrance to a child's development; in school, it can lead to misunderstandings with authority and peers, social ostracism, and failure, if left unchecked. Although they have normal hearing and intelligence, APD children often do poorly on tests. But first things first: the child must have his or her hearing tested. Children with APD ask, "What?"—even with perfect hearing.

How it is manifested

"Look out the door."

"Look out, the door!"

These four words could be misinterpreted by a child (or adult) with APD in several ways. When heard, the phrase has different meanings and implications. It could be everything from a polite command to an urgent imperative. Those with APD don't always "hear" the comma or the exclamation point. Jay Lucker, Ed.D., director and cofounder of NCAPD, uses the "door" example in seminars to demonstrate that, while a child with proper processing can distinguish the different meanings from the same four words, a child with APD might not be able to distinguish the stresses, pauses, nuances—the very auditory indicators that determine the tone and meaning of the sentence.

Pamela J. DeWitt, a pediatric audiological scientist working in Cork, Ireland, explains, "In processing sound, a listener detects the sound, determines where it is coming from, identifies it, separates it from background noise, and then interprets it. The disorder can be in any one or a combination of these skills. APD results in an inability to understand and manipulate information including speech and nonspeech sounds."

Dr. Lucker, an audiologist and speech-language pathologist, says that 5 percent of children suffer from APD but believes there are more who go undiagnosed. "More than half of all children with speech-language impairments and with learning disabilities have underlying auditory processing deficits in some areas of APD."

According to Dr. Lucker, there are many manifestations of APD. He describes three scenarios: In the first, a child looks at audiovisual stimuli and has "no automatic connection to sound." For example, the patient might only process the "kuh" phoneme for the letter "c," causing her great difficulty when confronted with the word *circus* in print. In the second scenario, she does not hear phonemic differences when spoken, which would affect her understanding of commands such as "Look out, the door!" In the third scenario, she has trouble paying attention to and remembering information presented orally, often because she cannot distinguish speech from background noise, such as air-conditioning, background voices, the whirring of machinery, outdoor sounds—in other words, the gentle hum of everyday life.

Linda, 12, a sixth-grader, was given an APD test where competing sentences were played in each ear. One voice, in the left ear, for example, would say, "My mother is a good cook," while the voice in the right ear would say, "Your brother is a tall boy."

Linda would repeat, "My mother is a really tall boy," laughing—but frustrated, knowing it was wrong. But it is what she heard.

Kathleen Page, M.A., a pediatric audiologist who operates Hearing Education, Assessment and Related Services (H.E.A.R.S.) in Smithtown, New York, who is Linda's audiologist, notices that patients with APD tend to exhibit the following problems in school:

- difficulty comprehending written or spoken language
- problems with following directions
- trouble taking notes
- problems with reading comprehension
- trouble understanding verbal math problems
- difficulty spelling and/or writing
- trouble recalling a story in proper sequence

Add to this the problems that occur outside the academic world:

- inability to communicate properly with peers and siblings, leading to social isolation
- misunderstanding nuances in people's speech
- difficulty comprehending movies, TV, and books
- anxiety, which might lead to illnesses such as irritable bowel syndrome or panic attacks

Priscilla L. Vail, M.A.T., author of the book *Words Fail Me: How Language Works and What Happens When It Doesn't*, describes in detail how the nuances of language can greatly affect a child's social status. "Popularity," she says, "hangs by a linguistic thread."

Signs and symptoms

Children who have auditory processing deficits have problems with:

- auditory discrimination—an inability to tune out background noise and understand words in unfavorable acoustical settings
- auditory memory, which might be deficient, causing difficulty in remembering what was heard
- inferring (understanding sarcasm or irony); they might take things literally
- incomplete sentences, which might be hard to comprehend
- following directions, comprehending abstract information, keeping organized
- conversations, or movie and TV plotlines, that are difficult to follow
- behavior, which might mimic that of a child with ADHD
- speech, which can be severely impaired or just plain quirky. APD affects their expressive and receptive language

Trouble signs/APD checklist from Judith W. Paton, audiologist, San Mateo, California:

- often asks "What?" or "Huh?"
- talks or likes TV louder than normal
- often needs remarks repeated
- difficulty sounding out words

- "ignores" people, especially if engrossed
- unusually sensitive to sounds
- asks many extra-informational questions
- confuses similar-sounding words
- difficulty following directions in a series
- speech developed late or unclearly
- poor communicator
- memorizes poorly
- hears better when watching a speaker
- problems with rapid speech

Cause

First identified in 1954, the disorder was originally called "auditory perceptual disorder." As with many types of neurological disorders, including autism and ADHD, no one knows what causes APD, but there are several theories. One of the most commonly held, and one that Ravichandran Sockalingam, Ph.D., Au.D.(C), MAudSA-CCP, and senior lecturer in audiology in the Department of Communication Disorders at the University of Canterbury, Christchurch, New Zealand, subscribes to, is that many APD kids had chronic childhood ear infections. Many had language development delays or disruptions. Some experts believe the cause is environmental, such as lead poisoning or other toxins. There are those who claim APD is caused by vaccinations (a popular autism theory as well) and many experts such as California audiologist Paton believe it's hereditary, also pointing out that sometimes these children have siblings or other close relatives with LDs.

As in the case of audiologist Teri James Bellis, Ph.D., chairperson of both the Department of Communication Disorders at the University of South Dakota and the ASHA Working Group on APD, there is medical evidence that head trauma also causes APD. Dr. Bellis herself has APD, which developed several years ago after suffering head trauma in a car accident.

As APD becomes more widely discussed, parents around the world are sharing anecdotal similarities in their children, matching symptoms with each other about things they would never have thought about before—OCD, ADHD, early hospitalizations, high bilirubin count in infancy, a cousin with autism (there's a school of thought that has suggested that APD is part of the autism spectrum, particularly PDD–NOS catch-all; Dr. Lucker says that theory is simply not correct), a droopy right eye, café-au-lait birthmark, low height percentage, snoring, tremors, jaundice after birth, ear infections, antibiotic use, allergies, short-term memory deficit with long-term memory acuity, and more. They are desperate for answers.

Diagnosis

Diagnosis of APD can be problematic, as it is sometimes confused with ADHD. A child can have both. Audiologist Page says that one way to get around this obstacle is to first rule out ADHD: "If [medicines like] Strattera or Adderall make the problem worse, look for APD."

NCAPD's Lucker maintains that "there are [so] many confounding variables involved in our present auditory processing measures, including most standardized and accepted measures, that it is difficult for most people to extract from the test findings what are the specific auditory processing deficits faced by a child."

Jack Katz, Ph.D., an audiologist and member of the Advisory Board for the National Association of Future Doctors of Audiology (NAFDA), disagrees, saying diagnosing APD is a cinch. "In one hour, most audiologists who use the Buffalo model [test] cannot only say if there is or is not APD," he says, "but also what categories of APD are present and what can be done to help the person in a relatively brief period of time."

"How many audiologists know the model?" Dr. Lucker asks in response. He adds that, unless they are specifically looking for APD, many audiologists either say that the patient has a learning problem and recommend the child to a psychologist or say nothing is wrong with the patient.

Even if many audiologists do not diagnose APD, primary care physicians such as pediatricians and psychologists should be able to suspect it and give referrals to audiologists familiar with APD, according to Page.

Though proper diagnosis can begin earlier, adds Page, the problems can still be related to the brain's ongoing development which ends between 15 and 16 years of age, with some of the symptoms naturally correcting themselves. Most experts, along with parents of APD kids, insist that the earlier the child is diagnosed, the better: they suggest that parents not wait until academic and social problems begin spiraling. While hints of the disorder can appear as early as in preschool, most audiologists recommend testing for APD between ages 7 and 8. Many parents of APD kids, on the other hand, say that is too late.

Dr. Sockalingam is an expert in APD. He also practiced as a clinical audiologist in Canada, Australia, and Singapore, mostly with indigenous populations.

"Until recently, there was no consensus on the definition of APD. There are many reasons for that," he says. "One of them is the fact that APD is not even taught in a lot of the audiology programs in North America. There are not many practitioners who diagnose or treat APDs. It is highly prevalent in children … but we don't have the numbers … not yet anyway."

However, the U.S. is taking the lead in the diagnosis and remediation of APD in the English-speaking world, Dr. Sockalingam says, and the best specialist to diagnose the disorder is an audiologist, although neurologists and psychiatrists, when evaluating input-based LDs, may also provide a diagnosis.

Parents should watch out for those concurrent disorders, warns Jennifer L. Smart, Ph.D., and Andrea S. Kelly, Ph.D., of the University of Auckland, Faculty of Medical and Health Sciences, Audiology Department: "Each child presents differently. Some things parents should consider are comorbid disorders, for example, dyslexia and APD; Asperger and APD; ADD/ADHD and APD, etc. What then becomes difficult with comorbid disorders is identifying each particular disorder and not confusing one for the other. For example, ADD/ADHD can negatively impact APD test results and, therefore, identify APD when, in fact, it was [the child's] inability to attend to the test battery. Of course, a multidisciplinary or interdisciplinary approach for diagnosis would always be ideal. Parents should consider that there might be more than one difficulty or disorder affecting their child's behavior, academics, and/or social life."

The ASHA guidelines should be followed for a diagnosis, says Dr. Smart and Dr. Kelly, and those guidelines should include "a test battery approach including tests of temporal processing (frequency pattern test, random gap detection test), dichotic tests (dichotic digits), monaural low redundancy (compressed and reverberated words), and binaural fusion (masking level difference test)."

Melanie Herzfeld, Au.D., who practices in Woodbury, New York, and was the first to suggest that Linda might have APD, states, "Before attention is paid to auditory processing, first we need to make sure the auditory peripheral mechanism is working, and that means a standard hearing test by an audiologist. Too many times failures in school can actually be linked to an undiagnosed hearing loss, so we have to rule that out first."

Treatment

"There is no one-size-fits-all approach to coping with APD," says Dr. Bellis, whose book *When the Brain Can't Hear* has entire chapters devoted to coping strategies for various types of APD. "It requires development of an individualized, deficit-specific approach to management and treatment that can only be developed via appropriate diagnosis," she says.

Appropriate APD treatments and modifications for a child's IEP may include:

- coping strategies such as visual learning and looking for visual cues (body language, lip reading)
- an FM system for auditory training (teachers use a small microphone to transmit directly to the student's headphones or hearing aid)
- speech-language therapy with an APD expert
- alternate (quiet) testing sites with extended times
- preferred seating
- note-takers
- less homework, so the student can learn the work, as opposed to having hours of fruitless study
- tutoring

- all school/class announcements, homework, and test instructions fully repeated and explained; depending on school district policy, offer a resource room where the child is provided with extra help
- psychological and/or occupational therapy services, often offered to repair social problems and teach the subtleties of child peer-to-peer speech and social interaction

In almost every case, a transdisciplinary approach—involving, for instance, a psychologist, speech therapist, and audiologist—is necessary.

Speech disorders are often the manifestation of a child's APD problems: sometimes cluttered, convoluted, long-winded, and dotted with spoonerisms or slips of the tongue ("Can I show you another seat?" becomes "Can I sew you another sheet?"); or stories with no obvious beginning, middle, and end. Unfortunately, processing is often not what school speech therapists look for or even think about. For the most part, they are concerned with articulation and, as many parents complain, averaging out scores. So APD is often misdiagnosed and goes unchecked for years, with disastrous results. The irony is that, while the audiologist determines an APD diagnosis, the speech therapist is supposed to help correct the processing problem. Audiologists like Dr. Herzfeld say that parents who suspect APD or are completely confounded by the idiosyncrasies in their child's speech, hearing, or processing should insist that their school district provide an audiologist to test for APD, and then have an expert in APD handle the speech therapy. There are many good ones out there; you just have to find the right one.

"Districts need to be educated regarding the value of having an audiologist perform tests and when to refer a child for APD testing," maintains Dr. Herzfeld. Another audiologist, who practices in New York and asked not to be named for fear of reprisals from the school district where she works, was more adamant: "Not testing the child for APD is educational malpractice."

Page takes it a step further and suggests that, when a child displays APD symptoms, ADHD and visual processing testing should also be considered. "They often go hand in hand," she warns.

The clarion call of all APD experts is that symptomatic children need to be tested. There is also a controversial movement afoot to test all children for APD, which some professionals, including Dr. Herzfeld, call "a waste of resources." But what everyone agrees on is that, when an APD diagnosis comes in, the school needs to attend to the child immediately.

"Parents should put pressure on the schools to provide high-quality services," says NAFDA's Dr. Katz. "It is very cost-effective to get so much benefit for a child, with relatively little investment in time and money. SLPs [speech-language pathologists], psychologists, teachers, and parents are most critical [in working with an APD child], in my experience."

"Most of the transdisciplinary team is found in the school system," adds Dr. Bellis. "Therefore, families should use those resources first and foremost, as they are free. Also, many university clinics may provide fee-based or no-cost services."

Unfortunately, the road to recovery is not an easy route. Some schools do not provide the adequate resources necessary for an optimal interdisciplinary approach. Linda, the young APD student, for example, was on the honor roll. But that achievement took her six hours of studying each night as well as a continuous struggle, trying to figure out what a teacher really meant or what an assignment was really supposed to be. Because she did well in school, her district refused to provide services—until Linda began spiraling down academically, mentally, physically, and socially. Her parents, now active in APD matters, have spoken to many parents across the country whose children have had identical experiences: being misdiagnosed by school speech therapists and denied services by school districts, and falling down in all aspects of their lives. Although Linda wasn't diagnosed with APD until later in her childhood, many other children are being diagnosed earlier, thanks to APD's emergence from the ADHD and LD spectrum.

As more and more people start hearing about the disorder, many will see themselves and their children as having it. That makes sense to Herzfeld, who suggests that, "while many people begin to hear these descriptions, they identify their own difficulties, but in a child who can't develop adequate compensatory techniques, real auditory processing failure is evidenced. But when we isolate and identify these difficulties—deficits in auditory memory, auditory closure, filtering—then it needs to be examined."

Self-esteem will be a necessary salve in the treatment process—in order to implement the necessary coping strategies, in order to succeed in the learning exercises, and in order to move on. Or, in Dr. Lucker's words, "I see a future in which children with auditory processing deficits can succeed without struggling, without giving up, and without feeling, 'I am stupid.'"

There are also programs like Fast ForWord, Earobics, and Lindamood Bell that have proven helpful. Other things that many parents have found helpful are vocabulary enrichment, auditory integration therapy, speech therapy, and a well-developed IEP, which will provide the child with accommodations in school including note-takers, preferred seating placement, and quiet-room testing.

Prognosis

There is no cure for APD, but through APD-focused speech-language therapy, remediation, occupational therapy, and school accommodations, children with the disorder can greatly improve. The biggest problem with APD is that it often gets misdiagnosed for or confused with other disorders, so parents should make sure they see the correct doctors who provide the proper testing and treatment.

Sources and resources

American Speech-Hearing-Language Association (www.asha.org)

Teri James Bellis, Ph.D., *When the Brain Can't Hear: Unraveling the Mystery of Auditory Processing Disorder* (New York: Atria, 2003).

Karen J. Foli, *Like Sound through Water: A Mother's Journey through Auditory Processing Disorder* (New York: Atria, 2003).

Dr.Jay Lucker (Dr-j.net)

National Association on Auditory Processing Disorders (www.ncapd.org)

Priscilla Vail, *Words Fail Me: How Language Works and What Happens When It Doesn't* (Rosemont, NJ: Modern Learning Press, 1996).

AS

Aarskog Syndrome

Terms used in this chapter: AS (Aarskog Syndrome)

Did you know?

There is a reason that rare genetic disorders have been included in this book: they might not be as rare as current statistics indicate. Disorders such as AS, also known as AaSS (Aarskog-Scott syndrome) or FDGS (facialdigitogenital syndrome), might be rare, indeed, but AS is also believed to be highly underdiagnosed because of the sometimes mild nature of its manifestations.

AS, named after Norwegian pediatrician and geneticist Dagfinn Aarskog, M.D., and American pediatrician and geneticist Charles I. Scott Jr., M.D., was first described in 1970. AS is one of those rare inherited genetic disorders associated with short stature passed on from mothers mostly to male children that presents itself with unique physical characteristics—often in the face, fingers, and toes, causing changes in bones and cartilage, affecting their size and shape. While it affects mostly males, females may exhibit a milder form.

Even though the child's symptoms may be slight and the disorder not diagnosed, it is still important to know that the child carries the gene because early intervention can help with physical aberrations that might show up later in life. Also, carrying the disease through other generations is a risk: male offspring of female carriers are at a 50 percent risk of being affected with AS; daughters, at a 50 percent risk of being carriers.

Signs and symptoms

These signs and symptoms are not present in all AS children, but if your child has enough of these, the possibility of AS is worth investigating. If your child has only a few of these signs and symptoms, it does not mean he or she does not have AS.

- abdominal pain
- ADHD (attention-deficit/hyperactivity disorder)
- broad big toes
- broad forehead
- broad thumbs
- cleft lip
- cleft palate
- crease below the lower lip
- cup-shaped ears
- curving of fifth finger toward fourth finger (clinodactyly)
- delayed but normal sexual development
- delayed growth spurt in adolescence
- delayed tooth growth
- downward-slanted eyes
- drooping eyelids (ptosis)
- excessive accumulation of fluid in tissue spaces or body cavities (edema)
- face abnormalities
- floppy ears
- front-facing nostrils
- head abnormalities
- heart problems
- high nasal bridge
- hyperextension of the knees
- infertility
- inguinal hernia
- interstitial pulmonary disease
- ligament problems
- limb edema
- liver problems
- long, large rectum and sigmoid
- lymphatic fluid builds up in soft tissue of body such as arms and legs (lymphedema)
- mild mental deficiencies in one-third of those affected
- misaligned teeth
- obstructed blood flow from heart to lungs (pulmonary stenosis)
- protruding navel

- round face
- scrotum surrounds the penis ("shawl" scrotum)
- seizures
- short neck
- short stature (obvious between ages 1 and 3)
- short toes and fingers (brachydactyly)
- single crease in palm of hand (simian crease)
- sinus abnormalities
- small nose
- small, wide feet
- small, wide hands
- sternum aberrations
- sunken chest
- underdeveloped mid-portion of face
- undescended testicles
- upper portion of ear folded over
- webbing of fingers and/or toes (syndactyly)
- webbing of sides of neck
- wide groove above the upper lip
- wide-set eyes (hypertelorism)
- widow's peak

Cause

AS is a genetic disorder that is X-linked, but whether it is recessive or dominant remains in question (the prevailing theory is that it is recessive, but new studies indicate it is dominant). The gene responsible for AS is FGDY1 in band p11.21 on the X chromosome.

Diagnosis

The diagnosis is usually made from a physical exam, by observing the distinctive physical characteristics, and then with follow-up X-rays of the face, head, and skull. Since the FGDY1 gene and abnormalities within that gene have been targeted by researchers as the cause of AS, genetic testing for mutations in this gene may be available.

Treatment

While AS has no known cure, surgical and orthodontic procedures may help certain conditions associated with the syndrome. Those procedures include surgery for cleft lip or palate, inguinal hernias, syndactyly, and undescended testicles. Growth hormone treatment does not work for children with AS.

Prognosis

Parents should remember that the long list of signs and symptoms are factors that could *possibly* show up, so, depending on the symptoms, the prognosis varies. In some cases, several aspects of this disorder change for the better over time. For example, there is delayed sexual growth, but that usually normalizes. Although infertility is listed as a symptom, for the most part, affected males can eventually reproduce. Even the problem of the short stature of children with AS diminishes after puberty. Unless there are accompanying psychiatric problems, those with AS usually have normal social and peer relationships and interactions. Even the distinctive facial characteristics decrease with time.

Sources and resources

Aarskog Syndrome Parents Support Group,
    contact: Shannon Caranci
    62 Robin Hill Lane
    Levittown, PA 19055-1411
    email: shannonfaith49@msn.comc
Children's Craniofacial Association (800-535-3643; 214-570-9099) (www.ccakids.com)
MAGIC Foundation for Children's Growth (www.magicfoundation.org)
National Organization for Rare Disorders (NORD) (www.rarediseases.org)
NIH/National Arthritis and Musculoskeletal and Skin Diseases Information
    Clearinghouse (www.niams.nih.gov)

AS

Angelman Syndrome

Terms used in this chapter: AS (Angelman syndrome); ASF (Angelman Syndrome Foundation); LD (learning disability); MR (mental retardation)

Did you know?

AS (Angelman syndrome) is a genetic disorder that was first described in 1965 by British pediatrician Harry Angelman, M.D., who initially referred to it as the "happy puppet syndrome"—because of the cheerful countenance and jerky movements of the children who were afflicted with it—a moniker eventually rejected by parents.

    With AS, everything appears normal at birth, from developmental growth to head size, but delay begins to show itself between ages 6 to 12 months. According to the ASF, the most common age for diagnosis is between 3 and 7 years—that is a late age range when it comes to intervention.

AS occurs in about one in 15,000 births. A Swedish study showed an AS prevalence of about one in 12,000, and a Danish study suggested a minimum AS prevalence of about one in 10,000.

Since AS has been difficult to track, the conventional wisdom is that the rate of prevalence is most likely much higher than indicated by current statistics. Unfortunately, many AS children, according to the ASF, have been misdiagnosed as having CP (cerebral palsy) or ASD (autism spectrum disorder). The syndrome is also not easily recognized at birth or infancy because the developmental problems have not really presented themselves at that point.

Despite their severe disabilities, AS children are very loving and, regardless of how profoundly the syndrome affects them, these children can get their happy demeanor across to loved ones.

One of the most curious aspects of AS is that distinctive happy demeanor. It is not understood why laughter is such a big component of AS children. There has not been any scientific study that has shown a defect in the brain that would cause the frequency of laughter they display. It is believed that AS laughter is an expressive motor event, according to the ASF ("Facts about Angelman Syndrome," subsection "Laughter and Happiness"), which reports that, in an AS child, "most reactions to stimuli, physical or mental, are accompanied by laughter or laughter-like facial grimacing":

> The first evidence of this distinctive behavior may be the onset of early or persistent social smiling at the age of 1–3 months. Giggling, chortling and constant smiling soon develop and appear to represent normal reflexive laughter but cooing and babbling are delayed or reduced. Later, several types of facial or behavioral expressions characterize the infant's personality. A few have pronounced laughing that is truly … contagious and "bursts of laughter" occurred in 70 percent in one study. More often, happy grimacing and a happy disposition are the predominant behaviors.

While AS children are known for their laughter, they do not possess only one emotion—they have a wide range, although it seems as if happiness is the principal one.

As with most other Alphabet Kids, many manifestations of symptoms fall into a spectrum, and you can have an AS child who displays fleeting happiness and who cries and screams as much as he or she exhibits laughter.

Signs and symptoms

- balance problems
- broad, flat nose
- curvature of the spine (scoliosis)
- delays in fine motor skills
- excessive drooling
- fascination with water
- feeding problems during infancy
- fold of skin of the upper eyelid that partially covers the inner corner of the eye (epicanthic fold)
- frequent laughter
- hand flapping
- happy demeanor
- high forehead
- holds flexed arms up while walking
- hyperactivity
- increased distance between eyes (hypertelorism)
- lack of muscle coordination (ataxia)
- lack of or minimal use of words
- LDs
- lighter hair and fairer complexion than family members
- long face
- MR
- pointed chin
- protruding tongue
- receptive and nonverbal skills less impaired than verbal skills
- seizures
- sensitivity to heat
- short attention span
- severe developmental delay in milestones such as sitting, walking, toilet training
- sleep problems
- small head
- smiles often
- sociable
- squinting or crossed eyes
- stiffness and jerky, uncontrolled movement of limbs
- sucking and swallowing problems in infancy
- unstable gait
- very excitable
- walks with feet far apart and flat, out-turned feet

- weak verbal skills
- wide mouth
- widely spaced teeth

Cause

Penn State Children's Hospital reports the science behind AS in this way ("A to Z Topics: Angelman Syndrome"):

> *Researchers have found a very small deleted area in chromosome 15 in patients with Angelman Syndrome. This deleted area contains genes that are activated or inactivated depending upon which parent the chromosome was inherited from. The Angelman Syndrome gene is called UBE3A and is present on both maternal and paternal chromosomes. When this gene is turned on, AS does not occur. However, when it is turned off or missing, AS does occur. In patients with AS, a missing UBE3A gene only occurs in the chromosome given by the mother. When the paternal contribution is turned off by similar mechanisms, the result is PWS (Prader-Willi syndrome).*

> *For this reason, it seems that the UBE3A gene is turned on only on the chromosome inherited from mother. Researchers have also found that AS is caused when a child inherits both chromosomes 15 from the father. This condition is called paternal uniparental disomy (UPD). In this case, both chromosomes have turned off UBE3A genes on them. There is a control region, called the Imprinting Center (IC), that can control or turn on or off the action of the UBE3A gene. Mutations in the area of the IC can also cause Angelman Syndrome.*

The National Institute of Neurological Disorders and Stroke (NINDS) states that AS can also be the result of mutation of a single gene. Eighty-five percent of AS is caused by the maternal deletion of chromosome 15. Although AS is not typically inherited, familial occurrence has been reported, but, according to the National Center for Biotechnology Information, "most families" have a low recurrence risk.

Diagnosis

While a pediatrician should be the first practitioner to evaluate your child fully to determine if there are any other underlying medical conditions, the AS child will benefit from seeing a developmental specialist who is familiar with AS. The most accurate diagnosis will come from genetic testing.

Although AS has been difficult to diagnose in the past, this situation is changing as more information is being disseminated to the public and awareness increases. Even more so, diagnostic testing has become more accurate and more children are being diagnosed. It doesn't mean more children are getting AS, just that more children are being accurately diagnosed.

Treatment

Many early intervention therapies are encouraged and are quite effective, such as physical therapy for mobility, fine motor concerns and joint stiffening, along with speech and occupational therapy.

Although AS children are often hyperactive, it is usually not recommended that they be given sedatives or other hyperactivity drugs. Many AS children outgrow their hypermotor activity.

There are also concerns about anesthesia for AS children because some intravenous and inhaled anesthesia activate gamma-aminobutyric acid-A receptors in these children. Special care has to be taken with surgery.

Prognosis

There is no cure for AS because it is a genetic condition. However, aspects of it can be treated, such as the use of melatonin for sleep problems and anticonvulsants for epilepsy. Because there is a wide range of severity with AS, there is an equally wide variety of prognoses. Those who are more mildly impacted will have the ability to raise their level of self-care, while, for those more profoundly affected, the chance of speaking, communicating, or walking will be greatly diminished.

As AS children grow to adulthood their epilepsy, sleep disorders, and incontinence often lessen or stop completely, although girls with AS sometimes have a spike in these areas when reaching puberty.

While AS is permanent, it is not degenerative—the symptoms do not gradually deteriorate. AS adults usually have a normal life span and generally good health. They can learn to dress themselves (as long as the clothes don't involve much fine motor coordination, such as having zippers or buttons). AS adults are able to use eating utensils and can perform simple household tasks.

Sources and resources

The Angelman Syndrome Foundation (www.angelman.org)
Angelman Syndrome Support and Education Research Trust (www.angelmanuk.org)
Canadian Angelman Syndrome Society (www.angelmancanada.org)
International Angelman Syndrome Organisation (www.asclepius.com/iaso)
National Center for Biotechnology Information (www.ncbi.nlm.nih.gov)
National Institute of Neurological Disorders and Stroke (www.ninds.nih.gov)
Penn State Children's Hospital (www.hmc.psu.edu/childrens)
Prader-Willi Syndrome Association (www.pwsausa.org)

AS

Asperger Syndrome

Terms used in this chapter: ADHD (attention-deficit/hyperactivity disorder); AS (Asperger syndrome); ASD (autism spectrum disorder); CBT (cognitive behavioral therapy); *DSM* (*Diagnostic and Statistical Manual of Mental Disorders*); HFA (high-functioning autism); IEP (individualized education program); LD (learning disability); NINDS (National Institute of Neurological Disorders and Stroke); PDD (pervasive developmental disorder); PDD–NOS (pervasive developmental disorder–not otherwise specified)

Sound familiar?

Betty Marie is 16. She can really be annoying.

First, you must call her Betty Marie. "It is not Betty," she says matter-of-factly. "It is Betty Marie."

She lectures everyone. She doesn't speak to you; she talks "at" you. She will stare straight into your face, not always into your eyes, as if there is no space between the two of you. But if you infringe on her space, she freaks out. And she holds grudges.

Most of the time she won't laugh at your jokes; when she does, it seems forced and eruptive. Her mother, Elizabeth, says that if Betty Marie tells a joke, it is usually totally inappropriate to the situation.

Those who know her say Betty Marie is deadly serious, rarely smiles, and seems very sad. She has only one friend, Karen, from childhood, who has stuck by her, inexplicably. They share a love of male rock stars. Betty Marie would like to one day marry Justin Timberlake.

Betty Marie knows every detail about every male rock star she obsesses over—every detail.

Socially, she is an outcast. She dresses straight out of the 1950s and is uncomfortable conforming to social norms. She finds it impossible to make social conversation. A self-described "nerd," Betty Marie is at the top of her class academically. Her IQ, she is quick to tell you, "is MENSA level." Elizabeth says her daughter's academic achievement "assures a fast track to a great college." She is a whiz at math, languages, and the computer. She taught herself Greek and Latin. She is a superb musician.

Betty Marie fights with her parents constantly and also with her younger brother and married sister. But nobody realized until a few months ago that she has a medical condition and wasn't just "being difficult," as Elizabeth describes it.

Recently, Betty Marie's young cousin was diagnosed with autism, and her aunt recommended that Betty Marie be evaluated. A diagnosis came quickly.

"The doctor took her whole history, tested her, observed her, sent her to other specialists, and the diagnosis was fast and concrete. It's a shame we didn't know this when she was younger because they said we could have changed some of her behaviors through therapy and had a better life together," says Elizabeth.

Betty Marie has AS—Asperger syndrome.

Did you know?

Betty Marie has AS and so, it is believed, did Albert Einstein, Thomas Jefferson, and Charles Darwin. The odd kid down the street probably has it as well.

Even Heather Kuzmich, who was a contestant on *America's Next Top Model* in 2007, has AS. Like the other young women on this popular television reality show, she was tall and beautiful. Unlike the other contestants, and against the expectation of what a model should be, Heather was stiff, uncomfortable when others touched her, and introverted. Highly intelligent, she was unable to repeat simple lines for a commercial. Although she frustratingly posed in profile as opposed to facing forward and couldn't walk down a runway without hunching over with an awkward gait, she captured that emotionless countenance that is gold for models. She was consistently voted the fan favorite and was the front-runner throughout much of the series, until she was finally eliminated because of her obvious nontraditional-model AS traits.

Heather is admittedly odd, but her not-so-unusual behavior prompted a journalist colleague to comment, "If she's got Asperger's, then a lot of people I know have Asperger's." And he could be right.

AS is perhaps one of the most misunderstood of all the disorders in the autism spectrum (a range of mainly communication and social interaction developmental problems). One reason is that many AS children simply appear "odd," and because of their normal physicality, they seem typical enough, except for a few obvious behavioral quirks—like avoiding eye contact or having intense eye contact. Often referred to as the "nerd disorder" or "little professor syndrome," AS children are usually described as just "weird," "socially inept," "quirky," or "eccentric." Unfortunately, the disorder is so much more than an eccentricity.

First identified in 1944 by Dr. Hans Asperger, an Austrian pediatrician, AS is one of five autism-related PDDs: autism, RS (Rett's syndrome), CDD (childhood disintegrative disorder), and PDD–NOS are the others.

AS, which had been undiagnosed or misdiagnosed for decades, became an official diagnosis only recently, when it was finally included in the 1994 edition of the *DSM-IV.* Between three and seven per one thousand children have the syndrome, according to the widely accepted Gillberg and Gillberg 1989 epidemiological data, but most AS advocates and experts believe the rate is much, much higher than that data indicates. Dr. Jim Vacca, department chair of special education and literacy at C.W. Post College, in Greenvale, New York, says, "The incidence of Asperger's could be more than one in three hundred. I know there's a high frequency."

Also, the estimate that four times as many boys as girls have AS is in dispute because conventional thought is that girls who have developmental disorders are often underdiagnosed.

Brenda Smith Myles, Ph.D., associate professor at the University of Kansas, is the author of many books on autism and is an expert on autism in girls. She says, "We 'train' girls to be conversational, quiet, affectionate, and obedient," so it is difficult to read through those behaviors and see the autism. "It appears that many girls with AS manifest anxiety, depression, and other 'hidden' symptoms that are not easily detected, as compared to boys who tend to manifest more overt behaviors," she explains. "Whether this is related to how we acculturate boys and girls or neurological differences is unknown. We need more studies of girls with larger sample sizes to pinpoint which behaviors are more evident in girls than boys. What is the warning? Listen to parents, conduct observations in 'real' environments, assess sensory issues. … Without intervention, girls are not likely to meet their potential and may have more significant challenges as adults.

"We should not be diagnosing in clinical settings," Dr. Smith Myles continues. "Our children and adolescents tend to look very good during short one-to-one sessions. Observations during extended, unstructured situations with same-age peers are most likely to yield valid information."

Children with AS display a wide range of symptoms, from mild to severe—and there are specific diagnostic guides that can help. Symptoms include deficiencies in social skills and interest in and need for routine, sameness, and habit, tendencies that often lead to difficulty with change, along with preoccupations and obsessions.

Though part of the autism spectrum, AS differs from autism. The core distinction between autistic children and AS kids is found in the young years, when they should begin to speak. The AS child, according to the text-revised *DSM-IV*, must show "a lack of any clinically significant general delay in language acquisition, cognitive development and adaptive behavior (other than in social interaction). This contrasts with typical developmental accounts of autistic children, who show marked deficits and deviance in these areas prior to the age of 3 years." Simply put, AS children speak on time or even early, and autistic children show speech delays or have loss of already established speech.

Temple Grandin, Ph.D., is a scientist, professor, best-selling author, and world-renowned lecturer who has autism. She knows what it is like to live with AS.

All AS children, Dr. Grandin cautions, have the potential to go undiagnosed because of the very nature of the warning signs for the disorder. "There is no obvious speech delay as there is with [classic] autism," she explains. But then, when children are older, the signs come: "By third or fourth grade, [Asperger's kids have] no friends; [they have] an area of strength [and they display] rudeness."

Girls in particular, Dr. Grandin warns, fall through the cracks. "Girls tend to be somewhat more flexible in their thinking. They get overlooked more often because they manage to fit in better than the guys."

How it is manifested

AS kids display their unique problems such as body-language awkwardness as they get older. These children are often uncoordinated and clumsy, with lumbering gaits, and exhibit difficulties reading social cues. When they speak, it is often *at* and not *with* the listener. They are often unaware of proper body distance and are usually "in the face" of the person with whom they are speaking. Sometimes they prefer not to converse at all. But when they do, their speech might seem rote or expressionless at times, and emotionless, lacking subtleties. They also take things literally, which can lead to disagreements, misunderstandings, and fights with their family and peers. And their facial affect, or expression, often appears flat.

Since many AS children have sensory issues, they dress according to comfort and not style, and their preference in clothes often adds to their oddness and to the labels of "nerdy" or "weird." This had been a sore subject for Heather on *Model*—the other contestants, and even the judges, had accused the potential model of "having no fashion sense."

Sensory overload issues are a main characteristic of these children, as they are often sensitive to sound, taste, smell, light, and/or touch. Their sensory issues might determine some of their unique behaviors, such as eating only crunchy foods because they like the texture or becoming anxious and frustrated in a room with certain lighting or acoustics.

"The sensory problems can be extremely debilitating," explains Dr. Grandin. "Extremely. And I think there needs to be a lot more research done on that because those sensory disorders prevent people from functioning in a job. How do you function in a job when the fluorescent lights look like a discotheque or a cell phone hurts your ears like a dentist's drill?"

Another main characteristic is that these socially uninhibited children will say exactly what's on their minds, without regard to social implications. They might find humor in things the average person won't or might be literal and not find the humor in a subtle witticism that all their peers are laughing at. They just might not "get" a very obvious joke. They are often mistaken for impolite or rude. There are painful social implications for these children.

"When I was in high school," Dr. Grandin recalls, "I used to get teased all the time, and it was absolutely, totally, terribly awful."

AS kids sometimes seem to lack empathy, and their interactions often appear one-sided. This leads to the inability to form proper friendships and often invites bullying and teasing. Many AS children are isolated and friendless. But, again, remember that one aspect does not necessarily fit all children with the disorder. There are AS children who can initiate and maintain friendships or not exhibit the usual AS obsessive interest. That said, it is often the AS child's preoccupation and full immersion in specific topics like trains, dinosaurs, movies, baseball, and the minutiae surrounding those topics that is a strong identifier for the disorder. The main character of the film *Rain Man* has mistakenly been an iconic role model for AS for years, but as AS has become more highly researched and understood, that autistic-savant stereotype has been replaced by a wide spectrum of others who have the syndrome, including the seemingly normal but quirky child.

AS children usually have a normal-to-superior IQ, but parents should not misread the AS child. The "genius" aspect of AS could be one of the most misleading misconceptions about the syndrome—not all AS children are brilliant, as is the common perception; some are even mildly retarded.

"You can be Asperger's and be Einstein," says Dr. Grandin. "You can be Asperger's and be not smart, too. You're not going to be, like, totally mentally retarded. It's a continuum. It goes all the way from kids who can't speak, who are severely handicapped, all the way up to Einstein."

Many AS children are hyperlexic, possessing a precocious fascination with letters or numbers as well as with language and a specific topic of interest. Although the speech of AS children is often advanced, their social interaction may be diminished, often because of a deficient ability for pragmatic, or social, speech. So, they can have an extraordinary vocabulary but not necessarily know how to use it in a social sense. With their high-level, literal, and unsubtle speech, they are bound for trouble in a social context.

Unlike classically autistic children, who withdraw in physical interaction, AS kids might inappropriately hug or touch or even smother another person with attention.

By the numbers

As more of these awkward children are being drawn into the autism spectrum mix, the numbers for the rate of autism rise significantly. The autism rate is now one in 150, according to the U.S. Centers for Disease Control study, "Prevalence of the Autism Spectrum Disorders (ASDs) in Multiple Areas of the United States, 2000 and 2002," released February 8, 2007. (This document can be viewed in html simply by putting the title in a search engine.) Many of these children were not diagnosed or were misdiagnosed prior to this time, especially girls, but are now falling into the high-functioning—having better cognitive and learning abilities—part of the autism spectrum, whether through a diagnosis of HFA, AS, or PDD–NOS (the catch-all term for quirky, odd kids).

Where on the spectrum?

AS floats around the autism spectrum as experts attempt to figure out where it really belongs. Some experts, such as Uta Frith, author of *Autism and Asperger Syndrome*, say AS children possess "a dash of autism." Others argue it is one of the ASDs. It has also been classified as an NLD (nonverbal learning disability), part of the OCD (obsessive-compulsive disorder) spectrum, ADHD, and even a CD (conduct disorder). Others say that AS is no official disorder, but rather a description of weird kids with weird habits.

AS expert Tony Attwood, Ph.D., the author of *The Complete Guide to Asperger's Syndrome*, says that AS kids just have a "different, not defective, way of thinking." He notes AS children's different perception of the world around them and their own unique way of experiencing sensory events. He points out their strong need "to seek knowledge, truth, and perfection," but they do it differently than do more typical children. To AS children, the solving of the problem is more important than what others might think about them: they see details, as opposed to the whole.

Autism advocates favor the inclusion of AS (and PDD–NOS) in their spectrum because it helps raise their numbers, which benefits awareness and research dollars. Often, though, the autism side separates itself from AS when it comes to advocacy and reaping the benefits of those research dollars. There is even a movement among some AS adults who do not want to be labeled, treated, or "cured," who consider themselves not handicapped by their disorder. They even call themselves "Aspies," a term that infuriates some advocates who consider it demeaning for such a serious disorder.

But there are those, like Dr. Grandin, who thrive in their Asperger's traits, even saying that there is no difference between a unique person with a couple of eccentric habits and a person with mild AS.

Dr. Grandin says emphatically, "They're the same thing. And *nerd* is another word for Asperger's. *Computer geek* is another word for Asperger's. They are the same thing. And they're called geeks. They're called engineers. They're called musicians. It's the same thing."

Symptoms that seem benign (e.g., nerdiness) are considered a disorder when they negatively impact the child's wellbeing or ability to function in everyday activities— domestically, socially, academically. Autism is a spectrum disorder, and AS is not always about being slightly odd. It can also include severely impacted children, ones who make absolutely no eye contact, who drool, or who cannot/do not groom themselves. For the most part, though, AS is on the high end of the autism continuum.

Signs and symptoms

An AS child can have any combination of the following signs and symptoms:

- abruptness
- aloofness
- appearance of boredom
- circumstantial speech (adding nonessential details)
- clumsiness
- defensive to touch
- doesn't always reach conclusion when speaking
- does not provide background for comments
- early speech precociousness
- eccentricity
- egocentric conversational style
- fascination with letters and/or numbers (hyperlexia)
- flat facial expression
- high IQ—IQs can run the whole spectrum; IQs often fall in the above-normal range in verbal ability and in the below-average range in performance abilities

- inability to form friendships
- inability to loosen up
- inability to share enjoyment, interests, or achievements with other people
- inappropriate social interaction
- incessant talking
- insensitivity to others' feelings
- interest in narrow or unusual topics
- jumps from topic to topic
- lack of "common sense"
- lack of emotional reciprocity
- lack of empathy
- lack of fear
- lack of proper body language
- LDs
- learns extraordinary amount of specific facts about a subject (train schedules, TV schedules, baseball stats, world capitals, etc.)
- learns in rote manner
- little patience
- "little professor"-like knowledge
- monologue-like speech
- monotonic speech
- mood disorders
- naïveté
- no clinically significant delay in cognitive development
- no clinically significant delay in language
- no delay in self-help skills
- odd posture
- one-sided social interaction
- pedantic speech
- poor comprehension of facts
- poor eye contact
- poor fine and/or gross motor skills
- poor nonverbal communication
- poor social judgment
- poor speech inflections, pitch, and/or sound levels
- preoccupation changes every year or two
- preoccupation with certain topics and minutiae surrounding special interests
- preoccupation with parts of objects
- problem understanding jokes
- repeating words (echolalia)
- repetitive motor mannerisms

- repetitive questions
- resists change
- rigid behaviors and thought
- sensitive to smells, sound, taste, touch
- social isolation
- speaks out loud what he or she is thinking
- stereotyped patterns of behavior, interests, and motor mannerisms
- talks about minutiae
- talks "in-your-face"
- tangential speech
- temper tantrums
- uncoordinated
- visual-perceptual problems
- well-developed long-term memory

Cause

Despite new public awareness and research, what we know about AS—its prevalence, etiology, or hereditariness—is incomplete. Add to that how different each AS child is from the other, and you have one of the biggest questions in modern medicine.

The potential causes of AS are many, and all are being researched. They range from genetic and biological to environmental and social. There are many theories about diet and vaccines, age of the father and testosterone, mercury poisoning and other environmental toxins, and imitative modeling of family members. New research is focusing on a defective chromosome 16.

What is becoming a popular consensus, though, is that, despite the cause, the child must have a genetic predisposition.

Diagnosis

AS, like the other PDDs, involves problems, delays, and deficits that require various areas of diagnosis and numerous forms of therapy. The best diagnosis and treatment are from an interdisciplinary team, including pediatricians, neurologists, psychologists, psychiatrists, and behavioral, physical, occupational, and speech-language therapists.

It is important for parents to keep good notes on their child's developmental growth; it will help in establishing the diagnosis.

Clinical observation is one of the main diagnostic tools. Social pragmatics and physicality are the two obvious giveaways that a child (or an adult) might have AS.

The NINDS describes the AS child's inappropriate and peculiar social interaction:

They may engage the interlocutor, usually an adult, in one-sided conversation characterized by long-winded, pedantic speech, about a favorite and often unusual and narrow topic." Also, although they are frequently self-described "loners" who want to make friendships, their "wishes are invariably thwarted by their awkward approaches and insensitivity to other person's feelings, intentions, and non-literal and implied communications (e.g., signs of boredom, haste to leave, and need for privacy). More typically, autistic persons are withdrawn and may seem to be unaware of, and disinterested in, other persons."

The NINDS also points to physical clumsiness, stating, "Individuals with Asperger's may have a history of delayed acquisition of motor skills such as pedaling a bike, catching a ball, opening jars, climbing monkey-bars, and so on. They are often visibly awkward, exhibiting rigid gait patterns, odd posture, poor manipulative skills, and significant deficits in visual-motor coordination."

Although the disorder often manifests itself in idiosyncratic and eccentric behaviors, parents should not be misled into thinking that AS is not serious. As the NINDS reminds us, "The disorder is meant as a serious and debilitating developmental syndrome impairing the person's capacity for socialization, and not a transient or mild condition." Intervention is crucial, although it might not always be effective.

The first doctor to be seen should be the pediatrician, who will run a full physical examination to rule out other medical problems and then refer the child to a specialist, most likely a pediatric neurologist or pediatric psychiatrist. The medical team will assess the child's developmental history—speech onset and language patterns, specific interests, social interactions within the family and outside the family, emotional health, self-concept, and mood presentation.

Other assessments include neuropsychological functioning such as motor skills, executive functions, memory, visual-perceptual, visual memory assessment, manipulative skills, parts-whole relationships, visual-motor coordination, problem solving, and concept formations and facial recognition. The team will check your child's self-sufficiency and compensatory skills. There will also be IQ testing.

Many communication assessments will be conducted as well, such as verbal testing for articulation, comprehension, vocabulary, and language construction, and nonverbal testing of gaze, physical signs and gestures, and language subtleties such as humor, sarcasm and irony, and prosody (speech rhythms, volume, stress, and pitch). The coherence and content of your child's speech will also be evaluated. The team will also assess turn-taking, cue-taking, and social rules of conversation. How your child spends his or her leisure time and how the child reacts to unexpected situations will be observed, along with how he or she determines other people's feelings and intent.

Dr. Grandin has her own thoughts on diagnosis: "You can't diagnose this like diagnosing tuberculosis. It's not precise. These categories are not precise. It's a behavioral profile, like profiling a hijacker. And I'm being absolutely serious about that. It's not a precise diagnosis where they can do this medical test and they can tell you what genetic strain of TB you've got. That's precise. None of this stuff is precise."

Treatment

Despite the various professionals who can work with an AS child, there are few therapies that have been proven to help, although there are many anecdotal success stories.

AS children benefit from the following therapies: occupational, physical, speech-language, behavioral, sensory-integration, psychological, and social-skills. All types of skill building are encouraged. A well-planned IEP, with modifications that best suit the child's diverse needs, is essential for academic success.

It is important to work with AS children in the areas of empathy and social interaction, but it has been found that these children do not respond well to therapy that deals with self-awareness. Mostly, AS children are supported by services that are usually used by those with HFA, SID (sensory integration disorder), and the assortment of specific LDs, all of which can mimic or be concurrent with AS.

"It's like the Olympic rings and [how] they overlap a little bit," explains Dr. Grandin. "You'll have an area of intersection—that's the way it is with [comorbid disorders like learning disabilities] and autism."

In terms of school services, many advocates feel that securing an autism classification will provide the child with more services than will the usual "other health impaired" classification, which many ASD students had until recently.

Since AS children live by their strict and rigid rules and routines, these can be used to help them function better and formulate positive habits instead of negative ones, which is the cornerstone of behavior-based therapies such as CBT.

The types of specific approaches that can be useful for the AS child besides CBT include work on communications and pragmatic speech, one-on-one therapy, and social-group interaction. Therapists and teachers can use imitative modeling, repetitive drills, auditory supplements, and mirror training, as well as practice correction of ambiguous language problems.

Again, Dr. Grandin has the last word. It all starts at home, she says: manners, the strict way they were taught in the 1950s when she was a child, is what AS kids (and all children, she adds) need to learn. Once they have their manners set, they need to broaden their obsessions and interests and find friends with those same shared interests. That's how AS kids can best socialize. Once they make those relationships, they need the valuable skill of taking turns, whether it's involved with playing or speaking.

Prognosis

The prognosis for AS is good.

Depending on the severity of the disorder, a person with AS can lead a normal life. You know people who fit the bill, people who were probably never diagnosed with the disorder.

If AS children follow through with their obsession when they grow up, they will find enjoyment in their work. A young AS child plays with computers constantly, and he ends up as a computer programmer. Another is a precocious musician who becomes an accomplished composer. The girl who knew the Latin name for every animal becomes a vet. Some stay away from jobs where there is social interaction. Others go into fields where their focused interests are a benefit or where the environment is more "geek"-friendly, like a computer tech company.

Ongoing research on AS is being conducted by the NIH, NINDS, and the Learning Disabilities Association of America, in a partnership with the Yale Child Study Center, so there is promise.

Dr. Grandin says that about 75-to-80 percent of her generation of AS adults (she is in her fifties) are in the workplace. They settle into jobs like the tech field where they are comfortable, remaining undiagnosed or keeping their diagnosis quiet, for medical insurance reasons. Dr. Grandin thrives in her form of autism, saying, "I like the clarity of thought."

"If you cured Asperger's, you would have no musicians, you would have no scientists," she adds. "[You would have no] famous people like Mozart, Van Gogh, Darwin, Carl Sagan, Thomas Jefferson, Einstein.

"I wouldn't want to be not autistic."

Sources and resources

If you suspect your child has Asperger syndrome, great places to start are *The OASIS Guide to Asperger Syndrome* by Barbara Kirby and Patricia Romanowski Bashe (revised edition, 2005) and *The Complete Guide to Asperger's Syndrome* (2006) by Tony Attwood. Dr. Temple Grandin's books and videos are also recommended, especially her wonderful biography, *Emergence: Labeled Autistic* (1996).

Asperger's Disorder Homepage (www.aspergers.com)

Tony Atwood (www.tonyattwood.com.au)

More Advanced Individuals with Autism, Asperger's Syndrome, and Pervasive Developmental Disorder/MAAP Services for Autism and Asperger Spectrum (www.maapservices.org)

National Institute of Neurological Disorders and Strokes (www.ninds.nih.gov)

Online Asperger Syndrome Information & Support (OASIS) (www.aspergersyndrome.org)

"Prevalence of the Autism Spectrum Disorders (ASDs) in Multiple Areas of the United States, 2000 and 2002," published on February 8, 2007 by the Centers for Disease Control (www.cdc.gov).

See the "Autism" contacts and the mental-health contacts under "General Resources" for more sources and resources for this chapter.

ASD

Autism Spectrum Disorder

Terms used in this chapter: ABA (applied behavior analysis); ADHD (attention-deficit/hyperactivity disorder); APD (auditory processing disorder); AS (Asperger syndrome); ASD (autism spectrum disorder); CBT (cognitive behavioral therapy); CDC (Centers for Disease Control); *DSM* (*Diagnostic and Statistical Manual of Mental Disorders*); ICD (*International Classification of Diseases*); IEP (individualized education program); OCD (obsessive-compulsive disorder); PDD (pervasive developmental disorder); PDD–NOS (pervasive developmental disorder–not otherwise specified); SID (sensory integration disorder)

Sound familiar?

—When 7-year-old Matthew gets a haircut, one of his parents has to hold his upper body down, while the other holds his lower body. He speaks only about five words, and the one he uses here is "No!" The barber has to buzz Matthew's head because the process has to go fast. Agitated, Matthew attempts to put his shorn hair back into his head whenever he gets his hands loose. His mother thinks he feels as if his hair is being pulled out of his head. Matthew reacts strongly to sound and touch. He starts to cry as soon as his parents drive the car into the barbershop parking lot and keeps crying throughout the haircut. But when the shearing is done, he's fine. He looks in the mirror, plays with his new haircut, and admires himself. He's friendly and happy again, until, of course, there is a noise or his routine changes. He can spend a day uninterrupted on the Internet or watching Blue's Clues *on TV, and he's making great progress. While he speaks just a few words—"up," "juice," "out," "pretzels," and "remote"—he reads books out loud and now says "Mommy."*

—Oliver, who just turned 5, would cry so hard when he was a baby that he'd stop breathing. It was one of the first signs that something was wrong. Not responding to people around him was another. After years of intensive therapy, he now runs to his grandpa and hugs him when he visits. Oliver greets his cousin with "Are you ready to rock?" whenever he sees her because she once said that to him in passing, a year or so ago. He likes only crunchy food and ice cream that is pink. He is obsessed with entertainment-production company logos and trains. His mother says that he has microvision and can spot the most miniscule train in a magazine, one that she needs a magnifying glass to see. He lines up all his train videos perfectly on the stairway in his house. He is also a computer whiz. He recently went on the Amtrak website and booked a trip to Santa Fe. Oliver, who operates on overdrive, scampers around his house on tiptoes. He possesses a great sense of humor and a gigantic smile, which creates deep canyons of dimples. Oliver currently repeats everything he hears. He recently began spontaneously telling his mother that he loves her. While he says this at appropriate times, his mother's not quite sure he knows what he's saying.

—*Lorelei, 12, has always been an enigma. Her babbling and speech stopped shortly after a vaccination when she was 9 months old and returned after she was 3 years old. She always "passed" as an average kid to her teachers, falling through the cracks because her testing was always in the "average" range. The fact is the average score was attained from very high highs and very low lows in developmental testing. Red flags were ignored. Like many girls, she was continuously being misdiagnosed. She doesn't like to be touched; she has difficulty with expressive, receptive, and pragmatic social speech and has a hard time making friends. She has a flat expression some of the time but is highly expressive other times. She often speaks as if she's reading from a script. She memorizes dialogue from her favorite TV shows and constantly repeats what she has memorized. Although friendly when she wants to be, she doesn't always make eye contact. But what confuses Lorelei's parents is that at times she acts like a completely typical child.*

—*Eydís, who lives in Iceland, is 13 years old. Her mother, Sigrún, first noticed that there was something wrong when Eydís was about 14 months old.*

"She didn't need me around," says Sigrún, "not even if she hurt herself." Eydís was brought to a specialist when she was 2 because she had stopped using the few words she had learned earlier, but the specialist told Sigrún not to worry. It was six months later when an audiologist agreed that there was something wrong. They were sent to the State Diagnostic Center. At 3, Eydís was finally diagnosed— her IQ was close to 50, and her speech was at a 1-year-old level. She has low muscle tone, and her fine and gross motor skills are not good. It was difficult to teach her to talk, but, by the time she was 5, she started to use words to express herself. Eydís has been in speech, occupational, and physical therapy on and off since her diagnosis. She attends a regular school with a special class for children with autism. Socially, she does not function well and does not like to talk to people or play with other kids. When she meets her classmates outside of her neighborhood, she becomes frightened because they are out of their normal context. She always talks about moving to Denmark or England because no one would recognize her there. Because of this anxiety she is on medications. She takes music lessons, plays the piano, and practices swimming with a group of handicapped children. She loves horseback riding. Eydís has a good sense of humor, and loves Mr. Bean, The Simpsons, Lazy Town, *and many other TV shows. She likes to read books and play with Bratz dolls, but the computer is her favorite activity. Eydís is a happy child, says Sigrún.*

—*As a child, Drew looked as if he could be a model. Now, at 9, his many medications have made him overweight. He has a few quirks: he likes to wear as many clothes as he can pile on, and he likes to eat—constantly. He started to speak only several years ago and is now probably at a 6-year-old speech level. He exhibits violent behavior by throwing tantrums, running away from his parents, screaming, thrashing, biting, scratching, and kicking, and he once tried to drown himself in a pool.*

—*Alastair, from Scotland, is now 21. His parents first noticed problems when he was about 18 months old, although he had been a very passive baby. He developed stilted and over-formal language, and behavior that was very disruptive, and he was unable to cope with change or choice. He had very little success socially and often was aggressive toward other children. He was not diagnosed until age 11. He was discovered to have a "spiky" IQ—very poor planning and organizational skills, but very high intellectual skills.*

Alastair went through mainstream school with little extra support, but his teachers were aware that his difficulties were not within his control and that he was not just being a naughty boy. He was very successful academically at secondary school and is now in his third year at the University of St. Andrews, studying computer science. He receives a lot of support from the university. He lives in a catered hall and receives help with organizational issues.

Alastair has become very interested in politics and is an active member of the Liberal Democrats. He was a constituency candidate for the Scottish Parliament elections in May 2007.

—Nika Louise, of Namibia, was born on November 17, 2000. Her mother, Karen, first suspected that something was wrong a few months after Nika turned 2. Karen brought her daughter to many specialists, who said Karen was "overreacting."

Nika had no speech at that time and poor eye-contact. There were frustration tantrums, her play was not typical, and she'd place everything in a line.

The young girl loves structure, although she is now able to start making changes to her routine. She still has very limited speech, although her receptive vocabulary is very large. She is very happy and displays and understands basic emotions. She will seldom play with other children; when she does, it is parallel play. She has recently started to engage occasionally in play with her sister, and she knows how to tease. Nika communicates only with people she knows and only if she wants something. She will use some words or point to what it is she wants. Her parents sometimes use sign language as a cue, but Nika does not sign back.

Nika is obsessed with books and is preoccupied with the alphabet; she will write it over and over.

Karen is very frustrated with the school system in Namibia, which, she says, "openly discriminates against these children. There are no government programs to put these children through schools (special or otherwise). Parents of children like Nika must fend for themselves."

—Maha Helali's son, Mostafa, is a 16-year-old Egyptian. As a child, Mostafa didn't sleep much and refused most foods except breast milk. But he reached developmental milestones, such as walking and talking on time. He would sing, recite nursery rhymes, and draw very detailed drawings like a mosque with minarets with a crescent on top. "Wow, a gifted child!" Maha thought. But by his twentieth month, Mostafa changed tremendously.

He began talking less and less. He seemed preoccupied and tended to daydream. He drew within himself and lost most of his speech by 24 months. Speech therapy didn't help. At 3, he became hyperactive and his love of repetition became more pronounced: he would draw the same pictures or pace the same area of the room.

Mostafa has "hyperhearing," Maha says, which was one of the reasons he couldn't sleep. "The boy was hearing beyond the walls; he was hearing his own body system." Mostafa traveled the world for treatment—first to England and then Belgium, and later the U.S.

At 10, Mostafa developed instrumental language, but he didn't use it unless he needed to. At 11, he moved from an intensive program to a prevocational program to help with his communication, daily living skills like hygiene and grooming, work-related skills like following schedules, and practical tasks like cooking and gardening.

At age 13, Mostafa began exhibiting obsessive-compulsive characteristics. He became obsessed with shoes. He likes them in all shapes, sizes, textures, and colors. Most of all, he fixates on new ones, especially ladies shoes with pointed toes and high heels.

Now, at 16, Mostafa still requires individual care. He is unable to care for himself without a lot of pre-verbal prompts and relies on others to guide him to meet his basic needs. His vocational training includes carpentry, weaving, and gardening (which he enjoys most). His domestic independence training includes shopping, cooking, doing laundry, and cleaning. He sight reads some words, but his concept of numbers stops at the number 5. He has been given responsibilities in the family; he takes the garbage out every evening, he shops with his companion, he dusts the furniture. His favorite chore is washing dishes because he gets engrossed in the sensation of the liquid soap on his hands.

Mostafa now likes receiving guests at home, which is very different from when he was younger and would put his shoes on to indicate he wanted to leave the house and the houseguests.

—Carl is 14, and he is considered a genius, always has been. His thing is dinosaurs. He might even know more about them than some paleontologists, say his parents. When he was young, he was like a little professor and he read scientific college academic books well beyond his age level. He can't make eye contact, and does not have any close friends. When he speaks to you, his tone is flat, awkward, and often inappropriate, and he exhibits in-your-face body language.

—Sanjoy is 8 years old, from a small town in West Bengal, India. He doesn't speak, doesn't have any social interaction, has repetitive actions, and makes no eye contact. His mother was told he was mentally retarded and will never be able to go to school, so Sanjoy has had no intervention or exposure to school until recently. Being nonverbal, he expresses his need by taking his mother's hand or giving her raw materials to request what he would like to eat. For example, if he wanted to eat roti (Indian bread), he would give her flour; or if he wanted curry, he'd give lentils for the choice of curry he wanted. He distinctly knows what the food is made from and what and where it is placed in the house.

He does nothing all day long. His mother has no idea what to do with him. She thinks he does not deserve to go to school. She is extremely busy doing household tasks and cannot give him time. She is happy that he is independent in most daily living activities.

—Susan is 6. She has never kissed her parents. She doesn't speak. She hates being touched. She rocks, flaps her hands, and sometimes bangs her head. She is not toilet-trained, and sometimes throws her feces. She does not respond to other children. She seems lost in her own world.

These are the children of autism.

There may be more of them than we thought.

Did you know?

On February 8, 2007, the U.S. Centers for Disease Control and Prevention released a stunning report, which stated that the U.S. autism rate in children is about one in 150— 6.6 per 1,000, up from a 2006 study figure of 5.5 in 1,000.

The study, "Prevalence of the Autism Spectrum Disorders (ASDs) in Multiple Areas of the United States, 2000 and 2002," a community report from the Autism and Developmental Disabilities Monitoring Network, was funded by the CDC, part of the U.S. Department of Health and Human Services.

While many autism advocates are thrilled with this validation of what they've been claiming for years, they also feel that the study is problematic in many ways. The research was conducted by reviewing medical and school records for 8-year-old children in fourteen states, leaving out regions such as New York State that are on the cutting edge of autism diagnostics.

Marshalyn Yeargin-Allsopp, M.D., a neurobiologist and chief of CDC's autism program, makes the study's parameters very clear: "This is not a nationally representative sample," adding that sites were chosen in a "competitive process, by a review panel." Maureen Durkin, Ph.D., a University of Wisconsin epidemiologist who led the Wisconsin part of the new CDC report, agrees, saying that the study is not demographically representative of the nation as a whole, but rather only sound for the specific state or county investigated.

One in 150!

This elevated rate doesn't come as a surprise to parents of autistic children, autism advocates, educators, and many health professionals, who have, for years, been claiming a higher incidence than reported in the original study; in fact, they believe the rate is even higher than that revealed by these new findings, closer to the study's New Jersey number: one in 94. But one in 150 is still a terribly disturbing number.

Evelyn Ain is the publisher of *Spectrum*, a U.S.-based magazine about autism and other developmental disabilities, and cofounder of Autism United. She is also the mother of Matthew (featured above), and she is not impressed with the study, which she calls "too little, too late." Not mincing words, she also calls it "a line of crap."

"This was not a fully accurate study," she argues. "Where's California, Texas, Florida, and New York? They couldn't count those states because it would have brought the number to one in ninety, or worse. It would have been too shocking."

Dr. Durkin says those states weren't included because "[they] had different methods of autism surveillance," but she believes that the rates for those states were "similar" to the CDC's results.

How it is manifested

Autism is the fastest-growing, serious developmental disability in the United States and other countries around the world. It is usually not diagnosed until after age 3, although early intervention is now the key thrust of advocacy groups, and children are being diagnosed years earlier. Many children with AS (Asperger syndrome), a form of high-functioning autism, especially girls, are not diagnosed properly until their teens.

It is easy to miss autism in girls for many reasons. Psychologist Shana Nichols, Ph.D., of the Fay J. Lindner Center for Autism in Bethpage, New York, explains that a girl's autism can easily be missed if conversational testing was brief, because girls are stereotypically trained in social conversation. But, she warns, when the testing runs longer than five minutes, the girl's "gaps in her social understanding will become evident." Don't compare girls to boys, she says, because "it's when they don't measure up to other girls" that autism might be indicated. Peers are most sensitive to these behaviors. "Other kids will notice it in the child's interaction," she says, and will pick up on a problem before a doctor might.

According to Autism Speaks, an advocacy organization for autism, more children will be diagnosed with autism this year than with AIDS, diabetes, and pediatric cancer combined.

It is important to remember that autism is a spectrum of disorders. A child might not have "classic" stereotypical symptoms, like muteness or hand flapping, and still be on the spectrum.

"No two autistic children are alike," warns Ain.

Arwa El-Amine Halawi, president of the Lebanese Autism Society and parent of an autistic teenaged son, agrees. "There is no child with autism like another," she says, adding that being a parent of an autistic child can be a positive experience. "Having a child with autism can teach us a lot," she explains. "[My son] teaches us the meaning of life; he teaches us how to be stronger to get over obstacles; he teaches us tolerance and genuine love."

But it is a struggle.

By the numbers

There's good reason to believe that these current revised numbers don't accurately reflect the actual high incidence of autism. Foremost, the studies were conducted in 2000 and 2002—years prior to the burst of awareness that has significantly raised autism spectrum diagnoses. In fact, it was in 2004 that the "Autism A.L.A.R.M." report distributed by the American Academy of Pediatrics was sent out to all pediatricians. There was a big push at that time toward spreading the word through its "Learn the Signs. Act Early" and "First Signs" public-education efforts. So it is easy to imagine how exponentially high the rise of autism grew *after* the current CDC study's completion.

Dr. Yeargin-Allsopp does have encouraging news: CDC researchers have already collected data for 2004 and are starting to collect data for 2006.

"It's about time someone finally did a broader, literal 'head count,'" says Patty Romanowski Bashe, M.S. Ed., an expert on AS and coauthor of *The OASIS Guide to Asperger Syndrome*, of this study. But, she warns, how a study gathers its statistics needs to be checked carefully.

"Remember, when you're looking at school records or other official counts [as they did in the CDC study], you're seeing only the children whose parents, doctors, or teachers referred them for evaluation," she explains. "Then from that group, you're certainly 'losing' some kids, because their parents didn't want the diagnosis, evaluators are reluctant to give a diagnosis at a certain age and want to 'wait and see,' or parents refused to have them placed in appropriate, nonmainstream school settings. Even if a child has a diagnosis, not every school district special-education committee will classify them under autism; they might choose a classification like 'other health impaired' or something else."

Dr. Durkin agrees, claiming that the Wisconsin numbers might be higher for just the reasons Bashe states.

"We were not able to review educational records [in Wisconsin]," Dr. Durkin says. "In previous research in Atlanta, 40 percent of the autism cases were identified only through educational records."

Because some areas had different types of records available than others, Dr. Yeargin-Allsopp admits, "It was like comparing apples to apples *and* apples to oranges," in some cases.

"We believe it is possible that the rates are, in fact, higher," says Dr. Ellen Giarelli, a coinvestigator of the Pennsylvania study. "This belief is based on not being able to review the records of all children in the study area who were eligible for such a review."

Even according to the CDC, the numbers of children receiving services for autism can't be accurately calculated because some children receive services for a specific need, like speech therapy, and do not have an official autism classification.

Whether the rate is one in 150, one in ninety, or one in seven, this increase in the number of children with autism is still a serious situation that needs to be addressed. For a disorder found in such a large part of a vulnerable population, it is surprising that there is such disagreement as to its etiology and whether the numbers are growing or just a result of refined methods of diagnosis.

"For some of us, this research study confirms what we already know," says Robert Krakow, a former member of the National Autism Association board of directors and a civil and criminal lawyer who specializes in vaccine-injury litigation. "The shockingly high numbers are going up in ways that indicate that the rate is truly rising, despite the fact that there is great debate on the theory that this is merely better detection, diagnosis, and awareness."

"For five years, I tried to tell everyone the numbers were wrong," says Krakow. "We think the numbers, however shocking they are now, are even higher. We've always believed it was an epidemic. It started in the '80s, rapidly increased in the '90s, and the CDC always tried to shade it. They have not done careful ascertainments."

Dr. Sydney Pettygrove, Ph.D., an epidemiologist and coinvestigator on the Arizona CDC study, stops short at calling this an epidemic because an epidemic occurs, he says, when "a condition is significantly higher [than] what you would expect based on previous experience." "The problem I see here," he says, "is our 'previous experience.' We don't have data collected in the same, rigorous way for earlier times." But this CDC study, Pettygrove's colleague Christopher Cunniff, M.D., says, can provide that "baseline."

"This *is* the baseline," says Dr. Yeargin-Allsopp of the study. And that's good news.

But to many autism activists, it *is* an epidemic. In New York, Krakow, Ain, and other advocates believe that their local statistics are similar to the CDC's New Jersey study, which claims one in ninety-four, and one in sixty boys.

But even that is surrounded by controversy because, as we have seen, girls are often misdiagnosed, or underdiagnosed, when it comes to neurobiological and behavioral disorders.

With stakes so high, there will always be controversy. There are some parents of high-end autistic children with AS, HFA (high-functioning autism), PDD–NOS, and older high-functioning children—the children many parents claim who make this a true spectrum—who say autism organizations use their children to boost up their numbers, but then don't address their children's needs.

But those advocacy organizations can also make a positive difference. Autism Speaks, for example, started by Suzanne and Bob Wright, former chairman and CEO of NBC Universal, started the organization in February 2005 after the diagnosis of their grandson Christian. The amount of awareness the organization has created has been amazing. It has been hailed by many as the impetus for getting worldwide attention focused on the disorder, and in the short time it's been in existence, it has also raised an enormous amount of research money and has sponsored numerous worthwhile programs.

Signs and symptoms

ASDs are lifelong neurobiological developmental disabilities. The behaviors might run from mild to extreme, but there are several consistently associated with autism, and they fall into three basic categories: interpersonal relationships; speech problems; and repetitive, ritualistic behavior.

Behaviors may differ widely among such children. For instance, autistic children might be nonverbal, or they might be extremely talkative. They might have trouble relating to others, but sometimes they can be very social. They might have an aversion to affection, or they might smother a parent in kisses. They might not play pretend games, or they can get lost in imaginary play. Some might have terrible tantrums, while others are docile.

Some symptoms, though, are common among children with ASDs. They often avoid eye contact, have difficulty comprehending other people's emotions, and have strong sensory reactions, so that they might not like being touched or being in a room with loud sounds. Even family and friends gently singing "Happy Birthday" can send them into a hands-over-ears panic. Despite common belief, they might be very interested in human contact but may not know how to interact appropriately. They might repeat or echo words and exhibit repetitive actions. When they want an object, they might not point to it or won't look in the direction someone else is pointing. They often have difficulty with change in routine, lose skills they once had, and find an interest that becomes obsessive. Children on the autism spectrum crave self-stimulation ("stimming") such as rocking, hand-flapping, making unusual noises, repeating words, and toe-walking. It is also believed that gastrointestinal problems are connected to autism.

CHAT, the "CHecklist for Autism in Toddlers," is a guide that was created for general practitioners to use at a child's 18-month exam. It was first published by Simon Baron-Cohen, Ph.D., and colleagues in 1992, and although it is not routinely used any longer, it is included here because it can serve as a guidepost for parents as somewhat of a screening—not diagnostic—tool. There are updated versions (M-CHAT, CHAT-23, and Q-CHAT) that are currently being tested.

In 1996, the *British Journal of Psychiatry* reported, in the article "Psychological markers in the detection of autism in infancy in a large population": "Consistent failure of the three key items from the CHAT at 18 months of age carries an 83.3 per cent risk of autism; and this pattern of risk indicator is specific to autism when compared to other forms of developmental delay." The checklist is printed below; the asterisk (*) before some questions indicates a critical question most indicative of autistic characteristics.

Checklist for Autism in Toddlers

Section A: Ask parent

Yes or No?

(1) Does your child enjoy being swung, bounced on your knee, etc.?

(2) Does your child take an interest in other children?

(3) Does your child like climbing on things, such as up stairs?

(4) Does your child enjoy playing peek-a-boo/hide-and-seek?

*(5) Does your child ever pretend, for example, to make a cup of tea using a toy cup and teapot, or pretend other things?

(6) Does your child ever use his/her index finger to point, to ask for something?

*(7) Does your child ever use his/her index finger to point, to indicate interest in something?

(8) Can your child play properly with small toys (e.g., cars or bricks) without just mouthing, fiddling, or dropping them?

(9) Does your child ever bring objects over to you, to show you something?

Section B: GP's observation

Yes or No?

(1) During the appointment, has the child made eye contact with you?

*(2) Get child's attention, then point across the room at an interesting object and say "Oh look! There's a (name a toy)!" Watch child's face. Does the child look across

to see what you are pointing at? [NOTE: To record yes on this item, ensure the child has not simply looked at your hand, but has actually looked at the object you are pointing at.]

★(3) Get the child's attention, then give child a miniature toy cup and teapot and say "Can you make a cup of tea?" Does the child pretend to pour out the tea, drink it, etc.? [NOTE: If you can elicit an example of pretending in some other game, score a yes on this item.]

★(4) Say to the child "Where's the light?" or "Show me the light." Does the child point with his/her index finger at the light? [NOTE: Repeat this with "Where's the teddy?" or some other unreachable object, if child does not understand the word "light." To record yes on this item, the child must have looked up at your face around the time of pointing.]

(5) Can the child build a tower of bricks? (If so, how many?) (Number of bricks …)

In the American Academy of Pediatric's "First Signs" awareness campaign of 2004, warning signs were provided:

- no big smiles or other warm, joyful expressions by 6 months or thereafter
- no back-and-forth sharing of sounds, smiles, or other facial expressions by 9 months or thereafter
- no babbling by 12 months
- no back-and-forth gestures, such as pointing, showing, reaching, or waving by 12 months
- no words by 16 months
- no two-word meaningful phrases (without imitating or repeating) by 24 months
- any loss of speech or babbling or social skills at any age

Again, it is important to note that these are just potential warning signs. A child can exhibit all of these behaviors or one—or completely opposite ones.

Newly diagnosed children include a broader definition of the autism spectrum, including those who are higher functioning or have milder symptoms or PDD–NOS, which has become a catch-all for hard-to-diagnose, atypical children like Lorelei, featured in the introduction to this chapter.

PDD–NOS is one of the five disorders on the PDD spectrum, which also include autism, AS, and two severe genetic developmental disorders, CDD (childhood disintegrative disorder) and RS (Rett's syndrome).

For many years, autistic children were stereotyped as having Susan's above-mentioned symptoms, perceived as rocking, silent head bangers. Now, there are children who are diagnosed as being on the wide autism spectrum who would appear "normal" to most outsiders.

It could be said that no other disorder has grown so fast in awareness as autism. It is a commonly held view that parents of autistic children sometimes know more about the disorder than do their doctors. Those parents began to spread the news, take control of their children's educational needs, and raise money for research into the possible cause factors: genetic, environmental, and vaccines.

Cause

As for the cause of ASDs, theories also range dramatically. Experts such as Jeff Bradstreet, M.D., founder of the International Child Development Resource Center in Florida, say it is medical; organizations like the New York-based Grassroots Environmental Education blame environmental factors; and others, like Patty Romanowski Bashe, say it's mainly genetically based.

Robert Krakow points out that the states covered in the CDC study that had the highest incidences of ASDs, such as New Jersey, were the states with the highest childhood vaccination rates. While some parents, advocates, and doctors believe vaccines are connected to autism, many studies and experts have indicated there is no connection. A compromise theory is that vaccines affect an already predisposed child.

Epidemiologist Dr. Pettygrove, the coinvestigator on the 2007 CDC Arizona study, suggests that maybe parents with autistic children moved to states like New Jersey for better services, and that is the reason their rates are higher. CDC's Dr. Yeargin-Allsopp says the higher rate can be explained because New Jersey has "more information in their records."

Diagnosis

Autism, as prevalent as it is, is still the subject of many debates. Some experts, like Dr. Bradstreet, don't think autism is a single disorder, but rather "autisms," as did many other specialists from around the world who were interviewed for this book. Perhaps autism is just a cluster of disorders such as SID, OCD, APD, ADHD, etc.

The U.K.'s National Autistic Society (NAS) reminds us that autism is "a spectrum of conditions." Not only do those conditions vary widely from person to person, NAS points out that it can vary in one individual, explaining that an autistic person's "difficulties" can change on a daily basis making him or her "more or less sensitive to particular things on different days."

While most professionals use the *DSM* and *ICD* as diagnostic guides, a growing number of parents of autistic children and experts in the field say the *DSM*'s and *ICD*'s criteria are immaterial.

"The *DSM* is totally irrelevant," says Krakow. "It's a classifications system that doesn't work." The ever-changing criteria in the *DSM* were determined by committee, as a guide, a way to rule out disorders. But that's not good enough for advocates like Krakow.

"You can come up with a different definition at any point," he says. "Look at what they did with homosexuality. Their criteria just suddenly changed."

Part of the diagnostic mystery is that there are no medical tests for autism. A diagnosis comes from empirical evidence such as clinical observations and family interviews. A developmental history is taken, speech and language are evaluated, psychological testing is given, and diagnostic tests for autism are performed.

If you have any concerns about your child's development, all experts advise that you get him or her help as early as possible.

Prognosis

Now that the staggering numbers have been released by the CDC, what needs to be done?

Dr. Durkin says that the report should have a positive effect. "I think it will contribute to a national consensus that autism is not an extremely rare condition," she says, "and that pediatric and educational services need to be enhanced to meet the demand."

Bashe, who has a 15-year-old son who has Asperger, says, "Treat autism as the real, serious, lifelong neurological disorder that it is.

"Pressure school districts to put evidence-based treatment plans and real experts on autism in classrooms and really help these kids to achieve their potential. I am a big fan of ABA for everyone [Bashe utilizes ABA in early intervention teaching. ABA is a method of breaking down a particular activity into its simplest parts and rewarding the child after he or she masters the part being taught]; there's room for other approaches as well, but the bedrock foundation must be behavioral. It's the only approach based on an application of scientific principles of human behavior. Focus on funding on helping children and families deal with the problems they have today."

"The most shocking aspect of this report," says Peter Pierri, executive director of the Smithtown, New York-based Developmental Disabilities Institute (DDI), "is that the CDC's analysis also found that delays in diagnosis were all too common—an average of at least a year and a half from the time parents first reported odd speech problems or other social deficits to the time of evaluation and diagnosis. It is frightening that many parents are waiting so long to have their children evaluated."

While everyone agrees that early diagnosis and intervention are crucial, parents and activists like Autism United's Ain are very concerned about the future.

"The number in this CDC study is very, very, very bad news," she says. "How are we going to take care of these children? Something has to happen in a major way. Where is the Department of Education? Where is the White House? Where's our president? The U.S. is 'helping' the world, but they're not helping our kids. We're talking at least one in 150. These children are falling through the cracks, minute by minute. We can't afford our [autistic] children now. What is going to happen when they are 21? It is going to be one big nightmare."

So, what can be done? "Get to work!" advises Bashe, who believes that getting the child into the proper educational setting is key. "But I mean get to work with the teachers who know what they are doing. Demand results, not just placement. Know that we can all do so much better.

"There are many concerns facing families affected by autism. The biggest one currently is what happens when these one-in-150 children start aging out of their school programs. What happens to them when they become adults?"

The Combating Autism Act of 2006, available on the Internet, might help that, with its $900 million in funding. But Dan Roland, development director of DDI, says where that money is spent is important. "Money for research is great, but more money needs to be apportioned for building capacity and programs," he explains.

As autistic children start aging out of school, parents are revisiting their wills and looking into living trusts, to secure their children's future when they become adults—but now, they need the right programs.

Robert Budd, chief administrative officer of Family Residences and Essential Enterprises, Inc. (FREE), a thirty-year-old agency serving "differently-abled" adults in one hundred sites on Long Island, New York, has been optimistically waiting for funding for an AS program for two years.

"I hope this [CDC] study highlights the vast need we've been experiencing as a provider of services to [the autistic community]," says Budd. "Any time facts can substantiate what people in the field are experiencing, it is very powerful. It is a very good step in the right direction."

Dr. Yeargin-Allsopp is also optimistic about the study, saying that it will lead to "early identification and services for large numbers of children and their families."

It better … for Matthew, Oliver, Lorelei, Eydís, Drew, Alastair, Nika, Mostafa, Carl Sanjoy, and Susan, and the counted and uncounted children like them.

Sources and resources

American Academy of Pediatrics:

"Autism A.L.A.R.M.," www.nomercury.org/science/documents/autism_alarm.pdf

"First signs Autism Campaign," www.dbpeds.org/articles/detail.cfm?TextID=148

Autism Speaks (www.autismspeaks.org)

S. Baron-Cohen, A. Cox, G. Baird, et al., "Psychological Markers in the Detection of Autism in Infancy in a Large Population," *British Journal of Psychiatry* 168 (1996): 158–63.

National Autistic Society, UK (www.nas.org.uk)

Spectrum Magazine (www.spectrumpublications.com)

See the "Autism" contacts and the mental-health contacts under "General Resources" for more sources used in this chapter.

B

BED (Binge-Eating Disorder)

BN (Bulimia Nervosa)

BED

Binge-Eating Disorder

Terms used in this chapter: BED (binge-eating disorder); CBT (cognitive behavioral therapy); ED (eating disorder); NIH (National Institutes of Health)

Sound familiar?

Martha, 16, can't wait to come home from school. She runs straight for the refrigerator and, as she says, "eats and eats and eats and eats."

"I talk on the phone with my friends, and they are always yelling at me because they hear me chewing on the other end," says the self-described "very pudgy" South Carolina high-school junior.

Her mother, Naolmi, says that Martha was always "out of control" with her eating. "When she was a child, she seemed like she didn't have that on/off switch when she ate," she says.

Martha would eat everything on her plate, mostly high-fat, greasy foods, and then go for the leftovers on everyone else's plates. "She'd live for dessert," says Naolmi, who eventually made stricter—and healthier—eating rules around the house.

When Martha first entered her teens, she was becoming depressed. She knew the overeating wasn't good for her. At age 13, at 5 foot 2, she weighed 210 pounds.

"I just couldn't stop," says Martha. "I wasn't even hungry most of the time. That was the weird part."

"We tried diets," says Naolmi, "but they seemed to make things worse. I would wake up at midnight and catch her eating salsa with her fingers, desperately scooping it out of the jar."

Soon Martha's parents began removing enticing food from the house.

"If she was going to binge, let her binge on fruit," says her mother.

The bingeing began affecting all aspects of Martha's life—academically, she began failing; socially, she became isolated; and psychologically, she had no self-esteem. As she recalls, "I had absolutely no happiness in my life. Especially with eating. I hated it, and I couldn't stop it."

Finally, at 15, Martha was brought for cognitive behavioral therapy (CBT) and group therapy. Both therapies made what Martha calls "a world of difference."

"I changed how I think about food—why I need it, why I think I need it. I now eat only when I'm hungry. If I catch myself grabbing for a piece of cake, I ask myself, 'Do you really want this?' I ask myself while I eat, 'Are you just finishing off everything on your plate because it's there or because you need it?' Most of the time, I realize I don't need it, and I don't eat it."

She has since lost what she calls "a serious amount of weight" and is very happy to be just "temporarily slightly pudgy."

She has built up her self-esteem, has supportive friends, and, most importantly, received a clean bill of health at her last doctor's appointment.

Martha has BED—binge-eating disorder.

Did you know?

Many children, and adults as well, have had bouts of overeating, whether overdoing it at a favorite restaurant, an after-school raid on the refrigerator, or downing a pound of candy at a trip to the mall. But BED is something altogether different.

BED is an ED that is characterized by uncontrolled periods of eating an unwarranted amount of food in a very short period of time. What makes it a disorder, as with other behaviors that can be considered normal at times, is when it meets certain clinical criteria and begins to have a negative impact on the child's life. Bingeing becomes a disorder when those periods of excessive eating become recurrent and cannot be controlled, and it is not associated with other manifestations of eating disorders such as purging, taking laxatives, strict dieting, fasting, overexercising, etc. Bingeing, which seems very much like bulimia, is different from that disorder because children with BED do not purge, as bulimics do.

Although overeating without purging, fasting, or exercising leads to obesity, don't be misled that children who maintain normal weight cannot have BED—they can. But overweight children with BED often bring the disorder along with them as they age and become obese adults. Early intervention can help prevent a future of bad physical and psychological health.

Although BED is not yet classified as a specific mental-health condition, it is believed by experts that BED is the most common ED.

The National Institute of Mental Health cites surveys that found between 2 and 5 percent of Americans experience binge-eating disorder in a six-month period.

Signs and symptoms

- avoids social activities
- anger
- anxiety
- being overweight
- binge eating for at least two days a week for six months
- boredom
- diabetes
- discernible distress over the bingeing
- eating an excessive amount of food within a short period of time
- eating enormous amounts of food even when not hungry
- eating until—and past—feeling uncomfortable
- embarrassment and guilt feelings over amount of food being eaten
- frequent episodes of out-of-control eating
- gallbladder problems
- heart problems

- high blood pressure
- high cholesterol
- lack of control or feeling there is a lack of control while bingeing
- poor self-esteem
- preoccupation with appearance
- rapid eating
- sadness
- school absences
- solitary eating
- weight gain

Cause

It isn't really known why children suffer from BED, but the NIH reports that "up to half of all people with binge-eating disorder have a history of depression." It is not known whether depression is a cause or effect of BED, but it is generally believed that negative emotions like anger, impulsivity, depression, and anxiety can induce BED. Again, we see the interconnectivity of the Alphabet Disorders.

Dieting could also bring on a binge-eating episode.

Of course, a child's metabolism and the chemistry of his or her brain have much to do with an ED such as BED, and researchers are currently pursuing those studies.

Diagnosis

A diagnosis of BED can be made by a child's pediatrician or a mental-health professional. The pediatrician will first conduct a full physical exam in order to rule out any other medical condition. The next step is a behavioral history and observation assessment of the child, including changes in weight, body-weight index, and vital signs. A blood test might be given to check electrolytes, cholesterol level, blood sugar, or the child's metabolism.

Treatment

What needs to be done to help children with BED is to interrupt the excessive-eating cycle. A new eating model is initiated, and the child's eating psychology changes: the goals are that the children aren't as hungry as they were formerly and that their distorted feelings about themselves and food are changed.

The best therapies are CBT and psychotherapy. CBT is a technique where patients are taught to remold their behaviors, replacing negative behaviors and responses with positive ones. It should help a BED child learn to control the urges for eating and, even more importantly, redirect the causes of those urges.

Individual, family, and group psychotherapy often prove effective methods of treatment, as do medications such as antidepressants. A doctor should be consulted when using any type of medication with a child. (See the "ED: Eating Disorder" chapter for more information.)

There isn't one specified treatment route for children with BED, and researchers are continuously trying to determine which type of therapy or combination is the most successful. But whatever the course, overeating isn't the answer—the child needs professional help.

Prognosis

Children with BED can certainly be helped, but, without professional treatment, they are susceptible to many complications and diseases. As anorexics suffer the complications of starvation, BED kids suffer the complications of obesity, which the NIH lists as diabetes, high blood pressure, high cholesterol levels, gallbladder disease, heart disease, and certain types of cancer. There are many psychological repercussions of BED, from severe depression to isolation, and the eating cycle and psychological disturbances become caught up in a vicious and stressful cycle of its own.

Sources and resources

Binge Eating Program/Western Psychiatric Institute and Clinic
    (http://wpic.upmc.com/EatingDisorderSvcs.htm)
National Institutes of Health, "Eating Disorders" (www.nih.gov)

See the "ED: Eating Disorder" chapter for more sources used in this chapter.

BN

Bulimia Nervosa

Terms used in this chapter: AN (anorexia nervosa); BN (bulimia nervosa); CBT (cognitive behavioral therapy); ED (eating disorder); OCD (obsessive-compulsive disorder)

Sound familiar?

Janis, now 15, has been bulimic for at least two years, she now admits. Her father says that he believes it has been much longer than that. Whatever the case, it's a miracle to the family that Janis has admitted to her problem and is allowing it to be addressed by medical and psychological professionals.

Janis' condition is simple. She thinks she's overweight (she is not), and she throws up or takes laxatives after she eats. She used to gag herself after each meal; now she can just vomit at will.

Her parents became alarmed at her weight loss and were savvy enough to realize Janis' view of herself was wholly off-base and inappropriate.

There was another key. Janis' mother, aunt, and grandmother each had battled an ED.

Janis' pediatrician was also very perceptive. He knew Janis had a problem.

At first, Janis denied it, but she could not explain away the visits to the bathroom after each meal, the erratic weight loss, the laxatives her mother found in her bedroom, and the sores she had in her mouth.

Her doctor took tests and found that Janis was having irregular heartbeats, and mouth, dental, and throat problems that indicated excessive vomiting.

Confronted with a supportive family and medical and psychological intervention, Janis began coming around.

She has gained weight and does not purge after each meal. Instead, she now sometimes uses diuretics, which is being addressed through therapy.

Janis has BN—bulimia nervosa.

Did you know?

BN, a fear of fatness, is a serious, chronic, binge-purge ED that often first appears in the teen years, but it can manifest itself at any age, even as young as 5. Probably the reason for the high BN rate in adolescence is due to the fact that younger, prepubescent, and preteen children are not necessarily knowledgeable and capable enough to purge and are less subjected to the pressures of being thin.

With BN, eating binges can occur several times a day. (Snacking throughout the day is not considered bingeing.) If the child eats amounts of food that seem to be larger than what his or her peers would eat or if the child seems to have no control over his or her eating, then it might be time for concern—for example, if the child eats an entire box of cookies instead of a few cookies. Bulimic children then try to mitigate their eating, and possible weight gain, by purging or using some other source to lose weight, such as laxatives, diuretics, etc. In between the bingeing periods, the bulimic eats very little, if any, food.

If left unchecked, BN can be a very dangerous disorder that is life-long and life-threatening. It affects mostly female adolescents, but it also affects males. Early intervention is very important in helping children with this disorder.

Abigail Natenshon, psychotherapist and author of *When Your Child Has an Eating Disorder: A Step-by-Step Workbook for Parents and Other Caregivers*, warns that "the most lethal of all the mental health disorders, eating disorders, kill 13 to 20 percent of their victims, 90 percent of whom are kids under the age of 20." But the good news, she says, is that "eating disorders are curable in 80 percent of cases where parents can detect disease in their child early and engage in the most effective treatment for both child and family."

These disorders can be tricky, Natenshon warns: "They are insidious, hardly appearing to look like pathology, but instead resembling self-discipline and self-control."

A child with BN, as with AN, can be putting his or her life in danger. Starvation can cause a string of life-threatening disorders (see the "AN: Anorexia Nervosa" chapter). Purging—vomiting—can cause stomach acids to be brought into the esophagus, causing great damage and sometimes even death. The use of diuretics, laxatives, and enemas can purge the body of essential electrolytes and minerals.

By the numbers

According to the National Institute of Mental Health, an estimated 1.1 percent to 4.2 percent of females have BN in their lifetime. The Mayo Clinic places the number of those with BN as between 1 and 3 percent of women, and one-tenth of that as men. In March 2007, it was reported by *The Scotsman* that one in every one hundred 12–25-year-olds in Britain has AN, and BN rates are highest among college-aged youth, where it is at a 4 percent rate.

Signs and symptoms

- abnormal bowel functioning
- acting mysteriously
- AN
- anxiety
- bloating
- cardiac arrhythmias
- chronic weight loss
- constipation
- damaged gums and tooth enamel
- dehydration
- dental cavities
- depression
- dry skin
- electrolyte abnormalities
- epileptic seizures
- esophageal tears
- excessive weight loss
- exercises strenuously after meals
- fatigue

- feeling of self-disgust
- hemorrhoids
- hoarding food
- inflammation of the throat
- irregular heartbeat
- irresistible cravings for food
- laxative abuse
- leaves for bathroom during and/or after a meal
- loss of control in terms of eating
- low calcium levels
- menstrual cycles in teen girls stops (amenorrhea)
- muscular weakness
- obsession with being thin
- pancreatitis
- preoccupation with dieting and weight
- purging
- recurrent episodes of binge eating
- secret weighing
- skips meals, followed by bingeing
- sores in throat and mouth
- sores, scars, or calluses on knuckles or hands
- starvation
- suddenly begins a strange eating pattern or stops eating certain foods
- swollen salivary glands in cheeks
- use of diuretics and/or enemas

Cause

There are an assorted number of causes for BN in children, including a low self-image, OCD, or a familial predisposition for anxiety or depression. There are also strong connections between BN and peer pressure, sociocultural expectations, and emotional crises.

Although there seems to be a biological connection, it appears that there is a strong genetic disposition for disorders like this, especially between mothers and daughters, and numerous twin studies support that connection. However, there has been no proved genetic link. The biological connection could be about serotonin, a brain chemical that influences such disorders as depression and OCD, which is thought to influence ED because it is connected to the regulation of food intake as well.

Sociological and cultural causes are also responsible for this disorder. Each generation gets inundated with more media images of a thin-equals-success mindset than ever before. And we're not talking about traditionally thin—it's all about being ultrathin, whether it is seen in young models, actresses, and athletes, and even singers. Images of bone-thin celebrities abound. Those kinds of images are all a vulnerable child who doesn't fit in needs in order to turn bulimic.

Diagnosis

If your child exhibits any of the above symptoms, he or she might be a bulimic. Your observation and those of friends and teachers can be the impetus to get the child the help he or she needs. The child's pediatrician will run a full exam to make sure there are no other underlying medical problems, and the doctor will probably refer the child to a mental-health professional who, through clinical observation, history, and psychological testing, will provide a diagnosis.

Unlike most other behavioral disorders, there are some medical tests that can help with the BN diagnosis.

Calcium levels can be tested and the "chem-20" test could indicate dehydration or imbalance of potassium, sodium, and other electrolytes. A dentist can examine the child to see if the acid resulting from the purging has affected his or her teeth—cavities, gum disease, and loss or erosion of enamel.

There are many other disorders with which BN can be confused, including AN, binge-eating/purging type; KLS (Kleine-Levin syndrome), a disorder characterized by hyper-sleepiness; MDD (major depressive disorder), with atypical features; BPD (borderline personality disorder); and BDD (body dysmorphic disorder).

Treatment

Treatment begins at home. Parents should not have a household that is obsessed with food, dieting, or body image. Children learn by modeling their behavior after that of their parents. The message parents should get across is one of high self-esteem, eating healthy foods, eating in moderation, and taking reasonable exercise.

Modeling behavior doesn't end with eating—a child who can assess conflicts and effectively problem-solve will know how to deal properly with the adversity of eating issues. Also, most ED organizations suggest that families who eat together—family meals—set a better environment for their children in terms of preventing eating disorders.

But what happens when the child begins to demonstrate symptoms of BN? The first key is to recognize that there is a problem. Most children with EDs attempt to hide their disorders.

Children, however, might not even realize that they have a disease and will most likely appreciate a parent's intervention. It shows that their parent loves and cares about them; for those children who realize they have a serious problem, this intervention might show them there is a light at the end of the tunnel.

Do not be intimidated into thinking you will upset your child or will turn your child away from you—it is your responsibility to take control of your child's future.

These BN children have a distorted perception, along with uncontrollable compulsions and obsessions, coupled with unmanageable anxiety and other mood disorders. The child is completely helpless, although it might not always seem that way to you. Even if this were an adult friend, they would need your intervention.

Educating your child about food, without lecturing, is important. Explain, for example, that traditional dieting is not the best way to lose weight. They can be taught that actually eating *more* food that is healthy might serve better than a restrictive diet.

As soon as signs begin to appear, seek professional help. While the child receives that help, remember that they still need great support from their family and friends.

Individual psychotherapy and family and group therapy are all approaches that can help a BN child. Working with a dietician or nutritionist can also prove very helpful. CBT has proved very effective with food disorders, as it replaces bad behaviors with positive ones and is relatively short-term. As you will learn throughout this book, medication, namely antidepressants, also has proved very effective in tandem with CBT in many psychological disorders. The correct combination of therapies is the key to success, and the good news is that it helps. All use of medications should be discussed with a doctor.

Sources and resources

The Mayo Clinic, "Binge-eating disorder" (www.mayoclinic.com)

Abigail H. Natenshon, *When Your Child Has an Eating Disorder: A Step-by-Step Workbook for Parents and Other Caregivers* (San Francisco: Jossey-Bass, 1999).

The Scotsman (http://thescotsman.scotsman.com)

See the "ED: Eating Disorder" chapter for more sources used in this chapter.

C

CA (Childhood Agoraphobia)

CAD (Childhood Adjustment Disorder)

CAS (Childhood Apraxia of Speech)

CBD (Childhood Bipolar Disorder)

CCS (Clumsy Child Syndrome)

CD (Childhood Depression)

CD (Conduct Disorder)

CDCS (Cri du Chat Syndrome)

CDD (Childhood Disintegrative Disorder)

CdLS (Cornelia de Lange Syndrome)

CLS (Coffin-Lowry Syndrome)

CMT (Charcot-Marie-Tooth Disorder)

COS (Childhood-Onset Schizophrenia)

CS (Cockayne Syndrome)

CA

Childhood Agoraphobia

Terms used in this chapter: CA (childhood agoraphobia); CBT (cognitive behavioral therapy); *DSM* (*Diagnostic and Statistical Manual of Mental Disorders*); *ICD* (*International Classification of Diseases*); OCD (obsessive-compulsive disorder); PD (panic disorder); PTSD (post-traumatic stress disorder); SAD (separation anxiety disorder); SPD (social phobia disorder)

Sound familiar?

Leif, a short but muscular long-haired, red-headed teen, used to love playing with his friends. But when he turned 14, his body began to endure an onslaught of hormonal changes, and that changed him forever, says his father, Gregory.

Leif had a "typical" childhood, growing up in a Los Angeles suburban community that looks like a set straight out of one of the nearby Hollywood movie lots. From house after house, all meticulously landscaped, you can hear the sounds of children splashing around in pools. Kids of all ages ride bikes in packs. There are impromptu baseball games on the street, and anything that can quickly gets adapted into makeshift skateboarding ramps. This was Leif's life, until something drastically changed.

No one knows what the particular incident was, or even if there was one at all, that set Leif's fear of going outside, playing with his friends, hanging out at the mall, going to McDonald's or a movie—even sitting on the front lawn with pals.

"He would have a total wave of fear run through him," Gregory explains. "And it would prevent him from doing anything. He could not walk out that front door to face the outside world."

Leif describes the "dark" experience: "I would walk around the mall with my friends, and all I could think about was my depression and my fear," he says. "I was obsessed with being outside of my safe zone."

He couldn't wait to go back to his poster-covered room and watch TV, play video games, listen to his iPod, and even do his homework. He says that he always had an undercurrent of anxiety and home was where he felt safest.

So what happens when Leif is invited to a movie with his friends?

"I start worrying about it well before I have to do the activity," he explains. "I come up with a million excuses. I get worried because it makes me so nervous and I anticipate the worst. I think I'm going to throw up or do something else weird in front of strangers.

"I'd just rather stay home."

Leif says the feeling is more one of "being trapped" than anything else, joking about being more comfortable on an open baseball field during a lightning storm by himself than in a closed restaurant with his friends.

Unfortunately for Leif, another trouble zone is middle school, always a chore for him to attend. But Leif's parents really dread next year: he is to begin high school and has exhibited extremely heightened anxiety several times when discussing it with his parents.

They realized that this was more than a passing phase and that he needed help. Leif's mother, Tara, knew firsthand what panic felt like. She has been phobic most of her life.

Preparing for his change of school—and because his problem is getting more and more severe, almost "paralyzing the kid," as Gregory says—Leif has begun behavioral therapy and is taking an anti-anxiety drug, Luvox, which his parents intend to be short-term.

His therapist is using cognitive behavioral therapy (CBT), desensitizing him to the situation through exposure to the stressor. "She [Leif's therapist] takes me through situations that make me nervous. Like, she'll act out with me, 'OK, you're leaving your front door now, you're walking down the street, you walk to the mall, you're walking in the mall.'"

Leif is thrilled about his small progress.

"I feel trapped. It's almost like being claustrophobic," he says, "but it's like now I have some hope."

Leif has CA—childhood agoraphobia.

Did you know?

CA is both an anxiety and phobia disorder. It is a fear of being trapped and being in places where, if a feeling of panic does occur, there might not be help available or it might be embarrassing to receive help. The fear causes avoidant behavior.

The misconception of agoraphobia being a fear of "open spaces," its literal meaning, must be corrected. Actually, there are many agoraphobics, like Leif, who *prefer* open spaces—it's the "getting to" the open space that's problematic. Agoraphobic children would rather stay in their safe zone than anywhere else.

While some agoraphobics panic about open spaces—an outdoor music festival, for example, would likely be a nightmare—most agoraphobia revolves around the fear of closed places like restaurants, movie theaters, malls, schools, and supermarkets. CA is the fear of being around people, particularly in large numbers, and being unable to escape.

The disorder is manifested when a child begins to avoid places or situations associated with anxiety. For an adult, it could include everything from meetings at work to driving a car on a crowded highway. For a child, it could be school, school trips, birthday parties, sitting in the middle of a row at the movies, or shopping in a crowded store with mom. For teens, it could be attending a concert or visiting potential colleges.

Anxiety is the key to CA. The anxiety condition escalates when the child fears going someplace where panic feelings have occurred. Once the disorder starts, anticipating the event causes unbearable stress, even if the event's stressfulness has diminished. While some children panic only during the stressful event, others have a general, constant sense of discomfort and anxiety.

What CA children fear most, whether they articulate it or not, is losing control and drawing attention to themselves. They fear embarrassing themselves in a public situation—throwing up, fainting, and acting irrationally. And much of the anxiety, panic, and stress come well before the actual activity starts—it is often anticipatory.

The *ICD*'s, American Psychiatric Association's, and the *DSM*'s main defining feature of agoraphobia is that the condition is expressed by anxiety about being in places or situations from which escape might be difficult or embarrassing or in which help may not be available in the event of having a panic attack or panic-like symptoms.

For young children who have school requirements, the disorder can leave them partially housebound; but for older teens who might not have those requirements, they might end up completely housebound. It can leave a child desperately coping with the disorder attempting very hard to appear "normal," adding even more stress and worry.

As opposed to other anxiety disorders that revolve only around a specific stressor, agoraphobia involves a cluster of types of stressors. Individually, the stressor might be understandably anxiety-producing, but massed together, they form a debilitating disorder. Normal stressors include going into tunnels, crossing bridges, driving in a car, being in a crowded restaurant, being brought into a different classroom, or standing on line at a store.

Children with agoraphobia, like adults, often need a companion to complete many tasks. Many, though, are afraid to display their panic in front of others, so a parent should not expect a CA child to come asking for help.

Agoraphobic children will do anything to avoid stressful or panic-inducing situations, from feigning illness to causing real harm to themselves or developing a sickness. Fights over attending school usually aggravate agoraphobic children's relationships with their parents.

It is almost guaranteed that a CA child has been plotting and planning all night, devising ways to keep from attending school the next day. Besides making up an illness or two, they make themselves physically ill, with a stomachache, diarrhea, nausea, dizziness, or a headache. If they are forced to go to school, family tension and a fight ensue, making the disorder worse; if they are allowed to stay home, their symptoms subside.

If a parent can get a CA child to school, he or she will probably refuse to take the bus if one is usually taken. They are in complete dread that they might do something embarrassing on the bus like throw up, lose control, or have to go to the bathroom. It's not the fear of the bus—it's the fear of *themselves* inside the bus. Even in school, there is a constant sense of dread, with these children often preoccupied with their anxiety.

Any change in school routine—substitute teachers, visiting another classroom, fire drills, assemblies, lunch, a trip to the library—provides the agoraphobic child with constant fear.

Signs and symptoms

- agitation
- anxiety or panic attacks
- becoming housebound for prolonged periods of time
- confusion
- crying spells
- dependence on others
- depression
- disorientation
- dizziness
- excessive sweating
- fear of being alone
- fear of being around others
- fear of being trapped, or in places where escape might be difficult
- fear of bringing attention to self
- fear of dying
- fear of going crazy
- fear of losing control in a public place
- feeling that the body or environment is unreal
- feelings of detachment or estrangement from others
- feelings of helplessness
- flushed skin
- headaches
- hot flashes
- lightheadedness
- irritability
- nausea
- near fainting
- numbness and tingling
- physical symptoms, many related to panic attacks such as breathing difficulties, chest pains, and chills
- rapid heart beat, palpitations
- rapid pulse
- stomach disorders
- temper
- trembling
- twitching
- vision problems

There are subtle but well-defined distinctions between agoraphobia and other anxiety disorders. Similar disorders include:

OCD: This disorder is characterized by unwanted, intrusive thoughts and fears about specific activities and uncontrollable behaviors in an attempt to satisfy those fears. OCD is exhibited when a child refuses to go to a baseball game because he or she is afraid of being contaminated by dust stirred up when the players run. Agoraphobia is the child's fear that he will be trapped at the game and exhibit embarrassing behavior out of his fear.

PD: Don't get agoraphobia and panic attacks confused—they are not interchangeable. A panic attack is a potential symptom of agoraphobia, but not all panic attacks involve agoraphobia. A panic attack is a separate disorder from agoraphobia, an episode during which a child feels intense fear or discomfort. The child experiencing a panic attack exhibits at least four of the physical symptoms listed above. The attack has a sudden onset and typically peaks within ten minutes. It can be unexpected—not associated with a specific trigger.

PTSD: PTSD is characterized by avoiding stressors that caused problems—a child fears driving in a car because it's a reminder of a traumatic accident she experienced when she was younger. Agoraphobia would be the child's fear of being out of the safety zone of her bedroom and being "trapped" on a highway in an enclosed vehicle over which she has no control, in case she needed immediate help.

SAD: A child with SAD is afraid of being away from his parents or other trusted relatives. An agoraphobic child would add that fear to not being around trusted people in public.

Specific Phobia: Children with phobias fear a specific thing, like not wanting to go shopping because the child specifically fears mannequins. An agoraphobic child is afraid of the busy, crowded store.

SPD: SPD is about a child's fear of looking foolish in front of peers or being judged by them. In the agoraphobic child, anxiety and avoidance are directly related to a fear of having an anxiety or panic attack. The SPD child doesn't want to visit her friend because her friend intimidates her, while the agoraphobic fears visiting because she has a panic attack whenever she does.

Cause

Although CA has been researched for a long time, no single cause has been determined—but many factors are believed to influence the condition. Experts at the Mayo Clinic and others believe, as with many mental-health disorders, that the etiology is a combination of several factors, including genetic, brain biochemistry, cognitive, and environmental factors.

As in Leif's case, agoraphobia is a highly inheritable disorder. If one family member has an anxiety disorder, others probably will, too.

Diagnosis

As soon as a child begins exhibiting anxious or phobic-type symptoms that are beginning to have a negative impact on his or her life, it is time to bring the child to the pediatrician to start the diagnostic process with a full physical exam, in order to rule out any physical problems. The pediatrician should then refer the child to a pediatric psychiatrist or psychologist.

Treatment

As with other anxiety and panic disorders, there is no prevention or cure. But early intervention, as with almost all psychological and developmental disorders, can greatly relieve the condition.

Many types of therapies are used in treatment: assertiveness training, biofeedback, and hypnosis. An especially effective phobia treatment is CBT.

With CBT desensitization (Leif's therapy), the patient is asked to relax and think about what causes the anxiety. Breathing techniques are often incorporated, connecting physical sensations with psychological ones, and therapists work from the least fearful step to the most fearful (e.g., walking out of the home compared to walking through the mall). This type of exposure/desensitization has proven very effective for disorders that manifest in anxiety, depression, and panic, such as agoraphobia. It is believed that treating agoraphobia with this type of exposure therapy has reduced anxiety in at least 75 percent of cases.

Anti-anxiety and antidepressant medications are often effectively used with therapy to help relieve symptoms associated with phobias, for the preferred short-term or last-resort long-term use.

As with all anxiety and mood disorders, medications may be helpful, especially when depression leads to suicidal thoughts. These drugs contain a "black-box" warning about the potential relationship between antidepressants and suicide in young people. So it is of utmost importance for the parent to be well informed about these medications when speaking with the doctor and never to medicate the child without consulting a doctor (or maybe several) first.

Antidepressants slow the removal of essential neurotransmitters (chemicals that move signals between the brain's neurons). Antidepressants of choice currently include selective serotonin reuptake inhibitors (SSRIs; see the "SSRIs" section in "What You Need to Know" for more information). There are also other medications that you can discuss with your child's physician, but, again, always consult with a doctor before giving your child any medication. Foods high in serotonin that are carbohydrate based such as breads, pasta, and potatoes, and foods rich in the amino-acid tryptophan such as turkey, meat proteins, and fruits and mushrooms, can help improve the child's mental state.

Much can be done at home to help with CA.

Agoraphobic children have a difficult time articulating what causes their fears, what they are afraid of, or even admitting to a problem. They fear being shunned, often thinking they are crazy and will appear crazy to others. Tell them that you appreciate their situation and that their problem is common and treatable.

It is important to know that without the proper help, these children cannot just simply go on by sheer encouragement. When your child says, "I cannot do it," understand that he or she cannot. Do not say, "Yes, you can. You're not trying." Pressuring the child without proper therapy or medication will only worsen the condition.

With these children, the flight instinct is extreme; if your child insists, be prepared to leave places at a moment's notice. Do not force the child to stay in a panic-inducing situation, unless it has been prescribed as part of the child's therapy.

Sources and resources

Agoraphobics in Motion (A.I.M.) (248-547-0400); (www.aim-hq.org)

Anxiety Disorders and the caregiver (www.healthyplace.com)

Anxiety Disorders Association of America (www.adaa.org)

The Anxiety Panic Internet resource (tAPir) (www.algy.com/anxiety)

Council on Anxiety Disorders (706-947-3854)

Duke University's Program in Child and Adolescent Anxiety Disorder (www2.mc.duke.edu/pcaad)

Mayo Clinic (www.mayoclinic.com)

Mental Health America of Virginia/ABIL (Agoraphobics Building Independent Lives), Inc. (804-257-5591); (www.mhav.org)

NIMH (www.nimh.nih.gov/health/topics/anxiety-disorders)

Panic Anxiety Disorders Association (www.panicanxietydisorder.org.au)

Panic Anxiety Education Management Services (www.paems.com.au)

Self-Help Corner: Anxiety (www.queendom.com/webpsychclub/members_anxiety)

See the mental-health contacts under "General Resources" for more sources used in this chapter.

CAD

Childhood Adjustment Disorder

Terms used in this chapter: AD (adjustment disorder); CAD (childhood adjustment disorder); DSM (*Diagnostic and Statistical Manual of Mental Disorders*)

Sound familiar?

Todd, 10, tells his mother that he feels hopeless. Well, not in so many words. He actually tells her he sees nothing good in his future. And because of this, his hands sweat, his heart beats fast, and he can't really talk to people.

The young man, with his shock of blond hair and a gigantic toothy smile—on the rare occasions in the past six months when he does smile—refers to himself as "bent out of shape."

Todd says it's all because he moved from his childhood home in central Ohio to a suburban Chicago school district—one that is much better than the district he moved from. But to a 10-year-old, his mother concedes, the services that a school district provides mean nothing compared to what the child thinks he's leaving behind. His mother also understands his pain because she, too, for most of her life, has suffered from chronic depression.

Todd's family had to move. His father, a well-paid chief financial officer, was relocated, and there was no choice but to make that transition. Todd's father, by the way, has depression and anxiety that runs through his own matrilineal line.

Todd, an only child, felt completely uprooted. His crying bouts, which were in private, have now become uncontrollable and public, even in school—which is not good, because even Todd admits that his new erratic behavior is turning off peers and teachers. One teacher, in particular, has not been sympathetic and has a very contentious relationship with the formerly easygoing young boy.

Since the move, Todd has been depressed, agitated, and withdrawn. He has developed a twitch in his right arm and right eye, and he always complains of stomachaches.

Todd has developed some obsessive-compulsive symptoms, like constantly having his books in the same order in his knapsack and keeping the door to his room open exactly a measured foot wide.

Todd has just begun seeing a psychologist who has used cognitive behavior therapy with the young boy, teaching him how to replace negative feelings with positive ones. It has already begun to show positive effects. Just to take the edge off his anxiety, Todd was put on Zoloft and that has already started to reduce some of his anxiety and obsessive-compulsive symptoms.

Todd's parents are thrilled with some of the promising changes.

"Just talking to a professional who is sympathetic means the world to Todd now," says his mother. "He now has hope that he will make friends and a life [for himself] here.

"It kills us to see him suffering, but the prognosis is good, it's a temporary condition most of the time, and we see a light at the end of the tunnel."

Todd has been diagnosed with CAD—childhood adjustment disorder.

Did you know?

A mean teacher, an illness, a parent's remarriage, or a move to a new town can cause anyone stress. Life changes can make the most mature and stable of us feel shaky and insecure, but, if that stress makes a child overanxious, physically ill, hopeless, or depressed, three months after the onset of the stressor—an incident that causes the anxiety—it might mean the child has AD (adjustment disorder), and that he or she needs help.

Adolescents are particularly prone to ADs; it is an age group with an approximately 32 percent prevalence rate, almost three times as much as in adults. These incidents are generally short-termed episodes, lasting less than six months.

CAD is a severe, prolonged, negative response to normal stress that has occurred in the past three months and is not the result of another mental illness. The anxiety, depression, or inability to cope lasts longer than it should for a normal person and, in turn, causes impairment in several areas such as social relationships, academic performance, and, in the case of some adolescents, work ability. ADs are not caused by expected stressors such as grief caused by death of a loved one.

The symptoms develop within three months of the onset of the stressor, and while the disorder usually lasts up to only six months, it can become long-term if it is related to a long-term problem, such as that bad teacher, chronic bullying, or a move the child is just unable to become used to, as in Todd's case. With older teens, it could be a bad job or relationship or ongoing money problems.

A breakup with a boyfriend or girlfriend or even a best friend might not seem much to a jaded parent, but such an event could turn a child's life upside down. It is natural for this type of stressor to disturb a child, and the child's anxiety and depression over such an incident should be taken seriously. Remember, an AD is just that—a tough adjustment period, so it should be a brief problematic period that can be overcome. When it lasts longer than its prescribed time, and the symptoms are more severe than what should be expected, it is time to take action.

While a specific stressor might appear as just a small bump in the road, in a child with an AD, it might be blown out of proportion for several reasons, including a genetic predisposition, previous life experiences, or even hormonal changes. If one stressor disappears and the disorder improves, it can get all stirred up again if another stressor, especially a similar one, appears.

How it is manifested

The *DSM* recognizes six main types of adjustment disorders, and, while all related, each has its own set of warning signs and symptoms.

AD with depressed mood. Symptoms mainly include feeling sad, tearful, and hopeless, and a lack of pleasure in the things the child previously enjoyed.

AD with anxiety. Symptoms mainly include nervousness, worry, difficulty concentrating or remembering things, and feeling overwhelmed. Children who have AD with anxiety may strongly fear being separated from their parents and loved ones.

AD with mixed anxiety and depressed mood. Symptoms include a mix of depression and anxiety.

AD with disturbance of conduct. Symptoms mainly involve behavioral problems such as playing hooky or vandalism, aggressiveness and fighting, and, in older teenagers, reckless driving or irresponsibility when it comes to money.

AD with mixed disturbance of emotions and conduct. Symptoms include a mix of depression and anxiety as well as behavioral problems.

AD unspecified. Symptoms don't fit the criteria for other types of ADs but often include school problems, work problems for older teens, and physical problems. They also exhibit interpersonal problems with family or friends.

Signs and symptoms

- academic problems
- aggressiveness
- anxiety
- behavioral problems
- belligerence
- crying bouts
- cutting classes
- depression
- feeling desperate
- fighting with friends and family
- hopelessness
- inability to concentrate
- inappropriateness
- irresponsibility
- isolation
- over-assertiveness
- physical illnesses
- recklessness
- skipping school
- suicidal feelings
- vandalism
- withdrawal

It is important to note that children exhibit different symptoms of ADs than do adults. While adults usually present symptoms that are a bit more passive, such as depression, children present more by acting out—with conduct and behavioral disturbances. But it is crucial not to have the more aggressive behavior overshadow what might be lurking within—the more internal problems the child might be feeling, such as depression.

Cause

As with all anxiety and mental-health disorders, no one really has a definitive answer.

A 2007 report from the Mayo Clinic on ADs has as good an answer as anyone: "Researchers are still trying to figure out what causes adjustment disorders. As with other mental disorders, the cause is likely complex and may involve genetics, your life experiences, your temperament and even changes in the natural chemicals in the brain."

Diagnosis

The only way to make a diagnosis of CAD is by having a thorough interview with a mental-health professional, which will include a detailed personal history pinpointing the reason for the onset. There are no blood tests, nor are there any physical conditions to be met. However, an initial visit with a medical doctor to run a full physical will detect any physical disorder that might be similar to the symptoms that appear psychologically based.

For an AD disorder to be diagnosed, several criteria must be met, including:

- having emotional or behavioral symptoms within three months of the occurrence
- having serious symptoms involving severe distress or an inability to function well in daily life
- showing improvement of symptoms within six months of the stressful event's coming to an end

Treatment

There are two main types of treatment generally considered for CAD—psychotherapy and medications.

Psychotherapy, often preferred as the first course of treatment over medication, is effective in three forms—individual, group, or family therapy. Therapy provides insight into the stressor and develops positive coping skills. A good therapist will focus directly on the stressor.

As with all anxiety and mood disorders, medications can be very helpful, especially when depression leads to suicidal thoughts. But there is always a risk when treating children with medications really designed for adults, as are the drugs that are used most for disorders such as CAD. The types of drugs used are antidepressants and anti-anxiety medications and can be used for short or extended periods, depending on the level of the condition.

Antidepressants slow the removal of essential neurotransmitters (chemicals that move signals between the brain's neurons). The antidepressants of choice currently are the selective serotonin reuptake inhibitors (SSRIs; see the "SSRIs" section in "What You Need to Know" for more information).

Other drugs used are NDRIs (norepinephrine and dopamine reuptake inhibitors), which work on the dopamine levels, the most popular being Wellbutrin. Although SSRIs and NDRIs are the most popular, there are other medications that you can discuss with your child's physician.

In addition to drugs, there are foods that are high in serotonin and are carbohydrate-based such as breads, pasta, potatoes, and breads; and foods rich in the amino acid tryptophan such as turkey, meat proteins, and fruits and mushrooms. St. John's Wort is a herbal supplement that has been used for centuries to treat depression.

A doctor should always be consulted when considering drugs or herbal supplements for a child.

Prognosis

While CAD is considered a temporary disorder, it can certainly lead to more long-lasting concerns if left untreated.

Sources and resources

American Academy of Child and Adolescent Psychiatry (www.aacap.org)
DSM (*Diagnostic and Statistical Manual of Mental Disorders*)
Mayo Clinic (www.mayoclinic.com)
National Institute of Mental Health (www.nimh.nih.gov)

See the mental-health contacts under "General Resources" for more sources used in this chapter.

CAS
Childhood Apraxia of Speech

Terms used in this chapter: CAS (childhood apraxia of speech); CASANA (Childhood Apraxia of Speech Association of North America); LD (learning disability)

Sound familiar?

Joseph, a 5-year-old from Portland, Oregon, liked to talk a lot, but no one could understand what he said. His mother, Doe, said that she believed it was just a "developmental glitch that he would get over as he got older."

For two years Joseph was going to a speech therapist, but he wasn't making much progress. And then more red flags began to show up.

"His problems all seemed to be about speech," Doe says. "He was pretty good in math, but it was all about getting letters and sounds all wrong."

"There were other things we began to notice," Doe recalls. "Joey started having all these sensory issues—sensitive to noise and light and tactile things, like his clothes were very uncomfortable. He was a mess when he ate. He never seemed to know when he had food on his face and hands. We weren't sure what was normal and what wasn't. Joseph was the first new baby in the family, so there was no one to compare him to.

"We thought he was just talking baby talk. He was unable to put together the sequence of the sounds in a word. He knew what he wanted to say, he could say 'big' and he could say 'boy,' but he had trouble saying 'big boy.'"

Unhappy with the work of the speech therapist, Joseph's parents insisted he be assessed in school by an occupational therapist, who determined Joseph had some sensory integration and fine-motor problems.

"Joey was progressing well, but we knew it was time for more. We then got him assessed by a developmental pediatrician."

Through further, more-sensitive testing, it was revealed that the basis of Joseph's problems was his inability to sound out multisyllable words and multiword phrases and problems with word retrieval and sequencing thoughts.

"We started with a new speech therapist in school, and she was terrific," Joseph's mother says, happily. "She really zeroed in on Joseph's problems now that they were clearly identified."

At this point, Joseph was having difficulty pronouncing more-complicated words and phrases. He was also leaving letters off his words—sometimes he would say "dogs" and another time he would say "dog" for a group of dogs.

"We were a little annoyed that the first speech therapist wasted so much time with Joseph. The new therapist explained that the previous one probably didn't realize the root sequencing problem and she treated him for just articulation problems. She assured us that the therapy probably helped him at the time, but we weren't sold. What the new therapist was doing was working, and we could see immediate results—although he was worlds apart from the other kids in his class."

And now it was starting to affect Joseph socially.

"The older he got the more self-conscious he was getting about his speech," says Doe. "Even when he began improving, his expressive speech was impaired."

But that soon changed. By the time Joseph was 8 years old, his speech had improved in a big way, and he began opening up more socially. He stopped some of his therapies along the way as he progressed, and now he works with a special-education inclusion teacher on his language skills in the classroom setting.

"If you didn't know his history, you wouldn't realize that he was so greatly affected by this," says Doe. "Don't get me wrong, he still has several more mountains to climb, but we see that the flag at the top of the mountain is reachable."

Joseph has CAS—childhood apraxia of speech.

Did you know?

Apraxia, a motor-speech programming disorder, is diagnosed when a child has difficulty executing and sequencing the skilled motor movements needed for speech. It is known by several names: CAS (childhood apraxia of speech), apraxia of speech, verbal apraxia, developmental apraxia of speech, and verbal dyspraxia. The apraxic child finds it difficult to produce and combine phonemes (the smallest unit of speech sound) to create words, phrases, and sentences at will. These children hear the words but are unable to put the consonants and vowels together to form the problem syllables and words. They understand the words, and they know what they want to say, but they cannot execute the sounds and the movements properly to form the words. An obviously shaky hand unable to write legibly is not the only kind of fine motor skill there is—the inability to combine phonemes into words is a fine motor skill as well.

It is important to note the disorders CAS *isn't*, but can be comorbid with: oral motor weakness (dysarthria) and articulation problems (see the "SLD: Speech-Language Disorder" chapter), could be comorbid with CAS, but they are not the same.

It is also important to know what makes CAS different from regular speech delays. The main difference is that, in normally developing children, their expressive and receptive skills will develop at the same rate. In the CAS child, the receptive skills will be much more highly developed than the expressive. One problem many parents find is that sometimes results of their child's speech testing might be averaged out, the highs with the lows. That is a disaster waiting to happen. You will want the full results of all tests and subtests.

Parents should also remember that the discrepancy between expressive and receptive skills is just a sign, it is not enough on which to base a CAS diagnosis.

The speech process

This is how CASANA explains the speech process:

> The act of speech begins with an intention to communicate. Next, an idea forms, outlining what the speaker wants to say. The words for the desired message are put in the correct order, using the correct grammar. Each of the words is comprised of a specific sequence of sounds (also called phonemes) and syllables that must be ordered together. All of this information is translated from an idea and information about order of sounds into a series of highly coordinated motor movements of the lips, tongue, jaw, and soft palate.

> The brain must tell the muscles of these "articulators" the exact order and timing of movements so that the words in the message are properly articulated. Finally, the muscles must work properly with enough strength and muscle tone to perform the movements needed for speech.

> In typically developing speech, children make word attempts and get feedback from others and from their own internal systems regarding how "well" the words they produced matched the ones that they wanted to produce. Children use this information the next time they attempt

the words and essentially are able to "learn from experience." Usually once syllables and words are spoken repeatedly, the speech motor act becomes automatic. Speech motor plans and programs are stored in the brain and can be accessed effortlessly when they are needed. Children with apraxia of speech have difficulty in this aspect of speech. It is believed that children with CAS may not be able to form or access speech motor plans and programs or that these plans and programs are faulty for some reason.

Signs and symptoms

- anxiety, which aggravates symptoms
- child can move parts of mouth on his or her own, but when directed to do so they might not be able to
- deletes difficult sounds
- difficult to understand
- early words are missing sounds
- feeding problems
- fine motor problems
- fumbles for words and sounds
- gets stuck on a specific word (vocal perseveration)
- grunts instead of speaks
- inability to combine sounds
- inability to imitate others' speech
- inconsistent sound errors that are not age appropriate
- lack of early speech
- LDs
- multisyllables and longer phrases are more difficult than single sounds and short phrases
- no comprehensible vocabulary by age 2
- no cooing or babbling as an infant
- oral-sensory problems
- pointing instead of speaking
- produces few consonant sounds, speaks mostly in vowels
- receptive skills are significantly better than expressive skills
- shyness
- spatial problems

Cause

The cause of CAS is not known; however, genetic disorders or syndromes have been connected to the disorder. Acquired dyspraxia can be caused by muscle weakness that affects speech production (dysarthria) or language problems caused by damage to the nervous system (aphasia). Stroke and brain injury have been noted as well. Research has shown that children with developmental CAS often have parents with speech problems, so genetics plays a big role. A miswired brain can be inherited through generations.

Diagnosis

It is difficult to diagnose a CAS child younger than 2 years old—even, perhaps 3—although there might be enough signs to keep an early watch on the child and employ some early interventions. Other medical conditions should be ruled out at the start. It is recommended to have an audiologist test the child's hearing, in case hearing loss is a cause of the CAS.

The best person to make a CAS diagnosis is a speech-language pathologist, but a pediatric neurologist, occupational therapist, physical therapist, or pediatric or psychiatrist are also helpful. A developmental pediatrician might be able to help the child with more global issues beyond the speech problems.

CASANA warns: "Most preschool age language tests are not sensitive enough to detect subtle or higher level language deficits."

Treatment

CAS is usually treatable.

The best generally accepted ways to help the apraxic child is through speech-language therapy utilizing repetitions and drills, conversation with the child filling in blanks and finishing thoughts, and modeling speech after someone offering the proper prompts and cues.

Children can learn through the repetition of songs and rhymes and even the repetition of a sound they are comfortable with. Reading with the child and engaging him or her in a familiar story by leaving parts out and helping the child fill in the voids is a valuable therapy that can be done in a therapeutic setting or home.

Do whatever you can to help the child communicate, whether it is through sign language, imitation, gestures, or word approximations. And all verbal attempts by the child should be met with any type of positive reinforcement.

Here are some of the universal techniques and skills the therapist will utilize and teach:

- conversational turn-taking
- eye contact
- focus on speech sequences versus individual sounds
- motivational play that incorporates speech
- music—melody and rhythm

- positive feedback
- practice
- pragmatic/social skills
- repetition of sounds and sound sequences
- slowed rate of speech
- speech correction
- staying on topic
- targeted motor placement
- targeted speech production
- touch sensory cueing
- verbal cueing
- visual sensory cueing
- watching him/herself in the mirror or watching a visual representation of some aspect of his or her speech on a computer screen

Depending on the severity of the CAS, therapy, with a professional, can be suggested for as much as five times a week.

Prognosis

CAS kids in general have a positive prognosis depending on many factors, including the severity of their disorder, early intervention, treatment, and comorbid disorders. Children who do get better might have some residual problems such as pragmatic or social skill delays, slight peculiarities in their speech, and the emergence of LDs.

Sources and resources

American Speech-Language-Hearing Association (ASHA) (800-638-8255); (www.asha.org)

The Childhood Apraxia of Speech Association of North America (CASANA) (412-767-6589); (www.apraxia-kids.org)

See the "SLD: Speech-Language Disorder" and "LD: Learning Disability" chapters, as well as the mental-health contacts under "General Resources," for more sources used in this chapter.

CBD

Childhood Bipolar Disorder

Terms used in this chapter: ADHD (attention-deficit/hyperactivity disorder); BD (bipolar disorder); BPS (bipolar spectrum); CBD (childhood bipolar disorder); *DSM* (*Diagnostic and Statistical Manual of Mental Disorders*); *ICD* (*International Classification of Diseases*); IEP (individualized education program); NIMH (National Institute of Mental Health)

Sound familiar?

Ty was 14 years old when, suddenly, at a friend's birthday gathering at his local movie theater, he found himself panicked, his heart pounding out of his chest, and unable to breathe. The attack eventually subsided, but for the following few weeks, he had difficulty breathing in school, becoming lightheaded and almost fainting several times.

Overwhelmed by fear of these attacks, Ty became school phobic and depressed. Along with that, his behavior became uncontrollable. His mother, Nicole, says that the best way to describe him at that time is that he was "completely, totally flipping out" with wild temper tantrums, reckless and hyperactive behavior, and then periods of quiet and depression. These moods could change several times during the day. Ty's parents brought him to his pediatrician who said he believed Ty was having panic attacks, and sent them to a nearby psychiatrist for a second opinion—which was a confirmation of panic disorder. Nicole says that the "panic" symptoms were the only symptoms the doctor focused on and Ty was prescribed Paxil.

The Paxil seemed to help. Ty's panic was gone, and he felt better than he had in a long while. "Peace returned to our house," Nicole recalls.

But then Ty's mother began noticing other strange behaviors. Ty was becoming, what she calls, "very, very, very busy." He started writing songs. He would stay up all night, on his computer, writing scripts for his favorite TV show, Scrubs. *Eventually, he almost stopped sleeping altogether, maybe an hour a night. He became "super-social," says Nicole, and he started talking on the phone "all the time," seemingly without letting the person on the other end speak. He reprogrammed his iPod, rearranged his room, and began keeping extensive lists of "Things to Do." Even his speech became as rapid as his actions.*

"There were days where he seemed so full of himself like he could conquer the world," Nicole recalls, "and then in a matter of minutes he would be suicidal. He bought extravagant gifts, made plans for trips around the world, and then he couldn't leave his room." He also flew into violent rages.

His behavior began to trouble Nicole and her husband, so they brought Ty back to the doctor, who immediately pegged his behavior as mania. Their doctor told them that, once the panic symptoms were treated, it unmasked the untreated manic symptoms. He recommended a different psychiatrist, who not only looked at the big manic-depressive picture that Ty was exhibiting, but conducted a thorough family history and learned that Ty had a great aunt with schizophrenia, and an aunt with manic depression. Now, two years later, Ty sees a psychologist weekly and a psychiatrist every three months and takes medications to control his moods.

Ty has CBD—childhood bipolar disorder.

Did you know?

We can now add CBD to the list of disorders—autism, ADHD, anxiety, etc.—that are seeing dramatic jumps in prevalence statistics. And here is the problem: BD in children is an extremely controversial disorder, and the assertive diagnoses by doctors in the past few years, which has helped grow that statistic, has rocked the psychiatric world.

BD (classified as bipolar affective disorder in the *ICD*) or manic-depressive illness is a diagnosis based on a patient's extreme mood swings and overexcited behaviors and thinking. It has, until recently, been an exclusively adult disorder. But there are enough experts and psychiatric specialists (including the NIMH) who report that the disorder *is* found in children and is too often missed. But others say that widespread overdiagnosing of the disorder is the problem and that, when those newly labeled children are treated, often with powerful and unwarranted medication, there are too many bad side effects. These critics also claim that, when those diagnosed children grow up, they do not manifest the aspects of adult BD, which, to them, indicates a misdiagnosis of BD in childhood. Even more so, critics claim, this is a disorder promulgated by the big pharmaceutical companies who have been making extreme profits off bipolar drugs for children.

On December 13, 2006, in Hull, Massachusetts, police were called to the home of 4-year-old Rebecca Riley, who was found dead on the floor. She died of an overdose of medication, authorities say, and three months later in February 2007, her parents, Michael and Carolyn, were charged with murder for intentionally poisoning the young girl. The parents say they were only following doctor's orders. Rebecca, it turns out, was, in fact, taking prescription medications: Clonidine for ADHD and valproic acid and Seroquel for bipolar disorder, all prescribed by a Tufts-New England Medical Center psychiatrist who diagnosed the young girl with both disorders at 2½ years old!

The number of children diagnosed with BD has risen from less than 3 percent in 1990 to 15 percent in 2000, according to a September 2007 study published in the *Archives of General Psychiatry*. From 1994 to 2003, the number of children treated for bipolar disorder grew forty-times, says the study based on data from the National Center for Health Statistics survey of doctor visits. And it is believed that the rate has climbed dramatically since then.

BD, also known as manic depression, is a serious mental illness but one that is treatable. Since there are no epidemiological studies on the subject, it is not known how many children might be affected with the disorder. If the above-mentioned studies are correct, it would mean that 1 percent of children have CBD. It is known that BD affects up to 2 percent of adults, and statistics for those in a BPS can reach as high as 8 percent of the general population. The BPS includes bipolar I disorder (manic-depressive illness with or without psychosis); bipolar II disorder (episodes of major depression alternating with episodes of hypomania that are not severe enough to result in impairment of function); cyclothymic disorder, brief and attenuated episodes of depression and hypomania sometimes known as minor cyclic mood disorder; and BD–NOS (not otherwise specified), a catch-all for children with symptoms that appear to be CBD, but are not quite in line with official criteria.

It is believed that some children with ADHD, depression, or PD (panic disorder) might instead have early-onset BD or have the disorders running concurrently. On the other hand, it's important to keep in mind that ADHD, depression, and panic symptoms can also be temporary glitches in a child's development and might not mean anything more.

CBD is all about extremes: high highs and low lows. While in adults, mood changes take longer to switch, in children, mood changes can be more dramatic and more constant, in fact, occurring numerous times a day. Another difference between childhood and adult BD is that the euphoria found in adults is often manifested as irritability in a child.

The National Alliance on Mental Illness (NAMI) reports that approximately 7 percent of children seen at psychiatric facilities fit the criteria for CBD.

Signs and symptoms

- ability to go with very little or no sleep for days without tiring
- agitation
- bedwetting
- beliefs that defy logic
- crying spells
- defiant behavior
- delusions or hallucinations in extreme cases
- difficulty with relationships
- distinct changes in energy
- distractibility
- explosive tantrums
- extreme sensitivity to rejection or failure
- feeling suicidal
- feelings of inappropriate guilt
- feelings of worthlessness
- frequent absences from school
- grandiosity
- great creativity

- headaches
- hyperactivity
- hypersexuality
- impaired judgment
- impulsivity
- inability to concentrate
- inability to settle down
- inappropriate behavior
- involvement in excessive numbers of activities
- lack of interest in former interests
- lack of interest in play
- morbid thoughts
- muscle aches
- night terrors
- overly elated
- overly inflated self-esteem
- overly silly
- periods of wellness between episodes
- persistent states of extreme agitation accompanied by high energy or mania
- persistent states of extreme elation accompanied by high energy or mania
- persistent states of extreme irritability accompanied by low energy or depression
- persistent states of extreme sadness accompanied by low energy or depression
- poor academic progress
- poor communication
- poor judgment
- powerful food cravings, often for carbohydrates and sweets
- racing thoughts
- rapid speech
- rapidly changing and distinct changes in mood
- reckless behavior
- separation anxiety
- significant change in body weight
- sleeping disorders
- social isolation
- stomachaches

Cause

There is no one cause known for CBD, but there are factors that can bring on the disorder. Brain chemistry and genetics are the two most cited reasons.

C

CBD tends to be highly inherited, but, as with other Alphabet Disorders, a predisposition or other environmental factors seem to play a large part. BD cannot only skip generations, it can also manifest itself very differently within the same family. When one parent has BD, there is a 15–30 percent risk of his or her offspring being bipolar. When both parents have BD, the risk rises to 50–75 percent.

It has also been reported that people with BD have an average of 30 percent more of a certain type of neurotransmitter, signal-sending brain cells, called monoamines, according to University of Michigan researchers in 2005. These monoamines release the brain chemicals dopamine, serotonin, and norepinephrine, all of which are involved in mood regulation, stress responses, pleasure, reward, and cognitive functions like concentration, attention, and executive functions. One doctor on that study and similar follow-up studies, Jon-Kar Zubieta, M.D., Ph.D., says that the studies "describe increases in the density of monoaminergic terminals in BD, which differentiated this illness from healthy controls and patients with schizophrenia (with some overlap in the latter). No studies have been done in unmedicated patients ([it's] very hard to do in that group), but in general it would be expected that those alterations would be present before treatment (that specific marker does not modulate much at all with treatment)."

This, experts believe, explains why CBD also mimics conditions like ADHD and anxiety disorders. It also indicates that those who suffer from CBD are predisposed to the illness because of the way their brains are wired.

Also, sleep irregularities can greatly affect the body and mind. The chemical body clock that controls the important rhythms of sleep regulates the much-needed hormone melatonin, which, when deficient, can cause insomnia, which further disrupts the body's chemical balance.

Puberty is also a big trigger, especially with girls; their CBD can be greatly influenced by their menstrual cycle.

CBD is not always triggered by what's inside a child's body; sometimes outside influences such as a great loss, death, or other trauma may be what sets off a child's first episode of CBD.

Diagnosis

Unfortunately, there is no one particular medical or lab test that can determine a diagnosis of CBD, which is a difficult disorder to detect. It is estimated that, in many cases, it takes up to ten years for a proper diagnosis. There are several reasons for this delay, and most have to do with the very nature of the duality of the disorder. Many patients are observed in one particular emotional state of CBD—mania or depression. In most cases, they are usually treated for the depression because, when they are in the more elated state, it is not often perceived as a problem. But depression is often a red flag for parents. So, many children have been diagnosed with depression instead of CBD. Also, CBD is sometimes diagnostically confused with ADHD, anxiety disorders, or schizophrenia. Whatever the case, the minute a child talks about suicide, treatment should be sought.

After the child has had a full physical examination by his or her pediatrician to rule out any other physical concerns, the main diagnostic tool for CBD is a complete psychiatric and medical history taken by a psychiatrist to determine if the child fills the criteria requirements.

The best doctor for a diagnosis of a disorder like CBD is a board-certified psychiatrist. Parents can provide great assistance to the diagnostician by keeping good records of their child's mood shifts and other symptoms.

At the present, children have to meet the adult criteria for an official CBD diagnosis. But some doctors look to symptoms that pertain more to children. One aspect of the text-revised *DSM-IV* that is troubling to some in terms of ascertaining a CBD diagnosis is the requirement of having a persistent mood last at least four days. It is believed that children with CBD have their rapid-cycle mood change many times in one day. As with other disorders, more and more psychiatrists are adding their own criterion to aid in their diagnosis.

A therapist familiar with the disorder will make sure that the child does not manipulate the session by hiding his or her depressive side and only be high-spirited and charming during a diagnostic visit. A diagnosis will most likely come after a couple of visits, personality testing, clinical observation, and a review of the child's (and family's) history.

Treatment

As with most of the disorders described in this book, early detection, intervention, and treatment can save a child from a lifetime of problems.

While there is not one prescribed treatment for CBD, there are several therapeutic avenues that work in stabilizing mood and allowing for control of symptoms.

The CBD child must be under psychiatric care, and, as long as there is constant vigilance (continued treatment after symptoms seem to subside), a combination of psychological therapy, behavioral therapy, and medication can make a big difference. Cognitive behavioral therapy (CBT), based on modifying behaviors, has proven to be a very effective form of psychological therapy.

Lessening the stress in a child's life—at school and home—will also aid the child in his or her treatment.

In his book *Kids in the Syndrome Mix*, Martin L. Kutscher, M.D., goes into depth in the chapter "Bipolar Depression" about having compassion and providing support for these CBD children. He writes, "Remember, too, that punishing a bipolar child for a rage attack makes as much sense as punishing a child who has epilepsy for having a seizure. Do not punish children for behavior that is out of their control."

The medicine used for treating CBD children has created the biggest controversy surrounding the illness. Very few medications have been approved for pediatric use, and these medicines are now being blamed for severe side effects and even deaths, especially in children diagnosed as bipolar.

There are three main types of drugs—Lithium, anticonvulsants such as valproate or carbamazepine, and antipsychotic drugs such as Risperdal, Zyprexa, Geodone, Zeldex, Abilify, and the aforementioned Seroquel. Antidepressants and stimulants are also used.

Mood stabilizers are often considered crucial for a CBD child by proponents of medicating these children but, if a doctor prescribes a medication, it will be well worth your while to get a second and even third opinion. Even when it is agreed that a child should be put on drugs, it often takes a while to determine the best drugs or even a particular drug cocktail.

On one hand, there are those who are vehemently against giving such powerful drugs to children, especially for a disorder they don't believe actually exists. On the other side, proponents of pharmaceuticals for CBD children say you might just be saving your child's life using medication and that you should start the drugs as soon as possible, especially if the child is suicidal. So, you can see the dilemma parents of children with symptoms of CBD face.

No matter what side you take, be careful with medications. Even the NIMH, which supports the CBD diagnosis, reports in its 2000 fact sheet "Child and Adolescent Bipolar Disorder: An Update":

[There is] some evidence that using antidepressant medication to treat depression in a person who has bipolar disorder may induce manic symptoms if it is taken without a mood stabilizer. In addition, using stimulant medications to treat attention deficit hyperactivity disorder or ADHD-like symptoms in a child with bipolar disorder may worsen manic symptoms. While it can be hard to determine which young patients will become manic, there is a greater likelihood among children and adolescents who have a family history of bipolar disorder. If manic symptoms develop or markedly worsen during antidepressant or stimulant use, a physician should be consulted immediately.

There are also medications that children take for pain, cold, and allergies that can negatively affect a CBD child, so check with your doctor whenever you are considering any over-the-counter medication.

Psychotherapy is a very important part of treatment, but a parent might not be able to start the child in it until the child's mood has been stabilized. And even if the child's mood is stabilized, a child who exhibits BD symptoms might be resistant to therapy.

School accommodations are extremely important for kids with CBD. A parent should secure an IEP for the child, which can help modify everything from the number of children in the child's class to the type of children in the class. The child might need a one-on-one aide, homework modifications when he or she is in a depressive state, a room to retreat to if needed, psychological services, and other accommodations.

Prognosis

With the proper treatment, CBD symptoms can be effectively managed. Unfortunately, many CBD kids can spend most of their youth without being properly diagnosed, and in that case, there is usually not a very good mental-health prognosis. Untreated, CBD can lead to other personality disorders, substance abuse, academic failure, reckless or illegal behavior, and even suicide.

Though some studies have indicated mortality rates of up to 10 percent from suicide, if treated properly and successfully children with CBD can lead full, productive, and happy lives.

Sources and resources

Child & Adolescent Bipolar Foundation (847-256-8525); (www.bpkids.org)

Depression and Bipolar Support Alliance (800-333-3632); (www.dbsalliance.org)

Juvenile Bipolar Research Foundation (866-333-JBRF); (www.jbrf.org)

Martin L. Kutscher, M.D., *Kids in the Syndrome Mix of ADHD, LD, Asperger's, Tourette's, Bipolar, and More* (London and Philadelphia: Jessica Kingsley Publishers, 2005).

Carmen Moreno, Gonzalo Laje, Carlos Blanco, et al., "National Trends in the Outpatient Diagnosis and Treatment of Bipolar Disorder in Youth," *Archives of General Psychiatry* 64, no. 9 (Sept. 2007): 1032–39.

National Center for Health Statistics (www.cdc.gov/nchs)

National Institute of Mental Health, "Child and Adolescent Bipolar Disorder: An Update from the National Institute of Mental Health" (www.nimh.nih.gov/health/topics/bipolar-disorder/index.shtml)

See the mental-health contacts under "General Resources" for more sources used in this chapter.

CCS

Clumsy Child Syndrome

Terms used in this chapter: CSS (clumsy child syndrome); DD (developmental dyspraxia); *DSM* (*Diagnostic and Statistical Manual of Mental Disorders*); IEP (individualized education program)

Did you know?

One of the questions I was faced with when writing this chapter was what to call it, because this disorder goes by several names. While "clumsy child syndrome" is not the most affirming name for a disorder, it is the most descriptive and is popularly used. *Developmental dyspraxia* is a more accurate name, and I like it because it doesn't focus on the one aspect—clumsiness; but my final decision to go with CCS was made mostly because I think it will attract the people who need to read it—hence, its use here. However, parents should remember that this disorder has more serious implications than just childhood clumsiness.

Also known as DD or DCD (developmental coordination disorder) or, as the *DSM* calls it, specific developmental disorder of motor function, CCS is a learning disorder (different than an LD, learning disability) that involves the impairment of movement, although it can involve language, spatial, and thought problems as well. It is often considered a closely related disorder to SID (sensory integration disorder) and NLD (nonverbal learning disorder) and is often diagnosed as such, or vice versa.

Dyspraxia, which is the defining characteristic of CCS, is the difficulty with the entire sequence of a sensory-motor task from initiating it, planning it out, and then carrying it out.

CCS, which as far back as 1937 was called one of the six most common developmental disorders, affects up to as much as 20 percent of children, an overwhelming majority being boys. But that statistic is being challenged because girls have not been diagnosed with CCS, as it has long been stereotypically held that it is normal for girls to be uncoordinated or have spatial problems, while these difficulties are less accepted for boys. That thinking has changed, and girls are being diagnosed in greater numbers. Despite this increase, many CCD children still go undiagnosed or misdiagnosed.

CCS is obviously more than a child's striking out in a baseball game or every once in a while tripping over his or her own feet—it is about a pervasive and negatively impacting lack of coordination.

Signs and symptoms

- anxiety
- appearance of being clumsy
- avoids physical activity
- bad handwriting
- cannot do jigsaw puzzles
- delays in reaching developmental milestones such as rolling over, sitting, speaking, walking, standing
- difficulties in copying from the blackboard, combing hair, sorting shapes, throwing or catching a ball, waving hello or goodbye, walking up and down stairs, brushing teeth, multilevel tasking, structured activity or structuring activity, physical act of writing
- distracted
- does better in one-on-one instruction than in group instruction
- falls and trips often

- fine motor skills impaired
- gross motor skills impaired
- inability to perform a single, simple motor task
- multisensory problems
- not on same level as peers with simple, common physical activities like running, hopping, and skipping
- poor ability to learn instinctively
- poor art skills
- poor grip on writing utensil
- poor social skills
- problems following sequence in writing, math
- problems with spatial concepts such as "in," "on," "in front of," "on the side of"
- putting clothes on in wrong order (e.g., shoes then socks)
- short attention span
- slow, hesitant movement
- speech problems
- unable to follow assignments and directions
- unorganized
- weak memory skills

Cause

There is no known specific cause of CCS, but it is believed to be biological, involving the impairment of neuron development in the brain—a miswired brain. Dyspraxic children do not have any clinically diagnosed neurological problem that causes the disorder, although they might have the neurological impairment from another disorder. Dyspraxia can also be caused by brain trauma.

Diagnosis

The first thing a pediatrician will do is to conduct a full physical examination to determine if the dyspraxia is caused by any medical condition. To help diagnose CCS, the child's doctor will need a developmental history, listing all developmental milestones. There are a number of motor-skill screening tests that can also be conducted.

Treatment

A child should have an IEP set up so that he or she can receive school modifications, accommodations, and services. There are many types of specialists who help dyspraxic children: speech-language pathologists will provide therapy for the verbal aspect of the disorder (see the "CAS: Childhood Apraxia of Speech" chapter). Psychologists will help children with their social and self-esteem issues. An occupational therapist will assist with life skills and the child's motor development, including balance, visual-motor skills, perception, and fine and gross motor coordination.

Prognosis

Depending on the severity of symptoms, usually if developmentally dyspraxic children have the proper intervention (the earlier the better), they can end up overcoming many of their disabilities and lead a productive fulfilling life. Without those interventions, the prognosis is not good because of the untreated physical, mental, social, and psychological problems that will negatively affect the child academically, occupationally, and socially.

Sources and resources

Dyspraxia Support Group of New Zealand (www.dyspraxia.org.nz)
Dyspraxia USA (www.dyspraxiausa.org)

See the "CAS: Childhood Apraxia of Speech," "LD: Learning Disability," and "NLD: Nonverbal Learning Disorder" chapters, as well as the mental-health contacts under "General Resources," for more sources used in this chapter.

CD

Childhood Depression

Terms used in this chapter: AACAP (American Academy of Child & Adolescent Psychiatry); BD (bipolar disorder); CD (childhood depression); DD (dysthymia disorder); MDD (major depressive disorder); NIMH (National Institute of Mental Health)

Did you know?

Depression, the most common mental-health disorder in children, is an illness that affects the child's entire physical and mental well-being. It seeps into their thoughts and affects their physical health. Depression in children is the same as in adults—helplessness, sadness, and fatigue—but adults often have an easier time recognizing depression and addressing it when it affects them. It is often difficult for a child to express how he or she is experiencing the debilitating disorder.

The Eastern Maine Medical Center reports that depression affects three-to-six million children in America. It is believed that many go untreated because they cannot properly articulate what they feel.

The NIMH estimates that 2.5 percent of all children and 8.3 percent of all adolescents will experience some form of clinical depression. NIMH also reports that some estimates suggest as many as one in eleven children may experience some form of clinical depression before the age of 14. In childhood, statistics regarding depression break down evenly between boys and girls; but, in adolescence, girls by a 2-to-1 margin are reported with the disorder more often than boys. It is believed that many adolescent boys, as with adult men, do not seek help for depression.

The NIMH has also sponsored research indicating that, without proper treatment, CD tends to repeat throughout childhood, adolescence, and adulthood, with each episode becoming more severe, reports Kathleen Panula Hockey, MSW, an author and clinician, in a 2003 article, "What Is Childhood Depression, Really? Raising Depression-Free Children: A Parent's Guide to Prevention and Early Intervention," published by the Not Alone Web site. Hockey reports: "Depression in children has also been linked to eventual cigarette smoking, substance abuse, academic difficulties, physical and health problems, and suicidal behaviors. This is why intervention and relapse prevention is so important for children who have already experienced even a mild form of depression or exhibit depressive symptoms even though not diagnosed with clinical depression."

Clinical depression is different from the general terms "getting the blues" or "feeling down." It must interfere with the child's functioning in normal daily activities. Depression can be treated, and children who have it *must* be treated. If a depressed child does not get help, he or she will suffer throughout life, so it is important for parents to know the signs. There is one important indicator that a parent should know: if you suffer from depression, there's a good chance your child might.

There are several types of depressive disorders, including three main types:

MDD is a disabling episode manifested by a combination of symptoms that interfere with daily life and once pleasurable activities. It can occur once or, as in most cases, several times throughout a person's life.

DD is a long-term, chronic, yet less severe type of depression than MDD. It is not as disabling but does affect the ability to function. DD children are likely also to experience depression at some time in their lives. Between 1 and 3 percent of children suffer from dysthymia, although it is also believed that a great many children are not discussing their symptoms and problems, so they go undiagnosed and uncounted.

BD, also called manic-depressive illness, is not as common as MDD, but it is enjoying a period of disorder *du jour*. Awareness of this disorder is growing, as is the number of cases being diagnosed. BD is manifested by mood change cycles—high highs (mania) and low lows (depression). The BD child's energy level bounces (sometimes suddenly, sometimes gradually) from high-level activity to somber and quiet. Childhood bipolar disorder (CBD) is discussed in a previous chapter.

Signs and symptoms

- angry outbursts
- anxiety
- chronic pain
- clinging to parent
- decreased energy
- difficulty thinking clearly
- digestive disorders
- feeling "empty"
- feeling guilty
- feeling helpless and/or hopeless
- feeling inadequate
- feeling melancholy or sad most of the day, every day
- feeling tired
- feeling worthless
- feigning illness
- getting into trouble
- grouchiness
- having suicidal thoughts
- headaches
- inability to concentrate
- inability to experience pleasure or excitement even when doing activities that were pleasurable
- inability to make decisions
- insomnia
- irritability
- low motivation
- mania
- memory loss
- mood change
- oversleeping
- pessimism
- phobias
- poor judgment
- refusing to go to school
- restlessness
- self-destructive behavior
- separation anxiety
- serious weight loss or weight gain in a short period of time
- skipping social activities

- sleeping too much, too little, or not well
- sluggish or jittery movements noticed by others
- sulking
- tantrums

Cause

There is no one specific cause of CD, but there are several potential factors. A biological disposition is believed to be one of the root causes of depression, since it runs in families. But since the disorder also occurs in people who have no family history of depression, it can also be associated with changes in brain structure or brain function.

A psychological cause makes certain individuals predisposed for depression as well—children with low self-esteem and a negative view of the world are perfect candidates, as are anxious and overwhelmed children. It is not known, however, which comes first—whether the depression is caused by this psychological state or whether this psychological state is the forbearer of the depression to come. Other psychological factors that can trigger CD include loss of a loved one or pet, trouble in school, body issues, or any stressor.

Depression has a physical aspect. A severe illness or hormonal changes can set a child on the road to depression.

When the level of neurotransmitters, brain chemicals that carry signals through the nervous system, diminishes, it affects the ability of a person to feel good. This, in effect, causes depression.

The comorbid nature of these Alphabet Kids' disorders also plays into depression. According to the AACAP, "Youth under stress who experience a loss or who have attention, learning, or conduct disorders are at a higher risk for depression." The AACAP also warns, "Almost one-third of 6- to 12-year-old children diagnosed with major depression will develop bipolar disorder within a few years."

Dr. Eileen J. Stellefson, M.P.H., of the Medical University of South Carolina, researches eating behavior and mood, and she has reported that clinical depression can contribute to eating disorders. However, "on the other hand, an eating disorder can lead to a state of clinical depression."

Thus, it is likely that it is a combination of genetic, psychological, biological, and environmental factors that contribute to CD.

Treatment

Talk therapy and cognitive behavioral therapy (CBT), along with antidepressants monitored by a doctor, are very helpful in treating depression. It is not the kind of disorder—although sometimes, frustratingly, it can appear that way—where a parent can say to the child, "Just get over it," or "Pull yourself together." The child can't, without help.

First, the child should have a physical exam by his or her pediatrician to rule out physical problems. Sometimes illness or medications can mimic or bring out depressive symptoms. Once physical symptoms are ruled out, the parent should consider bringing the child to a psychiatrist or psychologist.

Keeping a detailed history of the child's symptoms and behavior, including duration and severity of depression, will help the doctor make a diagnosis. Also the doctor will need a complete family history; an effective form of treatment can be culled from the family's health background.

While some patients do fine with psychotherapy, others are successful with antidepressants, and the combination is often a good start. Medications that have shown great promise are selective serotonin reuptake inhibitors (SSRIs). (See the "SSRIs" section in "What You Need to Know" for information on these drugs.)

Some natural supplements have been found to be very effective for depression, such as St. John's Wort, hypericum, gingko biloba, echinacea, omega-3 fish oils, and ginseng. No herbal supplement should be taken without consulting a physician (not all physicians are open to their use). Again, all drugs and supplements *must* be taken under a doctor's guidance. Some supplements cannot be taken with other medications, such as St. John's Wort and antidepressants. Drugs and supplements should not be mixed and matched, and doctors must be advised of any supplements you might be interested in giving to your child, in order to assess its interaction with a drug.

There are some at-home and self-help ways to aid a child suffering from CD. The children must first realize that their negative thoughts and feelings are not reality, but rather are distorted views and perceptions. There are many "don'ts" and "do's" a parent should be aware of: Don't let the child become overwhelmed; don't let him or her spend extended periods of time alone; don't insist that the child change; and don't belittle his or her problems. Do keep the child busy; let the child confide in you; participate in activities that may make them feel good; have them exercise as much as possible, eat well, and sleep well. Most importantly, talk to your child: let him or her know that there is hope, that this is a very controllable disorder.

Prognosis

According to the NAMI, once a young person has experienced a major depression, he or she is at risk of developing another depression within the next five years. In addition, two-thirds of children with mental-health problems do not get the help they need.

The AACAP reports that suicide is the third leading cause of death for 15- to 24-year-olds (approximately five thousand young people in the U.S.) and is the sixth leading cause of death for 5- to 15-year-olds. The suicide rate for 5- to 24-year-olds has nearly tripled since 1960.

CD can be effectively controlled through treatment, and early intervention can save a child a lifetime of trouble—and their life.

Sources and resources

American Academy of Child and Adolescent Psychiatry, AACAP (www.aacap.org)
Eastern Maine Medical Center (www.emmc.org)
Kathleen Panula Hockey, "What Is Childhood Depression, Really?"
    (www.enotalone.com)
National Alliance on Mental Illness (www.nami.org)
National Institute of Mental Health (www.nimh.nih.gov)

See the mental-health contacts under "General Resources" for more sources used in this chapter.

CD

Conduct Disorder

Terms used in this chapter: ADHD (attention-deficit/hyperactivity disorder); CD (conduct disorder); IEP (individualized education program)

Sound familiar?

Debra always said that her son Mark jumped around constantly from the moment he was conceived. When her husband, Paul, an accountant, saw the bumps pushing out of his wife's pregnant belly, he proudly said "There's a great athlete in there."

When Mark began attending school, Debra now vividly remembers how she tried not to watch the phone as soon as he got on the school bus. A stay-at-home mom, she also recalls being intensely jealous of her neighbor, Susan, who had a fulltime job as a banker in their small town. Susan's child, David, an avid sportsman, was never in trouble, had plenty of friends; Susan never had to worry every time the phone rang.

By the time Mark was in kindergarten, he was already diagnosed as having ADHD. His preschool teacher said she recognized it within a week and introduced Debra and Paul to other children who seemed as easily distracted as Mark, who was unable to focus enough to watch a three-minute video. They were sad that their child was not "perfect," but they were really happy that there was a name for what made Mark so difficult. There were many others who had the same problem, and, most importantly, there was medication that could help him. Maybe Mark would start hanging out more with David, Debra hoped.

Mark's ability to concentrate, have playmates, and follow simple rules alternated between getting better and worse as he grew older. Doses of one or another medication were changed, and then different medications were tried. For several years, he was put on various combinations of drugs to help him slow down but stay awake during the day, and another medication to help him get "good" sleep.

By Mark's twelfth birthday, Debra and Paul were beginning to suspect that their son was taking too much medication for a condition he might not even have. Debra was called by the school administrators several times a month to hear about Mark's pushing kids into lockers or refusing to enter a classroom when ordered to or just standing in class and yelling rude and sometimes even crude comments about classmates and adults. For another year, Mark's pediatrician and the ADHD Center they went to for medical and therapeutic treatment advised Debra and Paul that this downturn was typical for ADHD boys entering their teenage years. But by the time Mark turned 13, Debra saw that the phone calls and detentions were coming almost daily, and earlier and earlier in the school day. The early calls were the worst because that meant she had to deal with his uncontrollable behavior all by herself, at home.

When Mark was almost 14, local police were called when they found him slashing tires on cars parked at the local hospital. Debra and Paul finally realized that a lot of Mark's behavior was mean, cruel, and deliberate, not necessarily the actions of an ADHD child who was too hyperactive to recognize social cues. They were afraid that Mark would end up in jail or worse. They feared that his behavior would seriously hurt someone else, and, sadly, they admitted that they were afraid of their own child.

There was one really odd thing about the tire slashing event. Mark was not alone at the police station. The wonderful student, great athlete, polite young David was finally hanging out with Mark—also slashing tires. It turned out David had been undergoing treatment for his conduct as well for the past year.

Mark was brought for a battery of medical tests and was found to be a perfectly healthy boy. However, a coincidental meeting with a parent from Mark's original daycare center, another boy who was diagnosed with ADHD, led Mark and his family to another psychiatrist. While the doctor said he could never be sure that Mark originally had ADHD, it was likely; but his current condition was something else, and there were specific treatments available.

Mark's current diagnosis is CD—conduct disorder/childhood-onset type; David's diagnosis was CD—conduct disorder/adolescent-onset type.

Did you know?

CD is believed to be one of those Alphabet Disorders that is more common than reported. Many children who suffer from this disruptive behavioral disorder—ODD (oppositional defiant disorder) and ASPD (antisocial personality disorder) are the other two—are often deemed to be "problem" children who spend more time in detention than class.

The vast majority of those who have CD are boys, but social workers and other professionals who deal with children facing legal problems think many girls have CD but are often misdiagnosed. Depending on the severity of their apparent lack of empathy, and determination to break social rules at school and/or at home, kids with CD can learn why they act out and can be helped to conform their behavior to continue with their education, fit in with peers, and have a successful life.

One key appears to be early identification, treatment that includes therapy for the child and family, and often some medication, at least at the start of treatment, to enable the child to accept that his or her previous behavior needs to be changed for their own benefit.

The more severe the symptoms are, without intervention, it is more likely these children will grow up into "self-medicating" adults, abusing drugs and alcohol and getting caught up in the criminal justice system. CD children usually commit petty crimes but continue to get in trouble because they cannot abide by rules imposed by a judge.

While there is controversy about the term *conduct disorder* (some believe it is an overbroad term or an excuse for bad behavior), mental-health professionals who diagnose children and teenagers can clearly see a distinct pattern. Because this disorder is similar to ADHD, a lot of these children showed many of the signs that called for a diagnosis of ADHD. Even a child who is not disruptive may have signs of CD. When looking back at a child's seemingly glowing childhood, his or her constant participation in an assortment of sports, and a continuous change of hobbies, a doctor may see that this was the child's own way of dealing with an inability to focus for any significant length of time. It appears that CD is caused by both genetic and environmental factors, and affected children and teens almost always have a family history of alcohol addiction, mood disorders, or ADHD. They also often have comorbid, or concurrent, illnesses such as ADHD or mood disorders, further suggesting the utilization of medication and therapy. In adolescent-onset CD, the same type of family history also is commonly found, but traumatic events like the loss of a loved family member, coupled with other negative conditions, may trigger this condition.

Signs and symptoms

- bullies anyone, from those smaller than the CD child to adults
- burglarizes homes
- commits acts of vandalism that could cause harm
- deliberately breaks family rules
- disruptive
- lack of remorse
- leaves home for a day or two without telling anyone
- overly hostile
- refuses to go to school or repeatedly sneaks out of school, starting before age 13
- says socially unacceptable statements in school, at home, or at public events
- stays out past curfew
- steals from family members
- threatens or even forces unwanted sexual activity on someone
- threatens people with a weapon

- torments pets or other animals
- uses threatening words or actual aggressive physical aggression
- verbally and physically cruel to anyone from a toddler to a parent

Cause

As noted above, there appears to be a genetic cause to CD because family histories almost always include someone with mental-health problems. Family members will describe grandparents who had dramatic mood swings or who acted just the way a person with ADHD would behave. Often, family members will remark that the child in treatment acts just the way one or more members of the family behaved.

Environmental issues are also involved. Dysfunctional families, and households with abusive activity or neglect, can be found in the history of one diagnosed with this disorder.

Because of its close relation to ADHD, children who are raised in relatively healthy homes can end up with CD. Either they may have actually had ADHD or were misdiagnosed, but their unruly behavior may escalate causing bad relationships with adults and peers.

Those diagnosed with the adolescent-onset version of this disorder have the same family histories as those who have had behavioral issues when very young. Through treatment, it is often learned that a very traumatic event or a series of emotionally painful events triggered a sudden onslaught of some of the above-listed symptoms. Family therapy often reveals certain acts the young teen did as a child that were viewed as benign, unique, or acting especially active or good to mask or stop bad behavior may have been early symptoms.

It is generally accepted that addiction and certain behavioral problems are caused by genetic inheritance or other life incidents that control specific activity in an individual brain. This significant scientific advancement has generally replaced the outdated notion that people choose to drink or deliberately misbehave simply because they choose not to follow rules.

Diagnosis

A child or young teen who is disruptive, cannot follow rules, begins to bully people, or refuses to go to school should always be examined by a pediatrician first to rule out any medical conditions, including hormonal problems. Blood tests as well as vision and hearing examinations should be conducted; an unruly child simply may not have been hearing directions about behavior. Allergy tests are highly recommended. Also, some doctors believe that Lyme disease may be a trigger for behavioral problems.

Most importantly, any head injury must be treated seriously. Many children are now advised by their pediatricians to avoid sports or any other physical activity for at least a month after one concussion. Behavioral problems can be caused by any injury to one's head, whether it happened in a hockey game, a car accident, or a simple fall off a swing.

At the same time, the child can be evaluated by a psychologist who will personally spend time talking with him or her. This doctor will usually give a battery of question-and-answer type tests and other psychological tests to see how the child completes tasks.

The psychologist will also want to talk to the parents or the person responsible for this child's upbringing. Generally, questions will be asked to learn about the events that caused the request for this evaluation as well as getting a family history. A psychiatrist might then be brought in because that is the specialist field where the doctor cannot only confirm the diagnosis but also determine if medication is needed as well as therapy.

Treatment

As part of the diagnosis of CD, a determination is made of whether the condition is mild, moderate, or severe. Early diagnosis is important, but, unfortunately, parents may think their child needs different medication for a previous diagnosis of ADHD or may be in denial that their child is more than just "mischievous."

Treatment can include individual weekly therapy sessions with the child, meetings with the child's caregivers, residential placement, medication, and much more intensive therapy, depending on the severity of the disorder. Often, if the child does not need residential treatment, a plan, usually designed through an IEP, is devised so the child's school provides treatment and proper placement. It is important that everyone working to help this child is working with the same plan.

Unfortunately, proper treatment can be very expensive if it is conducted outside the school, and parents who have insurance should be prepared to fight for coverage for long-term treatment.

Those who have the most severe type of CD may be in a juvenile facility, having been caught breaking a law. In these cases, parents need to work with a lawyer who knows about juvenile law to get their child evaluated quickly and placed in a treatment facility, instead of a juvenile-detention center.

Prognosis

A child or young teen with a CD diagnosis can grow up to live a happy, successful life. The more a child's caretakers are committed to be active and perhaps even change some of their own behaviors, if deemed a part of the causation, the better chance of success in overcoming this disorder. Treatment may take years, different types of medications may be needed, therapy sessions may be increased, or a change of therapists may be needed if the child does not "click" with his or her doctor.

The biggest problem is that, while advances may be made quickly, there are often setbacks. The child or the parents may be so dismayed by a setback they may want to give up. But, since quick mood changes and bad behavior are not unusual for kids who don't have any mental-health issues, it is to be expected that children who have this condition will find the need to rebel against treatment.

The good news is that a lot of research is being done in areas specific to the treatment for these children. By studying the actual activity of the brain, neurologists are researching the reasons some children are more prone to certain behaviors than are other children. Pharmaceutical companies are constantly working to find medications to help the brain correct itself without causing unpleasant side effects.

Many psychologists will tell you that there are no guarantees, and, obviously, those with a mild CD have a much better success rate with a shorter need for treatment than a young teenager with a more severe case. But even that teenager, with later-onset CD, can look forward to a better life if given the appropriate treatment.

Sources and resources

American Academy of Child and Adolescent Psychiatry (www.aacap.org)
American Psychological Association (www.apa.org)
Conduct Disorders Online (www.conductdisorders.com)
DSM (*Diagnostic and Statistical Manual of Mental Disorders*)
National Institute of Mental Health (www.nimh.nih.gov)
Nemours Foundation (www.nemours.org)
psychologytoday.com

See the "ADHD: Attention-Deficit/Hyperactivity Disorder" chapter and the mental-health contacts under "General Resources" for more sources used in this chapter.

CDCS

Cri du Chat Syndrome

Terms used in this chapter: CDCS (cri du chat syndrome); CDCSA (Cri du Chat Support Group of Australia); ICD (*International Classification of Diseases*)

Sound familiar?

When Mindy was born, she had a weak high-pitched cry, like a kitten. Her mother Margarette, 18 and unmarried, had no idea that distinctive cry would signal a devastating diagnosis. She was informed, "Your baby has chromosomal damage, and she will be retarded."

Mindy cried a lot as an infant and did not eat well, but, in terms of developmental milestones such as rolling over, walking, and talking, she seemed as if she was keeping up, although her speech was difficult to understand. She used signs and gestures and eventually developed three-to-six-word sentences.

As a child, Mindy was overly stimulated, easily upset, startled, and frightened, especially by sounds. Her biggest problems have been obsessions, skin picking, and temper tantrums that were due to her inability to communicate adequately. Margarette says that Mindy used hair pulling, pinching, and biting to communicate, but eventually learned better ways to make herself understood. But Margarette adds, "She was the happiest little child, full of mischief, and an overabundance of hugs and kisses."

Mindy was unable to read or write, but she could recognize some words and loved to draw. Physically she was often ill with upper respiratory infections, bronchitis, a constantly runny nose, and occasionally pneumonia. Constipation was also an ongoing problem. Mindy also has mild vision and hearing impairments.

Margarette described Mindy at 19 as a "beautiful, loving, grown-up young woman." Mindy has lived away from home since then and trained in living skills. "Her life is mostly a happy one," says Margarette, "and she enjoys a valued and respected position within her home, community, and family.

"When she was born and given such a dismal prognosis for the future, no one ever expected her to live this long or accomplish so much."

Mindy has CDCS—cri du chat syndrome.

Did you know?

Although CDCS—5P Minus syndrome, Le jeune's syndrome, or, as classified in the *ICD*, deletion of short arm of chromosome 5—has many symptoms and signs associated with it, there's one highly distinctive one. In fact, its name—*cri du chat*, French for "cry of the cat"—is derived from it. That telltale characteristic is a high-pitched, monotone, cat-like cry believed to be due to physical abnormalities and hypotonia, low muscle tone. Although the voice will naturally lower as the child grows, the characteristic high pitch often persists into adulthood.

The syndrome was first reported in 1963 by Jérôme Jean Louis Marie Lejeune, a French pediatrician and geneticist who also developed the karyotype, the chromosomal constitution of the cell nucleus.

The official prevalence rates for CDCS are generally believed to be as low as one in 50,000 and as high as one in 20,000. However, it is thought that there are many children who have CDCS but have not been diagnosed. They manifest fewer symptoms, are more developmentally sound, and lack many of the most distinguishing features of the syndrome. So, it is believed that the rate is higher than officially stated.

Signs and symptoms

- abdominal hernia
- abnormal angle of the base of the skull seen on lateral skull X-ray
- behavior problems
- better receptive language skills than expressive skills
- bowel abnormalities
- cat-like cry that is weak and monotone
- chronic constipation
- cleft palate (rare)
- coughing when swallowing
- deformities of the feet
- dental problems
- distinctive creases on the palms of the hands (palmar creases)
- downward slant to the eyes
- drooling
- epilepsy, in rare cases
- extra fold of skin over the inner corner of the eye (epicanthic folds), becoming less pronounced in adolescence
- face more elongated in adolescence
- failure to thrive
- feeding problems
- females have higher-pitched, monotone voice throughout life
- frequent ear infections
- frequent upper respiratory infections, such as aspiration pneumonia
- gagging when swallowing
- gastrointestinal abnormalities
- head remains smaller than normal throughout life, becoming more evident in the first years (however, it is not particularly noticeable to the layperson)
- heart problems, such as atrial and ventral septal defects
- high muscle tone (hypertonia) later in life
- high palate
- hip dislocation
- hyperactivity
- incompletely or abnormally folded external ears
- inguinal hernia
- kidney abnormalities, in rare cases
- lack of interest in eating
- low birth weight
- low broad nasal ridge
- low muscle tone (hypotonia) in infancy

- low-set, malformed ears
- minor hearing impairments
- minor skeletal problems
- misaligned eyes (strabismus)
- motor skills delay
- MR (mental retardation)
- nasal bridge higher in adolescence
- obsessiveness
- oral defensiveness
- partial webbing or fusing of fingers or toes
- portion of the short arm of chromosome 5 seen on chromosome analysis
- problems with intubation for anesthesia, in a small number of cases, due to malformations of the larynx and epiglottis
- reflux
- repetitive behaviors
- round face
- scoliosis
- self-harming behavior
- sensitivity to sound
- sensory defensiveness
- separated abdominal muscles (diastasis recti)
- short attention span
- single line in the palm of the hand (simian crease)
- skin tags just in front of the ear
- sleep disorders such as apnea
- small head (microcephaly)
- small jaw, receding chin (micrognathia)
- speech and language delays
- sucking problems for newborns
- sudden, transient, high temperatures without obvious infection or illness
- swallowing problems (dysphagia)
- tactile defensiveness
- visual problems
- widely spaced eyes (hypertelorism)

Cause

CDCS is caused by spontaneous deletion of a significant portion of genetic material from chromosome number 5. Children with larger chromosomal deletions are more acutely affected than those with smaller deletions. Besides spontaneous deletions, a less common inherited form is caused by rearrangements of genetic material on the 5 chromosome, called translocations.

Diagnosis

It might take a while to determine that a child has this genetic disorder because pediatricians might brush off the high-pitched cry as normal. It is usually that distinctive cry that gets a parent concerned enough to find a well-informed physician who recognizes the symptom. Once the leap is taken, there are many sources of diagnosis, including genetic testing.

A karyotype chromosome test can help, but it is the symptoms—the cat cry or the distinctive head and facial features—that enable a doctor to turn clinical observations into a diagnosis. CDCS can also be genetically diagnosed in utero, by sampling the fetus' cells. A more detailed genetic test, fluorescence in situ hybridization (FISH) analysis, may reveal a small missing piece of chromosome.

Treatment

Early intervention is very important. Effective therapies include physical, occupational, behavioral, and speech-language. Sign language, pictorial symbols, or other alternative methods of communication should be instituted as early as possible. The CDCSA reports that CDCS children "are usually keen to communicate" and are open to different manners of communication. The earlier a child begins communicating, the less frustrated he or she will become, mitigating behavioral problems associated with the inability to communicate and improving the child's quality of life.

Prognosis

The prognosis of CDCS cannot be determined with accuracy. With a mortality rate of about 10 percent in infancy, the remaining 90 percent live normal lifespans, barring serious health threats. The CDCSA reports that the oldest person with CDCS is in her 60s.

The CDCSA also reports on its Web site that "most people with cri du chat syndrome are capable of achieving a degree of independent self-care but require supervision and care for life. Some of those least affected by the syndrome are able to live independently (or with minimal assistance) in the community."

Sources and resources

Cri du Chat Support Group of Australia (www.criduchat.asn.au)
Five P Minus Society (www.fivepminus.org)
Cri Du Chat Syndrome Support Group/UK (www.criduchat.co.uk)

CDD

Childhood Disintegrative Disorder

C

Terms used in this chapter: ABA (applied behavior analysis); AS (Asperger syndrome); ASD (autism spectrum disorder); CDD (childhood disintegrative disorder); ICD (*International Classification of Diseases*); MR (mental retardation); PDD (pervasive developmental disorder); PDD–NOS (pervasive developmental disorder–not otherwise specified); RS (Rett's syndrome)

Sound familiar?

Carl had all the typical developmental milestones, with not one red flag in his development. By the age of 2, he was speaking in sentences and seemed like the other kids his age. At two months short of 3 years old, he just stopped. Stopped everything, says his father, John, a Minnesota history teacher.

Carl regressed in every area. He could no longer speak in sentences. In fact, he could no longer speak at all. He did not interact with anyone—family members, friends of the family, other children. "There were no human interactions at all," says John, who admits he does not like talking about his son's early years. "Carl's behavior became very 'autistic,' his father says about Carl's "stimming," or self-stimulating with rocking, spinning, flailing, hand-flapping, and rubbing his arms.

Carl lost his toileting skills, and his father says it seemed as if it was "overnight when he changed from an independent child to a fully dependent one."

John and his wife went from doctor to doctor, but none could explain what Carl's father calls "the bizarre events."

Carl, who cannot walk or speak or care for himself, is now 11. None of his skills has returned. He attends a program for the severely handicapped. He, according to his father, "seems like a severely autistic and mentally retarded child."

Their journey with Carl has been hard for his parents, but not as difficult as the time period when he lost most of his skills. Carl has two siblings, one older and healthy, and one extremely gifted and younger who is 8 and is believed to have AS.

Carl's father says, "I just can't ever discuss what happened to [Carl] without it being painful."

Carl has CDD—childhood disintegrative disorder.

Did you know?

CDD is a rare and very serious disorder that was described years prior to autism but has only recently been officially recognized. It is one of five disorders on the PDD spectrum—CDD, RS, AS, autism, and PDD–NOS.

The disorder is known by other names: HS (Heller's syndrome), DI (dementia infantilis), DP (disintegrative psychosis), PdisD (pervasive disintegrative disorder), or—as classified in the *ICD*—other childhood disintegrative disorder; and it is diagnosed when a child stops normal development between ages 2 and 4, and degenerates to a lower-functioning level.

All the typical milestones are present in the CDD child—they speak, walk, get toilet trained, and express acceptable social interaction—until they begin regressing. Then there is that terrible period, which might follow a serious illness, when they begin to lose their skills.

The many developmental skills they acquired—intellectual, speech, motor, toileting, and social skills—disappear. They develop repetitive behaviors similar to children with ASDs. They soon lose control of their bladder and bowels. They often regress to a severely mentally retarded state.

As with other PDD spectrum disorders, CDD can't be cured. Most CDD children require lifelong care.

Regarded as a rare disorder, it is generally believed that CDD has been frequently incorrectly diagnosed and might be more prevalent than statistics indicate.

CDD appears to affect more boys than girls, but as research continues, that might change, as it has with other similar disorders.

There are several different directions onset of CDD can take, from gradual to more sudden.

Signs and symptoms

- delay of spoken language
- difficulty with transitions or changes in routine
- failure to develop peer relationships
- hand flapping
- impairment in nonverbal behaviors
- inability to initiate or sustain a conversation
- inability to recognize, understand, or respond to social cues
- inability to respond to feelings of others
- inability to voluntarily move the body in a purposeful way
- increased frequency of electroencephalogram (EEG) abnormalities and seizure disorder
- lack of emotional reciprocity
- lack of play
- lack of social reciprocity
- lack of varied, imaginative, or make-believe play
- loss of ability to say words or sentences (expressive language)

- loss of ability to understand verbal and nonverbal communication (receptive language)
- loss of bowel and bladder control
- loss of expressive language
- loss of motor skills
- loss of play skills
- loss of self-care skills
- loss of social skills
- maintaining a fixed posture or body position (catatonia)
- normal development for at least the first two years of life
- preoccupation with certain objects or activities
- repetitive and stereotyped patterns of behavior, interests, and activities
- rocking
- significant loss of previously acquired or learned skills
- specific routines and rituals
- spinning around
- stereotyped and repetitive use of language

Cause

CDD has no known cause. It can occur abruptly and spontaneously, or it can take place over an extended time period. But some illnesses are generally known to be associated with the etiology of CDD:

- autoimmune response
- epilepsy
- genetic disposition
- lipid storage diseases: rare, inherited metabolic disorders, where there is a toxic buildup of excess fats (lipids) in the brain and nervous system
- subacute sclerosing panencephalitis: chronic brain infection caused by measles virus causing inflammation of brain that kills nerve cells
- tuberous sclerosis: benign brain tumors

Diagnosis

The best approach for diagnosis and treatment is an interdisciplinary one starting with the child's pediatrician and including a pediatric neurologist, pediatric psychiatrist, pediatric developmental and behavioral specialist, physical therapist, occupational therapist, and an audiologist.

The first thing a doctor will do is a developmental screening—the loss of acquired skills is the biggest red flag for this disorder. The doctor will then differentiate the symptoms from CS (childhood schizophrenia), autism, RS, AS, SM (selective mutism), ERLD (expressive-receptive language disorder), MR, and SMHD (stereotypic movement habit disorder).

Treatment for CDD is the same as for autism—ABA training (breaking down skill training into small, basic steps and tailoring therapy to the child's specific behaviors) as well as physical, occupational, social skills, and speech-language therapy. Unlike autism, which sometimes responds well to these therapies, the CDD child's loss of functioning will likely be permanent. But even in a worst-case scenario, behaviors can be modified.

The Mayo Clinic suggests the following tests as ways to assess CDD:

- CAT (or CT) scan
- MRI
- electroencephalogram (EEG), to test for seizures and measure the brain's electrical activity
- genetic tests, to see if this is an inherited disorder
- communication tests
- language tests
- lead screening to check for lead poisoning
- hearing test
- vision test
- behavioral assessment
- developmental assessment tests: large-motor skills such as walking, running, jumping, throwing, and climbing; fine-motor skills, using the hands and fingers to manipulate small objects; sensory skills, involving sounds, sights, smells, tastes, and tactile responses; play skills (imaginative, varied, purposeful, goal-directed); self-care skills such as toileting, feeding, dressing, and brushing teeth; cognitive skills including attention, following directions, thinking, concentration, and problem-solving abilities.

Treatment

Treatment for CDD basically mirrors that of ASD, and the linchpin for success is early detection and early intervention. Most effective treatments are behavior-based and highly structured, such as ABA. Several therapies are helpful, including speech-language, social skills, and occupational and sensory integration therapy.

Some parents use complementary therapies such as music therapy, gluten-free diets, vitamin and mineral supplements, and art therapy. It is important that the family develop coping skills so they can advocate for their child in a well-informed way and have healthy, stress-less family relationships. Support groups and therapy are highly recommended for families. If you cannot find a CDD group, you might try an autism support group.

Early intervention is essential for CDD.

Prognosis

The prognosis for CDD is not good. Unfortunately, there is no cure for this disorder, but medications can help problematic behaviors, and therapies can enhance these children's lives. Only 20 percent of CDD children regain some language. Sadly, the prognosis for an independent adulthood is not good for children with CDD. According to the Yale Developmental Disabilities Clinic, "The available data suggest that generally the prognosis for this condition is worse than that for autism."

Sources and resources

Mayo Clinic, "Childhood Disintegrative Disorder" (www.mayoclinic.com)
Yale Developmental Disabilities Clinic
    (www.med.yale.edu/chldstdy/autism/research.html)

See the "Autism Resources" section for more sources used in this chapter.

CdLS

Cornelia de Lange Syndrome

Terms used in this chapter: ADHD (attention-deficit/hyperactivity disorder); CdLS (Cornelia de Lange syndrome); CdLSF (Cornelia de Lange Syndrome Foundation); GERD (gastroesophageal reflux disease); *ICD* (*International Classification of Diseases*); MR (mental retardation)

Did you know?

Although she was not the first to report the syndrome, CdLS was named after Dutch pediatrician Cornelia de Lange, M.D., in 1933.

CdLS is one of several congenital disorders described by the *ICD* as congenital malformation syndromes predominately associated with short stature. Those who have it strongly resemble each other. CdLS children are distinguished by excessive physical hairiness that doesn't affect the disorder. However, these features help diagnose the disorder. Many of its signs and symptoms, some severe and some unimportant, are present from birth or soon thereafter.

CdLS children suffer from significant problems such as vision abnormalities, hearing loss, and gastrointestinal tract complications. They are also often speech impaired and suffer from MR, although mostly moderately.

There is a low occurrence rate for CdLS, between 2 percent and 5 percent, and it usually does not run in the family. The CdLSF says that the incidence rate "is unclear, but it is thought to be approximately 1 in 10,000 live births."

Despite all the potential problem areas for CdLS children, there are some areas of strength, such as visual-spatial memory and perceptual organization.

Signs and symptoms

- abnormal gaze
- absent speech
- ADHD
- aggression in puberty
- auditory processing problems
- bowel abnormalities
- burping
- bushy eyebrows
- cleft lip
- cleft palate
- constipation
- cross-eyed (strabismus)
- crowded teeth
- curling of the fifth finger (clinodactyly)
- developmental delay
- diaphragmatic hernia
- diarrhea
- discharge or tearing from eye
- drooping eyelid (ptosis)
- dry eyes
- erosion of teeth caused by stomach acids from reflux
- excessive body hair
- eye tremor (nystagmus)
- feeble or low-pitched cry in infants, which disappears by 12 months
- feeding difficulties
- gaseous distention
- GERD
- hearing loss
- heart defects
- heartburn
- hip problems
- inability to speak (oral-motor and verbal apraxia)

- intermittent poor appetite
- lack of sensitivity to pain
- language delay
- lazy eye
- LDs (learning disabilities)
- lifts chin or arches eyebrow to improve vision
- light sensitivity (photophobia)
- limitation of elbow motions
- long eyelashes
- low birth weight (often under 5 pounds)
- lower gastrointestinal problems
- lower hairline than other family members
- minimal speech
- MR
- nearsightedness (myopia)
- need for gastric tube for feeding
- oppositional behavior
- partial joining of the second and third toes
- periodontal disease
- poor appetite
- premenstrual syndrome (females)
- red eyes
- seizures
- self-injurious behavior
- severe upper-limb malformations (missing fingers, metacarpals, and long bones of the arm)
- short thumb placed closer than usual to the wrist
- short upturned nose
- shorter stature than other family members
- single palm crease (simian crease)
- slow growth
- small hands and feet
- small head size (microcephaly)
- small jaw
- small stature
- tactilely defensive
- thin, downturned lips
- thin eyebrows that frequently meet at midline (synophrys)
- undescended testicles
- unexplained pain episodes in puberty

- unusual body movements: wiggling and moving constantly, turning head to one side, or throwing head back due to severe gastroesophogeal reflux (Sandifer syndrome)
- vomiting
- webbing of one or more fingers (syndactyly)
- worsening behavioral problems in puberty

Cause

It is thought that CdLS is a genetic autosomal dominant syndrome, meaning that the chance of having a male or female child with the disorder is 50 percent if one of the parents is a carrier of the gene. It is also widely reported that a few rare families have more than one person affected.

However, CdLS isn't an inherited genetic defect in 99 percent of the cases—it is caused by a genetic mutation, a *de novo* disorder. It is not present in parents, but is a new mutation that manifests itself in one individual. One reason it is not passed on, the CdLSF suggests, is that those who have the disorder usually do not have children. For those who are concerned about passing on CdLS, genetic tests are available.

Diagnosis

Since the cause is unknown and there are no identifiable chromosomal markers to create a specific test for, the diagnosis is made on clinical observations and physical features. Monitoring poor fetal growth and limb abnormalities through ultrasound can help detect problems prior to birth. The CdLSF Web site, listed under "For more information," provides detailed information on what to look for in an ultrasound.

A genetic specialist is the medical professional who should be seen after a full physical exam by the child's pediatrician, and depending on the range of problems, physical, occupational, and speech-language therapists might be needed on the team, along with audiologists and eye specialists.

Treatment

CdLS cannot be cured. But its symptoms can be treated. Surgeries can correct certain abnormalities, including hearing, hip, and gastrointestinal problems. For hearing problems, sometimes hearing aids are of use; eye patches often help correct vision problems such as strabismus.

Puberty becomes problematic for CdLS adolescents, and birth control/fertility issues should be discussed with the medical team. Treatments include synthetic hormonal treatment, such as oral contraceptives or Depo-Provera injections, and surgeries such as tubal ligation or hysterectomy, depending on the severity of mental and physical impairment. That said, the CdLSF suggests that these therapeutic solutions be considered as early as age 2, but certainly prior to puberty, to reduce the risk of cancer.

Because CdLS children have strong visual-spatial memory and perceptual organization skills, using computers, tactile stimulation, and visual memory may be effective learning methods.

Early intervention is highly suggested to deal with speech and communication problems. The CdLSF has strong words about early intervention and speech therapy:

> *The decision to begin speech therapy should not be delayed. Some parents have reported they have been told speech therapy could not begin until their children were talking! Additional parents reported they were told their children could not receive speech therapy or learn to talk until the gastric tube was removed and their children were eating normally. This, of course, is not true. Some children who are talking have never received nourishment except through their gastric tube. However, when appropriate, it would be beneficial to work with a speech-language pathologist on feeding therapy so the oral mechanism functions as normally as possible.*

Some alternative methods recommended by the CdLSF for the speech-impaired include a communication board, American Sign Language, American Indian Hand Talk or Amer-Ind Gestural Code, Blissymbolics, Total Communication, pantomime, a manual alphabet, eye-blinking encoding, and electronic communication aids. For children with severe upper-limb malformations, gestural-assisted and neuro-assisted strategies are available. Regardless of the disability, says the CdLSF, "it is important that all individuals be taught some means of indicating 'yes' and 'no.' It will often be most beneficial when speech-language pathologists function as communication therapists rather than as speech therapists."

Gastrointestinal problems are prevalent with CdLS, and many tests can be prescribed to assess the condition—for example, blood tests, stool tests, and X-rays. There are simple treatments for GERD that include medications, diets, and elevating a child after he or she eats. Surgeries include laparoscopic Nissen fundoplication (reinforcing the valve between the esophagus and stomach) and a gastrostomy, an incision in the stomach to enable G-tube feeding and an outlet for stomach gases.

Many communication problems a CdLS child has are closely tied to hearing problems. Since CdLS kids have a small ear structure, testing them is sometimes difficult, so it is advisable to consult an audiologist or otolaryngologist who is expert in CdLS. An expert on CdLS infants is suggested for pharyngeal-esophageal tube implanting for middle-ear drainage.

When a hearing loss is determined, it is highly suggested that hearing aids be acquired as early as possible because hearing loss, no matter how slight, can be a fertile breeding ground for speech and language delays. The CdLSF reminds parents that hearing, for the

C

most part, does not improve, so that, if your child's hearing scores are improving at each six-month visit, something might be wrong with the test or tester. Proper tests by expert specialists should be a priority.

Soon after a child is diagnosed with CdLS, he or she should have an eye exam to detect what is not as visible as other CdLS symptoms such as misaligned eyes. The child may be nearsighted and the sooner he or she gets corrective lenses the better. The CdLSF suggests rechecking for nearsightedness every few years until puberty.

The CdLSF issues the following warning:

> *Individuals who develop recurrent red eyes, crusting on the eyelashes, itchy eyes, tearing, or eye discharge [should see an ophthalmologist]. Although the symptoms may mimic a blocked tear duct (nasolacrimal duct obstruction), they are more often due to blepharitis, an idiopathic condition in which the 20 to 30 glands normally present in each eyelid have suboptimal flow. Rather than surgical treatment for a tear duct problem, baby shampoo eyelash scrubs can often result in dramatic improvement of the blepharitis symptoms. Older children with self-injurious behavior can seriously damage their eyeballs. Any signs of self-induced eye injury should also prompt an ophthalmic referral.*

Mouth and dental concerns should be addressed early also. Cleft palate, common in CdLS, should be surgically corrected as soon as possible. That improves the child's ability to eat and speak and lessens the chance of ear infections, which can wreak havoc on hearing functions.

The CdLSF has many interesting suggestions regarding the well-being of these children, but the advice applies to children with any Alphabet Disorder. One bit of advice: If the child is to be anesthetized for any procedure, consider having a second procedure done simultaneously—for example, when dental work is done, a needed endoscopy can also be done.

Prognosis

The CdLSF advises, "It is expected that most children with CdLS will live well into adulthood; however, each child must be evaluated for life-threatening conditions such as heart defects, untreated gastroesophageal reflux and bowel abnormalities."

"There is no correlation between age and cause of death," reported CdLSF Medical Director, Laird Jackson, M.D., at a conference in the U.K. in January 2001. "Adults with CdLS can live well into the 40s and beyond." According to CdLS experts around the world, the disorder does not necessarily mean a shortened lifespan.

With early intervention, there is hope for improving the life of children with CdLS because the disorder is not progressive. Newly acquired skills will not be lost. Early intervention could be the key between your child's learning to speak or never speaking.

Sources and resources

Cornelia de Lange Syndrome Foundation/Australasia (www.cdlsaus.org)
Cornelia de Lange Syndrome Foundation/UK/Ireland (www.cdls.org.uk)
Cornelia de Lange Syndrome Foundation/USA (1-800-753-2357); (www.cdlsusa.org)
Fundoplication information: NIH (www.nlm.nih.gov)

CLS

Coffin-Lowry Syndrome

Terms used in this chapter: CLS (Coffin-Lowry syndrome); CLSF (Coffin-Lowry Syndrome Foundation); MR (mental retardation); NIH (National Institutes of Health)

Did you know?

CLS is a rare genetic disorder typified by head, facial, and skeletal abnormalities, MR, short stature, and low muscle tone (hypotonia). It was first described in 1966 by Grange S. Coffin, M.D., a pediatrician based in Berkeley, California, and again in 1971 by R. B. Lowry, M.B., F.R.C.P. In 1975, the two descriptions were combined as the same disorder. The NIH reports that CLS occurs in about one in 40,000 to one in 50,000 births, but notes that this might be underestimated. It affects males and females equally, but is believed to be more severe in males, with severe MR, since it is an X-linked mutation and boys have only one X chromosome. Girls still have one normal X-chromosome, so symptoms are milder.

CLS children are least affected in their emotional makeup. They are very loving, polite, social, affectionate, and outgoing, feeling the range of emotions from happiness to depression.

Signs and symptoms

- abnormal front-to-back and side-to-side spine curvature (kyphoscoliosis)
- abnormal MRI of brain ("white-matter" disease)
- abnormally prominent brow
- affectionate
- anxious
- appropriate social skills
- ataxia or rigid muscles
- aversion to being touched

- awkward gait
- bad bite (malocclusion)
- better receptive language skills than expressive ones
- brittle bones
- broad nose
- bulbous ends of bones of fingers and toes
- constipation
- daytime sleepiness
- delayed and impaired fine motor functions
- delayed and impaired gross motor functions
- delayed bone development
- delayed speech development
- developmental delay
- dislike of change
- down-slanting eyelid folds
- "drop attacks" or sudden spontaneous falls
- early loss of baby teeth
- emotional outbursts
- engaging personality
- enlarged tonsils
- exaggerated deep tendon reflexes
- exaggerated startle reflex (hyperexplexia)
- extreme reactions to pain (oversensitive/undersensitive)
- fainting spells
- feeding problems
- flat feet
- fullness of upper eyelids (ptosis)
- good memory
- hearing impairment
- hearing loss cluster in family
- heart problems
- high, narrow palate
- intact emotions
- intact social skills
- kidney problems
- lack of speech
- large ears
- large mouth with full out-turned lips
- large tongue

- larger than normal permanent teeth
- loss of muscle mass
- loss of strength
- low birth height for boys, usually in third percentile
- midline groove in tongue
- missing permanent teeth (hypodontia)
- MR
- narrow spaces between vertebrae
- normal birth weight
- normal gait eventually changes to wide-stance gait
- one leg drags behind the other when walking
- painful and dangerous bowel blockages
- progressive paraplegia
- progressive spasticity
- prominent forehead
- protruding nostrils (nares)
- puffy hands
- repetition of last word or words spoken by others (echolalia)
- repetition of phrases (perseverance)
- respiratory problems
- sensorineural deafness
- severe temper tantrums
- short, curved fingernails
- short, horizontal line in palm of hand below little finger (hypothenar crease)
- short, hyperextensible, tapered fingers
- short stature
- SID (sensory integration disorder)
- sleep apnea
- small, widely spaced, peg-shaped baby teeth
- snoring
- soft, elastic skin
- "soft spot" on head takes up to two years to close
- toilet-training delays
- tunnel chest
- underdeveloped upper jaw bone (maxillary hypoplasia)
- unusual prominence of the breastbone (pectus carinatum)
- unusually thick eyebrows
- uses alternative ways of moving than crawling

Cause

The NIH reports that 65 percent of CLS cases are caused by a mutation in the RSK2 gene (a growth factor regulator) located on the X chromosome. The effect of this mutation was only identified in 1996. How that defective gene generates the distinctive CLS symptoms is not known. The remaining percentage of cases have no known cause.

According to the CLSF, "About 70 to 80 percent have no family history of Coffin-Lowry syndrome and 20 to 30 percent have more than one affected family member." The CLSF continues, "The risk to the siblings depends upon the carrier status of the mother. If the mother has the CLS mutation, the chance of transmitting it in each pregnancy is 50 percent."

Diagnosis

Since more than ninety distinct mutations can cause CLS characteristics, making a positive diagnosis using genetic testing is very difficult. Your child's doctor will give your child a physical examination and observe his or her developmental growth.

Since the symptoms in infancy are often mild—especially in girls—and can be confused with many disorders, a proper diagnosis often takes a while. The child's distinctive short, tapered fingers are usually a main, trustworthy symptom for diagnosis.

Treatment

With no cure, there is also no prescribed course of treatment, but symptoms are treated through a team of specialists including physical, occupational, vocational, and speech-language therapists.

The CLSF suggests the following general good advice:

Since you see your child every day, you may notice that something is different before your family doctor will. You can keep an eye out for scoliosis by having your child stand in front of you, facing away from you, and then have him or her touch their toes. If there is any doubt, have your child examined by a physician. In CLS, scoliosis may be present as early as birth or as late as the teenage years, with the average being early grade school years. Unexplained falls may develop which are neurological in origin and may be controlled with various medications. Sleep apnea is common and if untreated, the chronic oxygen deprivation can cause cardiac problems, and loss of cognitive function. Fainting spells could be an indicator of a heart condition. If behavior problems occur, first rule out any underlying physical cause; for example, head banging may be an indication that the child is in discomfort from chronic ear infections. Bone degeneration may be prevented or onset forestalled by a high-protein diet.

Prognosis

There is no cure for CLS at this time, but depending on the severity of the disorder, the prognosis varies. Early detection and intervention certainly help to improve the prognosis. The CLSF reports that, even among some of the most severely affected, "most" of the children will learn to speak and will be toilet trained. They can also learn sign language.

Self-care skills can also be learned by CLS children. The CLSF says that most intellectually impaired children can be toilet trained by age 7 and that, with easy-to-manipulate and Velcro fasteners, many skills can be mastered. Clothes that are easy to pull on or pull over are helpful.

Intellectual skills vary with CLS children. They may have certain abilities but cannot properly use them. For example, they have good memories but do not know how to apply that skill.

Some aspects of the syndrome are progressive, warns the CLSF: "Facial coarsening and skeletal involvement become more pronounced with age. Some motor and coordination neurological problems do not express themselves until later in childhood and may result in decreased mobility. Bone degeneration may occur. Behavior problems may develop. Premature death is increased in individuals who have severe cardiac problems, respiratory complications, or severe progressive kyphoscoliosis."

Sources and resources

Coffin-Lowry Syndrome Foundation (425-427-0939); (www.clsf.info)
National Institute of Neurological Disorders and Stroke, "NINDS Coffin-Lowry Information Page" (www.ninds.nih.gov)

CMT

Charcot-Marie-Tooth Disorder

Terms used in this chapter: ADHD (attention-deficit/hyperactivity disorder); CMT (Charcot-Marie-Tooth disorder); CMTA (Charcot-Marie-Tooth Association); IEP (individualized education program); MS (multiple sclerosis); NINDS (National Institute of Neurological Disorders and Stroke); OT (occupational therapist); PT (physical therapist)

Sound familiar?

Yohan Bouchard was born in Grenoble, France, on March 9, 1993. When he was 2½ years old, his parents Gilles and Elizabeth moved to California.

In first grade, Yohan started to lag behind his classmates. As the year progressed, he demonstrated less stamina and physical endurance during playground periods; he was frustrated that he could not climb the monkey bars at school or climb trees.

Gilles began noticing a difference in his son's physical capacities. The sun and heat bothered Yohan more and more; the child complained of burning on the bottom of his feet; and walks and hikes became shorter and shorter, as Yohan complained of fatigue, pain, etc.

In the summer of 2000, Elizabeth noticed that Yohan's feet were changing. His Achilles tendon was extremely tight, his arches very high, and his toes curled inwards, with the pinkie forming a hammer toe.

In the fall, Yohan was brought to an OT and a PT, who helped Yohan stretch out his very tight hamstrings, calves, and Achilles tendons and learn to ride a bike, a feat with which he struggled immensely because of balance issues.

The PT found gait abnormalities, gross motor delays, difficulties with balance and posture, tightness in bilateral hamstrings, and gastrocnemius/soleus complex (tight calf muscles and Achilles tendon), as well as poor coordination on opposite sides of his body. The therapist insightfully recommended that Yohan be seen by a pediatric neurologist.

In November 2001, a brain scan and genetic blood test were taken and the waiting started. Within a week, the brain MRI came back positive for mild CP (cerebral palsy). In the meantime, Yohan visited yet another orthopedic surgeon, who suggested that he be serial casted (plaster casts were put on both legs up to his knees at an angle, to keep him stretched twenty-four hours a day). After ten days, the casts were replaced with others at yet a more severe angle, to force his Achilles tendons to lengthen. The surgeon proposed a tendon-lengthening operation, "a much easier and less time-consuming" alternative, but Elizabeth was reluctant to have any surgery done on Yohan.

After six weeks of casts, Yohan wore night splints to keep his tendons stretched out. Yohan was not doing well. He became anxious, angry, and withdrawn. He couldn't keep up with his peers on the playground, and he was terribly fatigued and anxious.

Falling behind with his studies, he couldn't keep up with the homework. He'd come home from school in tears, feeling overwhelmed in most areas of his life. He hated school and felt left out. His self-worth was at an all-time low.

Yohan moved to a new school, and things began to look up. His teacher noticed he had difficulties with sequential learning and organizational skills. Educational testing showed learning disabilities, weaknesses involving executive functioning, short-term auditory memory, and sequencing.

A psychiatrist diagnosed him with anxiety disorders including mild OCD (obsessive-compulsive disorder), social phobia, and ADHD. Yohan's anxiety was treated with medication, psychotherapy, and enrollment in a social-skills group. All proved somewhat helpful, providing support around his daily challenges. Most importantly, he became eligible for an IEP.

Yohan missed a lot of school because of doctor appointments and therapies. Also, Elizabeth says, "Kids can be quite cruel toward other children perceived to be weak or different in any way. He was teased quite a bit, not only because he could not keep up with [physical education] activities and was labeled lazy, but also because he was pulled out of class to receive extra help. He received OT in school and was allowed to have a cushion on his chair for posture stability and was allowed to take off his shoes in class to lessen pain. These tiny 'comforts' infuriated many of the other children as they did not comprehend why Yohan got these luxuries and why they were not privy to the same treatment."

In third grade, he had to be serial-casted again, having lost the flexibility gained by the first casting. Suddenly, Yohan's "invisible" disability became visible, and kids were intrigued and curious about the casts. The positive and empathetic attention he received from teachers and his peers was overwhelming, and Yohan gained popularity. However, these visual signs lasted only about six weeks and did not remain in the memory of most people.

Elizabeth gave a presentation at Yohan's school explaining his disorder and afterwards most of his peers embraced him, as they now had the knowledge to understand his disorder and special needs.

In fifth grade, Yohan moved to a private school, which Elizabeth says "focused on the development of the whole child." He repeated fifth grade, to relax in a no-pressure atmosphere and "enjoy his childhood."

Yohan is now 14. He is entering eighth grade and doing very well, despite an additional diagnosis of scoliosis. "It is not fair for any child to struggle with pain, anxiety, and physical limitations on a daily basis," says Elizabeth.

"I know that this disease has given Yohan ways to meet challenges head-on and to overcome barriers. He is intellectually curious, personable, empathetic, fun-loving, and endearing. For parents to think this of a 14-year-old, a teen, says something in and of itself. I believe that Yohan, with structure, will achieve his heart's desire."

Yohan has CMT1A—Charcot-Marie-Tooth disease, Type 1A.

Did you know?

CMT is one of the most common hereditary neurological disorders and one of the most common rare disorders. It is so common, in fact, says Pat Dreibelbis, director of program services at the CMTA in Chester, Pennsylvania, that "it can easily tip to the other side."

The NINDS and CMTA report that the disease affects one in 2,500 in this country. The NIH reports that CMT affects "about 1 in 3,300 people" worldwide. However, it is believed that many people mildly affected by the disorder—or who don't want to be labeled with a genetic disorder or who don't know they have anything wrong with them—are never diagnosed. So, the rate of prevalence for CMT is thought to be much higher than statistics indicate.

Dreibelbis states, "The comment that always comes up at conferences is that the number of [officially diagnosed] cases could in actuality be doubled." The first CMT prevalence study is now being conducted.

According to the CMTA, CMT is a "very strongly inherited" sensory, motor, and nerve disorder that primarily manifests itself as weakness and atrophy in the muscles of the legs, but it can affect other body parts. It is also known as hereditary sensory and motor neuropathy and peroneal muscular atrophy.

The disorder affects the body's peripheral nerves that lie outside the brain and spinal cord and affect muscles and sensory organs in the limbs. The primary difference between CMT and diseases like MS, caused by a central brain disorder, is that, in CMT, etiology is peripheral to the nerves. Although CMT is one of more than three dozen diseases represented by the Muscular Dystrophy Association (MDA), CMT is not a muscular condition but rather a nerve defect that controls the muscles.

The curious name, as with many diseases, comes from the doctors who first described the disorder in 1866: neurologists Jean Martin Charcot, M.D., Pierre Marie, M.D., and Howard Henry Tooth, M.D.

How it is manifested

CMT does not affect intelligence, but instead manifests itself as weakness in the foot muscles, a condition that moves to the calves and eventually the lower arms. The classic sign is the high arch in the foot, although the muscles can release and "puddle" on the bottom of the foot causing flat-footedness.

There is a distinctive walk—clumsy, high-gaited with a foot drop—associated with the disorder. This gait sometimes appears similar to disorders such as ataxia and MS. The CMT child often trips and falls. The high-stepping walk has the foot raised well above the ground ("stork leg"), and the feet slap down as they hit the ground.

CMT is progressive, and the symptoms wax and stabilize, so it is difficult to determine the ultimate severity. But CMT is not life-threatening—except in rare cases when it affects the respiratory system. Pain may accompany the disorder, and sometimes leg braces are required.

There are two main types of this genetic disorder: hypertrophic or Type 1 (which Yohan has) and neuronal, Type 2. Type 1 is the most common and involves the thickening of nerve fibers and disturbances in the myelin or insulating material, slowing down nerve signals. Type 2 involves the weakening of nerve fiber, but nerve impulses aren't dramatically affected, if at all.

CMT progresses very slowly, so it is difficult to pinpoint onset. Hypertrophic CMT appears before the age of 20, usually in adolescence. Neuronal CMT usually appears after 20.

There are several other forms of the disease: CMT3, or DSD (Dejerine-Sottas disease), begins in infancy, with severe muscle atrophy, weakness, and sensory problems. Children with CMT4 usually develop weakness in their legs and might be unable to walk as adolescents. With CMTX, which is linked to the X (male) chromosome, males inheriting one mutated maternal gene exhibit moderate-to-severe symptoms of CMT in late childhood or adolescence, while females who inherit one gene that is mutated from one parent and a normal gene from the other have less severe symptoms, ranging from mild to none.

The CMTA warns that the disease may become worse if certain neurotoxic drugs are taken.

Signs and symptoms

- arch in foot is very high (most distinctive symptom), but can also be unusually flat
- auditory neuropathy, in rare cases
- breathing difficulties, in rare cases
- burning sensation in hands and feet
- chronically cold hands and feet
- cocking of toes
- degeneration of motor and sensory nerves
- delayed skills
- depression
- difficulty with fine motor skills and manual dexterity such as using eating utensils, buttoning buttons, picking up small objects, turning doorknobs, using writing implements, zippering, everyday tasks
- diminished sense of touch
- dry skin in affected areas
- enlarged nerves that can be felt or seen through the skin
- foot ulcers
- frequent ankle sprains
- hair loss in affected areas
- hammer toes (middle toe joint bends upwards)
- hand tremors, which may indicate RLS (Roussy-Levy syndrome)
- high-stepping drop-foot gait, with foot raised well above the ground (stork leg); to prevent the feet from dragging on the ground and upsetting balance, the foot slaps as it hits the ground
- hip dysplasia
- inability to run fast or properly
- inverted heel
- late walking skills
- limited mobility
- loss of knee-jerk reaction
- loss of movement and feeling in arm below the elbow and in leg below the knee

- loss of the opposable pinch
- muscle cramping
- pain
- poor balance
- poor handwriting
- progressive muscle atrophy
- scoliosis
- sensitivity to cold
- severe weakness in feet, ankles, and lower legs
- severe weakness in wrists, hands, and fingers
- slowing reflexes
- swelling (edema) of feet and ankles
- thin calves (lower legs may have "inverted champagne bottle" appearance)
- tingling in hands and feet
- toe blisters
- toe-walking, especially after age 3
- uncomfortable in standard shoes

Cause

Since CMT is usually inherited in an autosomal dominant pattern, if one parent has it, there is a 50/50 chance of each child inheriting it.

The NINDS provides the science behind CMT:

A nerve cell communicates information to distant targets by sending electrical signals down a long, thin part of the cell called the axon. In order to increase the speed at which these electrical signals travel, the axon is insulated by myelin, which is produced by another type of cell called the Schwann cell. Myelin twists around the axon like a jelly-roll cake and prevents dissipation of the electrical signals. Without an intact axon and myelin sheath, peripheral nerve cells are unable to activate target muscles or relay sensory information from the limbs back to the brain.

CMT is caused by mutations in genes that produce proteins involved in the structure and function of either the peripheral nerve axon or the myelin sheath. Although different proteins are abnormal in different forms of CMT disease, all of the mutations affect the normal function of the peripheral nerves. Consequently, these nerves slowly degenerate and lose the ability to communicate with their distant targets. The degeneration of motor nerves results in muscle weakness and atrophy in the extremities (arms, legs, hands, or feet); in some cases, the degeneration of sensory nerves results in a reduced ability to feel heat, cold, and pain.

The gene mutations in CMT disease are usually inherited. Each of us normally possesses two copies of every gene, one inherited from each parent. Some forms of CMT are inherited in an autosomal dominant fashion, which means that only one copy of the abnormal gene is needed to cause the disease. Other forms of CMT are inherited in an autosomal recessive fashion, which means that both copies of the abnormal gene must be present to cause the disease. Still other forms of CMT are inherited in an X-linked fashion, which means that the abnormal gene is located on the X chromosome. The X and Y chromosomes determine an individual's sex. Individuals with two X chromosomes are female, and individuals with one X and one Y chromosome are male. In rare cases, the gene mutation causing CMT disease is a new mutation that occurs spontaneously in the patient's genetic material and has not been passed down through the family.

Diagnosis

Since CMT is often inherited, there is not a wide leap in getting a diagnosis. The problem is with the spontaneous (*de novo*) case—as with Yohan's family—and then CMT is often not the first diagnosis.

Children inherit their parents' type of CMT but might manifest it at a different level of severity. There are many cases, CMTA's Dreibelbis says, where parents actually get diagnosed *after* their children. She notes also that many families believe the symptoms are just a unique family anomaly, and they say something like, "Oh, I just thought he had the Johnson family foot."

Diagnosis is based on family history and a physical exam. Electrodiagnostic nerve function exams such as nerve conduction studies and electromyography (EMG) are available as well as a nerve biopsy. And, of course, genetic testing can be conducted to confirm the diagnosis. While it is treatable, there is no cure for degenerative CMT. Fortunately, most cases are not too severe.

Treatment

Several types of therapies are effective: PTs, OTs, and orthopedists can address deformities caused by atrophy as well as the walking problems. The NINDS says that the preferred treatment for CMT involves muscle strength training, muscle and ligament stretching, stamina training, and moderate aerobic exercise. Strength training, NINDS adds, is most useful if it begins before nerve degeneration and muscle weakness progress to the point of disability.

Stretching reduces joint deformities resulting from uneven muscle pull on bones, and exercises including moderate aerobics help build stamina and endurance. Low-impact or no-impact exercises such as biking or swimming, rather than activities such as walking or jogging, which may put stress on fragile muscles and joints, are recommended.

Since so many problems involve the feet, it is wise to consult a podiatrist who can assist with foot, shoe, and mobility concerns. Ankle braces, high-top shoes, or boots to help prevent sprains by providing support during everyday exercise such as walking or climbing stairs are recommended. For weakness in hands and degeneration of fine motor skills, thumb splints are suggested. Some CMT children might need surgery to correct orthopedic deformities.

The CMTA says that it is important for people with CMT to have the proper footwear, as shoes are often ill-fitting because of high arches and hammer toes. Getting custom-made shoes is important. Dreibelbis says that podiatrists are often much attuned to diagnosing CMT, and it is suggested that those with CMT should have foot grooming (cutting toenails, removing calluses) by a podiatrist, because there is sensory loss in the foot.

Pain treatment is important, and the CMTA is adamant about its being recognized:

A ... problem related to CMT that needs to be addressed by a medical professional is the pain that some patients experience. Pain might be sharp and sudden or the gnawing, continuous ache of chronic pain. Some pain is associated with dysfunctional nerves that fire off sporadically and some can be attributed to weakened and poorly functioning muscles. Joints and ligaments in the feet and ankles are often painful because of the extra strain put on them by other muscles that have been rendered useless by CMT. Because the causes of pain vary, so will the treatments. No one, however, should be told that there is no pain associated with CMT, since pain is experienced in a very personal and individual way.

CMT individuals need to work hard to maintain their otherwise generally good health. They need to keep their hands and feet warm because of circulation problems and be careful when walking—or during any activity—because it might take them longer to heal if they fall or are injured. Wearing proper footwear, reports the CMTA, is crucial to their safety.

As with any degenerative disease or disabling disorder, depression and low self-esteem can manifest, so the psychological health of CMT children (and adults) is very important to address.

Prognosis

CMT patients have a wide range of symptoms, from severe to patients not even knowing they have a disorder. Depending on the severity, the disease's slow progression, and the treatment's effectiveness, the CMT child's quality of life can be good. CMT is not a fatal disorder, and most people who have it lead normal lives, with normal life expectancy.

Sources and resources

Charcot-Marie-Tooth Association (CMTA) (800-606-CMTA [2682]); (www.charcot-marie-tooth.org)

Muscular Dystrophy Association (800-344-4863); (www.mda.org)

National Ataxia Foundation (NAF) (www.ataxia.org)

National Institute of Neurological Disorders and Stroke, "Charcot-Marie-Tooth Information Page" (www.ninds.nih.gov)

Neuropathy Association (212-692-0662) (www.neuropathy.org)

COS

Childhood-Onset Schizophrenia

Terms used in this chapter: ASD (autism spectrum disorder); BD (bipolar disorder); COS (childhood-onset schizophrenia); IEP (individualized education program); PTSD (post-traumatic stress disorder)

Did you know?

COS is a severe, chronic psychiatric disorder that is characterized by hallucinatory symptoms and peculiar ways of thinking. It is a disconnection from reality that usually starts around 9 to 15 years old. It affects one in 40,000 children under the age of 13, mostly males. The prevalence increases in adolescence.

The symptoms of a schizophrenic child build slowly, but they eventually erode away the child's mental health. A schizophrenic child might start off being sociable and friendly and then will deteriorate as he or she grows older. Some might start off secure and self-assured and eventually turn shy, lack confidence, and become clingy. The child may begin to become more isolated and withdrawn into his or her own world of bizarre thoughts.

Schizophrenia is on the more severe end of a biologically related spectrum of disorders, with SPD (schizoid personality disorder) on the most mild end and STPD (schizotypal personality disorder) in the middle.

Signs and symptoms

- academic problems
- anxiety
- bewildered and bizarre thinking
- confusing dreams with reality
- confusing media such as TV and movies with reality
- delusional
- detached

- developmental delays
- diminished emotion
- diminished energy
- disconnected from reality
- disruptive behavior
- emotional expression is lacking or inappropriate
- extreme mood changes
- fearfulness
- hallucinations
- hearing voices
- illogical
- immobility
- irrationality
- isolation
- lack of personal hygiene
- little verbal communication
- paranoia
- problems maintaining friendships and peer interaction
- purposeless excessive mobility
- speech and language problems
- withdrawal

Cause

The cause is not known, but there are some strong suggestions borne out of research including a variety of biochemical, genetic, and environmental factors such as viruses, childhood malnutrition, and early childhood physical and psychological trauma affecting changes in the brain. It is widely held that it is the result of an aberration in early brain development. Areas in the brain associated with the neurotransmitter dopamine appear to be affected most often in schizophrenia.

Diagnosis

One problem with diagnosing COS is that it is often difficult to recognize in its early stages. The symptoms for children and adolescents with schizophrenia are sometimes different from the symptoms for adults.

Since children have rich imaginations, it makes for a problematic diagnosis when a child presents with behaviors that can be considered both normal and symptoms of schizophrenia. There are also many other Alphabet Disorders that are easily confused with schizophrenia, including BD, schizoaffective disorder (a mix of schizophrenia and mood disorder symptoms), severe anxiety disorders, severe major depression with psychotic features, PTSD, substance abuse disorders, brain disorders, personality disorders, and ASDs.

Treatment

Parents should first bring their child to the pediatrician so the child can be fully evaluated medically. The next step would be a referral to a pediatric psychiatrist. If schizophrenia is suspected, a specialist in the field should be seen—someone who is experienced in diagnosing and treating a schizophrenic child. Follow-up will include psychiatric therapy, medication, and an IEP for school that will map out academic and therapeutic services and modifications specifically designed for your child. Psychological therapies that involve the family as well as the individual child are often suggested.

Treatment may well involve hospitalization and enrollment in a special school that deals with COS.

Medications are often used with schizophrenic children and might actually be prescribed before an official diagnosis is given to alleviate the psychotic episodes the child might be exhibiting that might be disguising a true diagnosis. Antipsychotic drugs, neuroleptics, are the medication of choice for schizophrenics. They help to suppress psychotic behaviors by regulating the brain's production of the neurotransmitter dopamine. Risperdal, currently the drug of choice, was finally approved in 2007 for treatment of adolescent schizophrenia. All medications should be discussed with a doctor, and, for good measure, an additional specialist for a second opinion. These medications often have very strong side effects.

Prognosis

COS is a serious disorder with no cure, but it can be controlled. The earlier this lifelong disorder is diagnosed and treated both medically and psychiatrically, the better the prognosis.

Sources and resources

National Alliance for Research on Schizophrenia and Depression (800-829-8289); (www.narsad.org)
Schizophrenia.com (www.schizophrenia.com)

See the mental-health contacts under "General Resources" for more sources used in this chapter.

CS

Cockayne Syndrome

Terms used in this chapter: CS (Cockayne syndrome); G-tube (gastronomy feeding tube in the stomach); NG-tube (nasogastric feeding tube through the nose); RNA (ribonucleic acid)

Sound familiar?

Tim and Haylee were only 18 when their son Ian was born on December 29, 1997. Ian Walker was 6 pounds, 8 ounces, and 19 inches tall. Haylee and Tim took Ian home the next day, a snowy Tennessee Tuesday.

Ian hardly ever cried, although he had feeding problems that eventually got so bad he'd vomit every time he was fed.

At that time, the doctors said the young parents should just keep an eye on him, since he was gaining a little weight. At his four-week check-up, the doctors mentioned that Ian hadn't gained a pound and his head hadn't grown much, "but it should catch up," Haylee says she was told.

Ian was started on reflux medicine, which never helped. He was also diagnosed with an underactive thyroid, and he began medicine for that.

At 4½ months, Ian was holding his head to the left side and couldn't turn it to the right by himself. His legs also seemed to be very tight. At 8 months, he still couldn't keep any of his food down. He was hospitalized for observation, an NG feeding tube was placed in his nose, and a CAT scan was performed.

"The pediatrician came in and said his scan wasn't normal and that Ian was going to be retarded," recalls Haylee. "He put it so nicely."

When Ian was 9 months old, he had several procedures—the placement of a gastronomy tube (g-tube—a feeding tube in his stomach) and surgery to alleviate chronic reflux. "He was cut from his breastbone to the top of his belly button and was acting like it didn't hurt," says Haylee.

An MRI, along with CAT scan results, showed that Ian's brain was underdeveloped, had abnormal white matter, enlarged ventricles, and other abnormal findings.

Ian's diagnosis was microcephaly, Dandy-Walker variant, and CP (cerebral palsy). The neurologist told the young parents that their young son "would probably be a vegetable and not live very long."

Geneticists performed numerous tests, all coming back normal. One geneticist said Ian's condition was "a fluke" and shouldn't happen again.

Ian started on Botox injections, which helped his muscle tone, and began to walk for a few steps using a walker. He also sat up by himself for about three weeks.

"All our 'little fluke' wanted was to be held and have people to talk to him," says Haylee.

During this time, Ian was still vomiting, often dry heaving.

At 1 year, Ian seemed well. His vomiting became just a part of their lives. "He wasn't a vegetable!" Haylee declares.

For a year, Ian saw many GI doctors, but none offered help. He was often hospitalized for dehydration. Even a cold would send him to the hospital. One GI doctor even expressed anger that Haylee and Tim had brought Ian somewhere else for a second opinion.

Ian was exhibiting other strange symptoms. His penis appeared very small and one of his testicles had gone back up into his body and was stuck, so surgery was performed to redo Ian's circumcision and lower his testicle. His muscle tone was getting worse, and Botox was no longer helping. Through all this, Ian remained happy, even enjoying the hospital stay. He was a great sleeper and never complained about anything.

When Ian was 2, his liver enzymes began to rise. He scratched constantly and made himself bleed. They tried medications and numbing lotions, but Haylee says, "He would claw himself to pieces."

Ian's feet were always cold and would turn bluish-purple—more symptoms doctors couldn't explain. His growth had also slowed, so the endocrinologist started him on growth hormone. As if the caretaking for Ian wasn't high maintenance enough, his parents now had to administer nightly injections.

Ian developed vision and hearing impairments. He had a lazy eye and wore a patch on the good eye to strengthen the weaker one. This didn't help at all. Ian was also very sensitive to the sunlight and would hide his eyes whenever he was taken outside.

"He also had begun sleeping with his eyes open ... creepy!" says Haylee. "They never shut on their own."

Ian was found to have moderate to severe hearing loss, but doctors felt it was more of a processing problem than a hearing one.

His liver enzymes were still rising, so Ian was brought to Vanderbilt University Hospital, 3½ hours away. A liver biopsy was conducted: it showed nothing wrong, and the family was sent home with some medicine and told it was a virus.

During this time, Haylee became pregnant and had a miscarriage.

Ian's third year was better than his second, with fewer hospital visits. Haylee learned that the moment he seemed sick she should stop feeding him and start Pedialyte (for diarrhea and dehydration) and medications. But he was still scratching, with scars all over his face from digging at it so much. He had to have surgery again to remove an underdeveloped testicle; they were told leaving it alone could cause cancer. His vision was getting worse and surgery couldn't fix it. His muscle tone in his legs was getting very bad. He was still vomiting a lot. And this year was better than the previous one! But still through all this, Ian never cried and was happy.

"So we just went on with life and didn't think much about his outcome," Haylee remembers.

Haylee became pregnant with Gage shortly after Ian's third birthday. It was something for Haylee and Tim to look forward to. A month before Ian's fourth birthday, Gage was born.

Ian was becoming much thinner, with sunken eyes. He hadn't gained weight or grown very much in length despite receiving growth hormone.

Ian's fourth year was the roughest. He slept fourteen-to-eighteen hours a day; if awakened before he was ready, he'd throw up and fall asleep wherever he was. His scratching and muscle tone were becoming worse. They cut his feedings down to what he needed to stay hydrated, so he wouldn't be so sick. His liver function was still haywire, and he became jaundiced. Haylee says he "looked like a lizard ... his eyes went outwards."

Ian's muscle tone had become so bad that his hips pulled out of their sockets, so he needed surgery to loosen the muscles and pop his hips back into place. For the first time in four years, his thyroid medications needed to be upped. But there was still no conclusive diagnosis.

"No one ever said, 'Your kid is in liver failure, he might die soon,'" says Haylee. "No one ever told us that he was that sick. We didn't notice, I guess, because we were with him every day and didn't notice how much he had changed. It is amazing what parents don't notice."

The family celebrated Ian's fifth birthday with a big party, five days after his birthday. "He had one of his best days in months," recalls Haylee. "He hardly threw up and was so happy.

"We were all at home, and we were cleaning the house," Haylee remembers. "He was sleeping all day. I cut his feeding pump off and changed his diaper around noon and ran him some bath water. I told my husband to go ahead and give him his bath. Next thing I hear is, 'Oh God ... Haylee!'

"I went upstairs thinking maybe Ian had gotten out of his bed or threw up everywhere. He was gone." Ian passed away on January 3, 2002.

"It didn't seem real," says Haylee. "We had always kept it in the back of our minds [that] he wouldn't live forever, but never thought it would actually happen or happen that soon. We were in shock. He looked like he was just sleeping. We called 911, and I changed Ian's diaper and took off his PJs and wrapped him in a blanket. I'm not sure why I took off his clothes. I was going to go ahead and bathe him, but the ambulance came. I'm not sure what I thought I was doing. When the ambulance came, they made us put him back in his bed where we found him so they could pick him up. They had us follow them to the hospital so that a doctor could pronounce him dead. Then they let us stay with him until the funeral home came to get him.

"I couldn't believe that he was really gone. He looked so peaceful, and he still had his eyes half open. We also knew that he was in such pain and he was in heaven and would never be in pain again. We felt sad that we would never get to hold him again or hear his beautiful sounds. But he was in such a better place and was perfect. We had his funeral, and I handled myself so much better than I thought I would. The owner of the funeral home let us come the day before and let me hold him one last time. That helped me so much."

A few months after Ian passed away, Haylee found out she was pregnant. She remembers feeling that something wasn't right during her pregnancy but didn't dare say anything. The doctors reassured her that the baby's measurements were normal.

Eden Elizabeth Carroll was born on December 2, 2003.

At birth, she looked like Ian, with a very small head, but still considered on the "normal" side. The following day Eden was sent for a CAT scan, which came back normal.

"So we thought, of course she looks like Ian, he is her brother," says Haylee.

Eden was a very difficult baby. She would scream, not cry, all the time. Nothing seemed to soothe her.

Eden's regular pediatrician visits showed she was "getting fat," but her head still hadn't grown much. At 3 months, her MRI showed pretty much the same thing Ian's had. And the routine started all over again—therapies and constant fruitless doctor appointments. But finally it was suggested that it was a genetic disorder.

"They still had no idea what my kids had and really didn't seem that interested in finding out," says Haylee. "They diagnosed Eden with a spastic paraplegic disorder that her symptoms didn't even fit."

Eden went through some helpful speech therapy, but at 9 months her growth slowed down. Lab tests showed elevated liver enzymes—the same problems Ian had, but starting earlier in life. A GI doctor blamed it on poor nutrition, so they put Eden on an NG feeding tube to see if she could gain weight, and she did. When she was 15 months old, doctors put a G-tube in her stomach, thinking that, if they got her overall weight up, her liver enzymes would come down. The GI doctor had Haylee quit nursing and put Eden on a formula that was easy on the liver. Eden quit eating food by mouth after she quit nursing. She began gagging on her baby food and would choke. On the upside, she did gain weight and grew taller. But her liver enzymes still failed to come down. So the GI doctor suggested that, since Eden's liver problems were starting earlier than Ian's, she probably wouldn't live as long as he did. He advised Haylee to let him know when they wanted hospice. Haylee was angry.

"That was not OK with us," she says. "We had no idea what she had, and they didn't care to try and find out."

Even visiting the well-regarded Johns Hopkins Medical Center didn't help. "We went on with our everyday lives and kept up therapy, and Eden learned how to army crawl and side-sit. Then, shortly after Eden's second birthday, her liver enzymes had gone up to over 600—normal is 30. So we were freaking out. We are very lucky to have a great pediatrician. She contacted Johns Hopkins, and they said, 'She needs to be here right now.' So we made the ten-hour trip once again and had her admitted to the hospital. They ran a battery of tests and asked lots of questions. The most popular question was, 'Are you and your husband kin?' We got asked that question a handful of times.

"They had no answers for us. They did testing on her heart, and it was normal. She had an ultrasound on her liver, and it was normal. A genetic ophthalmologist said Eden had bilateral cataracts, but she also had a pale optic nerve and retinopathy. She said she would look at her eyes again when she had her liver biopsy so she could see her while she was asleep. The eye doctor came out after seeing Eden's eye while she was sedated and said she had Type II Cockayne syndrome, a degenerative disorder. We then asked the geneticist what she thought, and she said, 'No, that's not what Eden has.' She said Cockayne had to do with skin cancer. So we went back to the hotel and looked up Cockayne syndrome on the Internet. We first saw photos of some of the kids on the Cockayne Share-and-Care Web site and one boy looked so much like Ian. We knew just from looking at the photos that this is what our kids have. We then looked at the symptoms and cancer wasn't one of them, but every symptom Ian and Eden have/had was there. They pretty much had every symptom listed. It was so eerie looking at this Web site and seeing my kids.

"So now we have a diagnosis, and even though the outcome is that the kids live an average of five years, it is still better than the doctors telling us she may not see her third birthday. I was so excited to

finally know what my kids have. Now comes the hard part of knowing exactly what happened to Ian and what is going to happen to Eden. This is an aging disorder, which explains what happened with Ian and how he changed so much. Now we look at Eden, wondering, 'When is it going to happen?'

"So Eden is 4½ years old now and is doing amazingly well—better than I could ever imagine."

However, Eden has begun scratching herself, and she doesn't like to sleep, so there are many sleepless nights.

Another mother who lost a child to Cockayne reminded Haylee to think of the sleepless nights this way: "One day you will be thankful you had those nights with Eden."

"We try to look at it that way," says Haylee. "Eden is such a joy to have and brightens up our day and can always make us laugh. I feel blessed to have her."

Ian had CS—Cockayne syndrome. Eden has CS. Gage is healthy.

Did you know?

CS, also referred to as XP (Xeroderma pigmentosa), is a rare genetic disorder that is recessively inherited (both parents must be carriers) in which children have characteristic pinched faces with beaked noses, low-set ears, sunken eyes, and bad teeth; they have short stature, appearance of premature aging, and sensitivity to sunlight. CS was first reported by British physician Edward Alfred Cockayne in 1946.

There are several types: Classic CS (CS type I) is the most commonly seen form. The first year of life is somewhat normal, with symptoms manifesting in the child's second year. In early-onset CS (CS type II), symptoms show up in the child's first year. There is also a milder type of CS, in which a child exhibits few CS characteristics.

It is believed that the incidence for CS is less than one case per 250,000 live births. But many cases are misdiagnosed or not diagnosed, so the rates are believed to be, in actuality, higher.

Signs and symptoms

- bad breath
- beaked nose
- bluish/purple feet
- calcium deposits in basal ganglia
- cataracts
- characteristic facial appearance
- choking or gagging
- chronic vomiting
- cold extremities
- congenital hypothyroidism
- contracted and tilted neck (torticollis)

- decreased tolerance for infection
- dry eyes
- dwarfism
- exaggerated round back (kyphosis)
- failure to thrive
- feeding problems
- freckling from sun
- global developmental delay
- happy personality
- hearing loss
- hip dysplasia
- less-than-normal muscle tension (hypotonicity)
- liver abnormalities
- loss of joint movement (contractures)
- loss of subcutaneous fat
- low growth hormone levels
- low-set ears ("Mickey Mouse ears")
- micropenis
- open eyes while sleeping
- pinched face
- pneumonia
- precancerous skin lesions from sunlight (actinic keratoses)
- premature aging
- progressive mental deficiency
- projecting jaw (prognathism)
- respiratory infections
- retractile testicle(s)
- rigid muscles (hypertonicity)
- salt-and-pepper appearance in retinas (pigmentary retinal degeneration)
- sensitivity to sun
- seizures
- severe acid reflux
- severe itchiness
- skin cancer from sun exposure
- small head (microcephaly)
- sunken eyes
- thinned corpus callosum in brain
- tooth decay (dental caries)
- unsteady gait
- ventricular enlargement without obstruction

C

- vision loss
- white-matter abnormalities in brain
- wide nasal bridge
- wide-set nipples

Cause

Research has shown that mutations in the ERCC6 and ERCC8 genes, which are involved with DNA repair, cause CS. This is involvement with a recessive gene; once a couple learns that one of them is a known carrier, they have a one in four chance of having a child with CS.

Diagnosis

Sometimes a child will have enough major characteristics of the disorder for an immediate diagnosis at birth, but, in most cases, problems develop over the years. Usually a major symptom such as blindness will bring the parents to a specialist who recognizes the disorder. But, as with Haylee and Tim, sometimes even with geneticists, specialists can miss the signs.

Because the syndrome is so rarely diagnosed, the time between first noticeable symptoms and a correct diagnosis can take years. Diagnostic tools include MRI and CAT scans, which can show brain and cardiac abnormalities.

Lab tests that are performed to determine CS include complementation testing identifying the affected gene; mutation analysis showing how genes are damaged; skin biopsies; and Ultraviolet tests. They include UV survival curve and RNA synthesis inhibition assay because cells and RNA in CS children are killed off easily by UV light, as is the RNA used by cells to help make essential proteins. Both tests use UV light to see how many cells are killed and how long it takes the RNA to repair itself. A doctor will explain the tests in detail.

Treatment

Specialists who can help the CS child include a clinical geneticist, audiologist, dermatologist, ophthalmologist, otolaryngologist, pediatrician, pediatric cardiologist, occupational therapist, physical therapists, speech-language pathologists, social workers, family counselors, and rehabilitation therapists.

There are many ways to approach the numerous varied needs of CS children: special-needs education, sign-language training, ankle and foot orthotics, hearing aids, feeding tube, covering windows with UV-blocking material at home (and in the car, which might require a permit) and school, using high-level sunscreen outdoors, incandescent lighting, UV-blocking clothing, minimum skin exposure, gloves, UV-proof sunglasses, wide-

C

brimmed hats, restricted outdoor daytime play, minimized sun exposure by keeping doors shut, and entering/exiting cars with little sun exposure.

Prognosis

According to the Share and Care Cockayne Syndrome Network, the oldest known CS patient is in his late 30s. Depending on the severity of genetic damage and ability to eat, a CS child has a median life expectancy of 12, according to a report by Suzanne M. Carter, M.S., and Suzanne M. Gross, M.D., of the Division of Reproductive Genetics at Montefiore Medical Center, Albert Einstein College of Medicine, New York.

But as you can see from Ian's story, the range is wide: Some children could die in infancy, at age 3 or 5. It is believed that CS children with cataracts have a more rapid progression of the disease.

Two promising directions in research include protein therapy, to replace the CS child's missing protein (similar to a diabetic's insulin shot), and gene therapy, replacing the damaged gene with a healthy one. Both therapies have their downsides along with benefits.

Sources and resources

Prenatal diagnosis of CS is not available in the United States, but is found at two European laboratories. For information, contact the following:
Alan Lehmann, chairman, Genome Damage and Stability Centre,
University of Sussex, Falmer, Brighton BN1 9RR, England;
Phone: 011 44 1273 678 120; Fax: 011 44 1273 678 121;
E-mail: a.r.lehmann@sussex.ac.uk
Montefiore Medical Center (www.montefiore.org)
Share and Care Cockayne Syndrome Network, Jackie Clark, president and executive director, P.O. Box 282, Waterford, VA 20197 (703-727-0404 or 865-435-9777); (www.cockaynesyndrome.net); (cockaynesyndrome@gmail.com)
The French Cockayne Association (http://cockayne.free.fr)
Xeroderma Pigmentosum Society (www.xps.org)

D

DGS (Developmental Gerstmann's Syndrome)

DPD (Dependent Personality Disorder)

DS (Down Syndrome)

Dyscalculia

Dysgraphia

Dyslexia

Dystonia

DGS

Developmental Gerstmann's Syndrome

Terms used in this chapter: AS (Asperger syndrome); DGS (developmental Gerstmann's syndrome); *ICD* (*International Classification of Diseases*); IEP (individualized education program); LD (learning disability); NLD (nonverbal learning disorder)

Sound familiar?

Susan Koniak didn't have it easy as a child. The chubby youngster with short, thick, dark brown hair and a big, round face was caught between two worlds. On the one hand, she was brilliant, reading like a demon and writing like a pro; by six years old, she was tested at a twelfth-grade reading level. On the other hand, she couldn't add, subtract, divide, or multiply and didn't know her left from her right. She didn't even know her pinky from her thumb. And that's the crux of her problems—her two hands.

One of Susan's most distinctive symptoms is finger agnosia or not having a sense of her fingers. She can't figure out where they are, and she doesn't know how to use them. If she goes to grab a plastic shopping bag, for example, she doesn't know how to fit her fingers into the handles.

When writing, she held on to the pen so tightly that it was like holding on for her life. Her grip was so tight it eventually damaged a tendon.

If she holds her hands 12 inches away from her face, she says, "They disappear."

Susan also has dysgraphia, an LD that is a deficit in the ability to write. Her writing on a piece of paper eventually begins to look like abstract art. But she can type fast.

Susan, unable to use utensils, ate with her fingers as a child.

She was also virtually lost in the physical space that surrounded her most of the time.

She didn't speak until her toddler years, well into her second year, and then started talking in sentences. But the term "toddler years" isn't a correct description of her first years. She hardly toddled. In fact, she was unable to crawl.

Susan's senses were overly stimulated, her motor skills were impaired, and her spatial skills were nonexistent. In fact, she ranked in the lowest percentiles when tested in spatial and perceptive skills. But in matrix reasoning, she ranked in the 99-plus percentile. She can't add simple numbers, spell the word "know" correctly, or use a comma in its right place—but she could read the most complex books (she leaves out word endings, however) and write complex poems and stories.

She was different from other kids, she says—in fact, she was kind of "spooky." Other children didn't like her when she was young.

That was Susan as a child. She was not diagnosed until she was 50. And she is happy, in a way, that this was the case. Up until then, she says she just "managed." But when the diagnoses came they were confused, contradictory, and never fully correct. She was misdiagnosed with disorders ranging from LDs to NLD. When NLD was suggested she knew it was wrong, because, despite her facility with language and trouble with space, her main strengths are nonverbal. She gets "a feeling" for the answer and then tries to put what she senses she "knows" into words. Unlike someone with AS, she is highly intuitive, reads people easily, has animated speech, good facial expression, and has "a billion friends." She is intuitive enough to have known, even as a child, that something wasn't quite right. And intuitive enough to know there are other children out there like her, for whom she has started a foundation, Sarah's Place, which can be found at www.sarahs-place.org.

She has a cognitive processing deficit, and although she told people she had dyslexia, because the term is familiar, it is not what she has. She has an interesting way of assessing her disorder.

"You can't be this impaired and not know there's something wrong in your head," she says. "How can you be both so smart and sort of retarded?"

Remember how she couldn't crawl as a child? She tried to crawl as an adult and was still unable to. In fact, she got vertigo because she says she was not seeing the whole picture, only part of the room. "No wonder I never wanted to crawl," she now says. She can't crawl, but she was a ballroom dancer.

When Susan walks, in order to feel secure spatially, she uses a blind cane to keep track of the ground.

She is very happy that she was able to develop enough skills to counteract her deficits and that she could bluff her way through most of her schooling. She believes that had she been properly diagnosed as a child, she would not have developed those skills.

"I'm worried about children who might have a lot to give and won't be able to give because they were not given the opportunity to expand their compensatory skills," she says.

Susan says that Dr. Tony Simon at the University of California at Davis M.I.N.D. (Medical Investigation of Neurodevelopmental Disorders) Institute uses her for research because she is so high-functioning and can articulate what she experiences. It is like getting insight into autism from someone with the disorder who can speak and has insight into the illness, she says.

So, let's recap. Susan can't do simple math problems; she has trouble reading word endings; she's distracted by punctuation on the printed page; she lacks the organizational skills to write an outline; she needs to be grounded when she walks; she can't crawl; she has a low threshold for sensory stimulation.

But she went to Yale and has become a well-respected lawyer and law professor. In fact, she says, she provided expert testimony before the Senate Judiciary Committee in the notorious Enron case.

Susan has been diagnosed with DGS—developmental Gerstmann's syndrome … which might or might not be the full story.

Did you know?

DGS is the diagnosis in children, but Gerstmann's Syndrome is the term used most often to describe a neurological disorder characterized by LDs such as dysgraphia, the inability to write, and dyscalculia, the lack of understanding of arithmetic rules; the inability to distinguish right from left; and a lack of sense of the fingers (finger agnosia). Josef Gerstmann, an Austrian neurologist and psychiatrist, first wrote about the disorder in 1924.

DGS is often misdiagnosed as one of its parts such as LDs. Depending on its severity, DGS might even go undiagnosed. It is often diagnosed as an NLD or missed altogether. The *ICD* describes it as an arithmetical skills disorder.

It is believed that problems with the brain's left angular gyrus, part of the left parietal lobe, which controls spoken and written language, is responsible for DGS, but there are other deficits as well generating from the right parietal lobe, including problems with knowledge of numbers and their relations, the manipulation of objects, and visuospatial processing. Finger agnosia is believed to derive from deficits in the right lobe as well.

Children with DGS can exhibit the full range of intellectual capacity.

Signs and symptoms

- balance problems
- difficulty with math functions
- finger agnosia
- inability to copy simple drawings
- inability to differentiate between right and left
- inability to discriminate between different fingers
- LDs
- poor handwriting
- poor spelling skills
- reading problems

Cause

The cause of DGS in children is not known, but it is believed that, since both parietal lobes are affected, the deficits occur during early brain development. Brain trauma, stroke, tumor, viral encephalitis, and toxic exposure are possible causes in adults.

Diagnosis

The child should first be examined by a medical doctor to make sure there is not another illness at play. Diagnosis for DGS is made through a complete neurological examination, psychoeducational testing, and clinical observation.

Treatment

There is no cure for DGS, but certain treatments can help. Unfortunately, DGS is often diagnosed late—when a child is in school—so early intervention, as important as it may be, is usually not a consideration.

Children with DGS can benefit from various therapies such as occupational therapy for social skills and dysgraphia (a disability dealing with writing) and speech-language therapy for dyspraxia (a motor-planning disorder). Also, working with a physical therapist, a psychologist, and an educational therapist are suggested. In school, many modifications can assist the DGS child, such as calculators and the use of word processors. A well-conceived IEP is essential.

Prognosis

Those on the high-functioning end of DGS, as Susan proves, can have a very successful life, albeit one wrought with several non-life-threatening dysfunctional symptoms.

Generally, many DGS symptoms seem to lessen with time, but it is believed that this occurs because the child has learned to compensate for their deficits, as did Susan.

Sources and resources

DSM (*Diagnostic and Statistical Manual of Mental Disorders*
ICD (*International Statistical Classification of Diseases*)
National Institutes of Health (www.nih.gov)
www.sarahs-place.org

See the "NLD: Nonverbal Learning Disorder," "LD: Learning Disability," and various LD chapters, as well as the mental-health contacts under "General Resources," for more sources used in this chapter.

DPD

Dependent Personality Disorder

Terms used in this chapter: DPD (dependent personality disorder)

Sound familiar?

Victor is 14 but acts as if he's 4. His parents complain that he cannot do anything without checking with them first. He doesn't want to go anywhere without them, cannot make a decision without their input, and constantly needs to be attended to because, as his mother says, "He can't do anything on his own."

Victor has been acting out like this for two years, although he always demonstrated less severe symptoms such as separation anxiety and insecurity. But now, this need for dependency has started interfering with every aspect of his life.

"It is terrible when your teenager cannot even eat a snack because he can't make up his own mind, and that he needs someone to guide him through every aspect of his day," says his mother, who suffers from depression and anxiety disorders. "I love him, he's my son, but he drives me crazy sometimes with his neediness. He drives his friends crazy, and he drives his teachers crazy."

Victor, a high-school freshman, was referred by his school psychiatrist to a pediatric psychiatrist at a local clinic. He was finally diagnosed there and already, in just four months of treatment, Victor is showing progress.

"[Therapy] has taken such a weight off the family, seeing Victor less anxious, more independent, and happy again," says his mother. "These personality quirks run in the family, but with Victor, it was the worst. It doesn't sound so terrible, but it is devastating watching your kid hurt so much."

Victor has DPD—dependent personality disorder.

Did you know?

DPD is a chronic anxiety disorder that manifests itself in helplessness, overreliance on others, and submissiveness. Children with this disorder have a great need to be nurtured and taken care of. They constantly need support and encouragement and assurances that all is going to be fine. Dependent on others for emotional support, they are unable to make decisions. DPD usually starts in childhood, although it manifests itself in adolescence.

Those with DPD are very needy for both advice and attention and can't seem to make up their minds, even about the most seemingly minor subjects. Children with DPD might be unable to decide what to eat, what to wear, and what to do in a social situation, depending totally on their parents' advice.

The problems are all-encompassing and pervasive and range across the spectrum of life's activities. DPD becomes problematic when its inflexibility impairs day-to-day daily living—when the need for others to assume responsibility moves further from age- and situation-appropriate needs.

Signs and symptoms

- anxiety
- avoidance of personal responsibility
- clinginess
- depression
- difficulty being alone
- does not disagree with others
- easily hurt by criticism
- fear of inability to care for oneself
- general fearfulness
- general neediness
- inability to make decisions, even simple ones

- inability to start projects
- intense fear of abandonment
- lack of self-confidence
- maintaining abusive friendships or relationships
- naïveté
- need for constant reassurance
- nervousness
- oversensitivity to criticism
- passivity
- pessimism
- placing the needs of caregivers above own needs
- preoccupation with being abandoned
- sense of devastation
- sense of helplessness when friendships/relationships end
- separation anxiety
- unable to meet life's ordinary demands
- willingness to tolerate mistreatment and abuse from others

Cause

No specific cause for DPD is known, but there are most likely biological and developmental factors involved. It is believed that children who have authoritative or overprotective parents can be more susceptible to DPD. Children whose parents have DPD are more inclined to have it as well. Whether it is inherited or learned, or a combination of both, has yet to be determined.

Diagnosis

The first specialist to consult is the child's pediatrician, who will assess the child with a full physical exam and help to determine if the child needs a mental-health specialist. If you believe the child's problem is greater than what the pediatrician suggests, seeing a pediatric psychologist or psychiatrist is advised. One thing that many experts agree on is for parents to trust their gut feeling.

Treatment

Psychotherapy is the most common form of treatment. Since low self-confidence is a big issue with DPD, the child might also benefit from assertiveness training. Cognitive behavioral therapy (CBT), which redirects negative patterns of thinking and behavior, replacing them with more positive thoughts and behaviors, is a very well-received approach to personality disorders. DPD also responds well to group therapy.

Anti-anxiety and antidepressant medications are often prescribed and have proved effective in conjunction with therapy to help the anxiety related to DPD. A short-term dosage is often used.

Antidepressants slow the removal of essential neurotransmitters (chemicals that move signals between the brain's neurons). The antidepressants of choice are SSRIs. (See the "SSRIs" section in "What You Need to Know" for more information.)

Other chemicals are also addressed with antidepressants and anti-anxiety drugs. NDRIs (norepinephrine and dopamine reuptake inhibitors) work on dopamine levels, with the most popular being Wellbutrin. Although these are the most popular, you should discuss other medications with your child's physician.

Foods that are high in serotonin and carbohydrates include breads, pasta, potatoes, and (amino acid) tryptophan-rich foods such as turkey, meat proteins, fruits and mushrooms.

Prognosis

With early intervention and proper treatment, DPD children can lead happy, productive lives. However, they may always be prone to anxiety or personality disorders.

Sources and resources

American Academy of Child and Adolescent Psychiatry (www.aacap.org)
American Psychiatric Association (www.psych.org)
American Psychological Association (www.apa.org)
DSM (*Diagnostic and Statistical Manual of Mental Disorders*)
Mayo Clinic (www.mayoclinic.com)
National Institute of Mental Health (www.nimh.nih.gov)
psychologytoday.com

See the mental-health contacts under "General Resources" in the appendix for more sources used in this chapter.

DS

Down Syndrome

Terms used in this chapter: CVS (chorionic villius sampling); DS (Down syndrome); IEP (individualized education program); MR (mental retardation); MSST (maternal serum screening test); NADS (National Association for Down Syndrome); NDSS (National Down Syndrome Society); PUBS (percutaneous umbilical blood sampling)

Sound familiar?

When Pamela's family found out she was pregnant, they were ecstatic; she was the first of the eight siblings and cousins to get pregnant. Her pregnancy was as normal as anyone's. She took prenatal vitamins and had all the appropriate tests, including a CVS, a preliminary test for DS, which came back negative.

Because Pamela was only 26 and not considered at risk, no further testing was done. The pregnancy was full-term, the sonograms were normal, the baby seemed healthy. At Pamela's last visit before giving birth, the obstetrician found that the umbilical cord was wrapped around the baby's neck, and he sent Pamela for an immediate Cesarean section. Her labor was only a few hours, but Pamela and her husband, Michael, were shocked when the happiest moment of their lives became the most confusing. The doctor held their brand-new baby girl, May, in his gloved hands, umbilical cord still attached to Pamela, lying cut open on the table, and callously asked, "Why didn't anyone tell me this baby had Down syndrome?"

No one had known. It was a possibility they had never considered, and one they were completely unprepared for.

To make matters worse, nobody came to see them afterwards to explain exactly what the disorder was or how it might affect the baby's childhood and adult life. Pamela says that the staff in the Port Jefferson, New York, hospital hadn't bothered to make her and her husband aware of complications they could face in the immediate future. Pamela and Michael left the hospital confused and disoriented. Pamela breast-fed her baby like any other nursing mom, all the time unaware that May was losing vital body weight. Down's infants have a condition called hypotonia, low muscle tone. The muscles in their arms, legs, neck, and throat are underdeveloped, making breast-feeding a sometimes futile attempt. The baby wasn't latching on, and wasn't getting the nutrition she needed.

Within days of bringing May home, Pamela and Michael took the baby to Stony Brook University Hospital, where May thrived—and they were educated by staff specially trained to deal with parents with DS infants. They were told that Down children sometimes have heart and hearing problems and are at risk for juvenile diabetes.

May was evaluated at 8 weeks, and luckily, early intervention began at 12 weeks. Today, at age 4, May's case seems mild (doctors say it is too early to label the severity officially). She receives speech, occupational, and physical therapy, is happy and healthy, and, amazingly, is on the same cognitive percentile as others her age. May is the perfect example of the benefits of early intervention.

The early intervention was crucial to May's "normal" development. Nowadays, her physical therapy has taken on a playtime feel. She jumps rope, walks on a balance beam, climbs through tunnels—she never even knows she's having therapy. And she's joined both gymnastics and ballet classes. But it is never clear sailing for parents of Alphabet Kids. At May's last evaluation, she tested so high on cognitive examinations that the state tried to take away her speech therapy, says Pamela, claiming the young girl was on track with other children her age. But Pamela and Michael made the case that May is doing so well because she has had therapy, and that they are fearful that she would fall behind without it. Ultimately, they won.

May has DS—Down syndrome.

Did you know?

DS, or Down's in the U.K., is the most common genetic disorder, and, according to the NDSS, it occurs in one of every 733 live births. It is a disorder with distinct physical characteristics and physical and intellectual development delays. Many of these children reach their developmental goals, but there are delays. For example, while walking skills develop between 12 and 14 months, DS kids usually learn to walk between 15 and 36 months.

DS, or trisomy 21, was named after the English doctor John Langdon Down and is caused by a chromosomal abnormality in which a triplicate of the 21-chromosome exists inside the human cells, instead of a duplicate as in the general population. This anomaly causes variable mental and physical disorders, including MR and delayed child development.

DS is a well-known disorder that has received a lot of attention in recent decades; with that renewed and expanded awareness came great strides for DS children. DS kids accomplish so much more than ever before—socially, academically, and professionally.

According to the NDSS, as the mortality rate goes down, and the age of parenting goes higher, DS will increase. The NDSS reports that "some experts project that the number of people with Down syndrome will double in the next 10 years."

Signs and symptoms

The symptoms of a DS child vary widely.

- affectionate
- cataracts
- celiac disease
- cheerfulness
- childhood leukemia (one transient form disappears spontaneously in newborns)
- cross-eyed (strabismus)
- distinctive facial appearance
- dry skin
- ear structural abnormalities
- early dementia or Alzheimer's disease
- excessive space between large and second toe
- fine motor skill delays
- first two neck bones not well aligned
- flat facial profile
- gross motor skill delays
- hearing loss
- heart defects
- high blood pressure in the lungs (pulmonary hypertension)

- hip dislocation
- hypothyroidism
- incomplete or partial dislocation of kneecap
- increased susceptibility to infection
- inner ear fluid buildup
- intestinal abnormalities, such as blocked small bowel or esophagus
- large tongue (macroglossia)
- lazy eye (amblyopia)
- loose joints
- low muscle tone (hypotonia)
- MR
- naïveté
- obesity
- recurrent pneumonias
- respiratory problems
- seizure disorders
- self-care skill delays
- single deep crease across the center of the palm (simian crease)
- sleep apnea
- small hands and feet
- small mouth
- small nose
- small skin folds on the inner corner of the eyes (epicanthic fold)
- sterility in males
- stubbornness
- teething problems
- tendency for infection
- upward slant to the eyes
- vision problems
- white spot on iris of eye

Cause

In 1959, it was determined that an extra partial or complete 21st chromosome results in the characteristics associated with DS.

The cause of these extra chromosomes is not known, but there are factors that can be attributed to DS. There are three types of DS: trisomy 21 (the most common, found in 95 percent of DS cases), mosaicism, and translocation.

The NDSS describes the three types:

In **trisomy 21**, because of a cell-division error, children with this disorder have forty-seven chromosomes instead of the usual forty-six in each cell. The failure of paired chromosomes to separate is called nondisjunction.

In **mosaicism**, the nondisjunction takes place in an initial cell division after fertilization, causing forty-six chromosomes in some cells and forty-seven in others. The least common form of DS, mosaicism accounts for only 1-to-2 percent of cases.

Translocation, which accounts for 3-to-4 percent of cases, occurs when part of chromosome 21 breaks off during cell division and attaches to another chromosome, usually chromosome 14. While the total number of chromosomes in the cells remains forty-six, the presence of an extra part of chromosome 21 causes DS characteristics. This inherited form can be of concern if the father is a carrier.

According to the NDSS, the following age of the mother versus incidence of Down ranges from age 20, where the incidence is one in two thousand; age 28, one in one thousand; age 34, one in 450; age 40, one in one hundred; age 49, one in ten.

While MR is often associated with DS, some DS children are not retarded at all, although most have IQs that range from mild to MR.

Diagnosis

It is important to note that prenatal screening such as MSSTs and a sonogram can give an idea of the risk assessment of having a DS baby. However, MSSTs are not accurate for the most part because they are run usually between fifteen and twenty weeks into the pregnancy and detect about 60 percent of cases, many with false-positive results. These tests, to be more accurate, should be run with ultrasound screening.

But some tests can give an (almost) 100 percent diagnosis. The more accurate DS diagnostic procedures include CVS, amniocentesis, and PUBS. These procedures have an accuracy of 98 percent and 99 percent, respectively, although there is a small risk of miscarriage. Amniocentesis is usually performed between fifteen and twenty-two weeks of gestation, CVS between nine and fourteen weeks, and PUBS after eighteen weeks.

These tests are, of course, carried out prior to birth, but, unfortunately, most DS children are not diagnosed until after birth. And then the child is often diagnosed through clinical observation of characteristic traits.

As with other genetic disorders, a karyotype blood test is performed for a definitive diagnosis.

Treatment

Two words: *early intervention.*

DS children should receive physical, speech-language, and developmental therapies. They should also be seen by a pediatric cardiologist and pulmonary specialist. Since such a high percentage—up to 50 percent—of DS children have heart defects, echocardiograms should be performed on newborns. Eight percent to 12 percent of DS kids have gastrointestinal tract abnormalities present at birth. Most of these ailments, along with leukemia, are treatable or are correctable through surgery. An audiologist and ophthalmologist should be seen early so that hearing and speech problems don't get out of hand.

NADS has some suggestions on getting help:

Many states [in the U.S.] provide free early-intervention services to kids with disabilities from birth to age 3, so check with your child's doctor to determine what resources are available in your area.

Once your child is 3 years old, he or she is guaranteed educational services under the Individuals with Disabilities Education Act (IDEA). Under IDEA, local school districts must provide "a free appropriate education in the least restrictive environment" and an IEP for each child.

Where to send your child to school can be a difficult decision. Some kids with DS have needs that are best met in a specialized program, while many others do well attending neighborhood schools alongside peers who don't have DS. Studies have shown that this type of situation, known as inclusion, is beneficial for both the child with DS as well as the other children. Your school district's child study team can work with you to determine what's best for your child, but remember, any decisions can and should involve your input, as you are your child's best advocate.

Today, many children with DS grow up going to school and enjoying many of the same activities as other kids their age. A few go on to college. Many transition to semi-independent living. Still others continue to live at home but are able to hold jobs, thus finding their own success in the community.

DS is a worldwide concern. In India, Sujatha Jagadeesh, M.D., a geneticist and pediatric dysmorphologist, is worried about children receiving the proper treatment: "We don't have proper statistics [for] Down's in India. It is becoming better in urban areas but still lagging badly in rural areas because priorities there are different—the priorities in rural areas are infection prevention, immunization, and promoting hygiene and nutrition. Intervention therapy for a Down's child is way back on the list."

Also in India, Rekha RamaChandran, Ph.D., a parent of a DS daughter with trisomy 21, addresses cultural concerns that need to change: "The parents in India ask only one question when they meet us: 'What sin have I done to have this child?'

"They also want to know, 'Will my child go to special school or can we see our child in regular school?' 'Will my child be married and can they have children?' 'Will society accept them?'

"India is still a very conservative country. People find it difficult to accept slow learners. We also have the extended-family system, and they still consider the woman responsible for the birth of a child with challenges. Guilt, blame, fear, and torture are the normal routines that women face."

In Malta, things have changed over the past decades for the better for DS children. According to Professor Alfred Cuschieri, head of the Anatomy Department, University of Malta, and chief advisor to the Down Syndrome Association of Malta, "The ... concerns of Maltese families today—are they doing all they possibly can for their disabled child? They will leave no stone unturned! They participate in associations and self-help groups. Everyone contributes voluntarily and generously to the voluntary institutions who work for the education and welfare of disabled persons."

Israel has a DS birth rate of about one in nine hundred, and Ariel Tenenbaum, M.D., who heads the Down Syndrome Medical Center, at Hadassah Mt. Scopus University Medical Center in Jerusalem, says, "In medical terms, [DS children] get good medical treatment in Israel. Our center tries to detect medical problems as early as possible, and to prevent those that are preventable. In Israel all the population is fully medically insured by law. Israel is a small country, so all the hospitals and doctor's offices are near and approachable. Also, we have a very high rate of number of doctors and other medical professionals compared to the population size.

"But Down syndrome is universal," he reminds us, "and the problems are very similar all over the world."

Prognosis

With recent medical advances, individuals with DS are enjoying longer life spans—as of 2007, it is generally reported that 80 percent of DS adults reach 55, with many growing older, well into their 70s.

Even for associated disorders such as heart defects (50 percent of DS kids have heart defects), there is promising news. Congenital heart defects associated with DS children are now surgically corrected, leading to general better health. Oncology advances have made acute megakaryoblastic leukemia, the leukemia that is up to 20 times more apt to strike kids with DS, a highly curable disease.

Children with DS have a more promising future than ever before. According to NADS, "It is important to remember that while children and adults with Down syndrome experience developmental delays, they also have many talents and gifts and should be given the opportunity and encouragement to develop them."

Sources and resources

Down Syndrome Research and Treatment Foundation (DSRTF) (650-468-1668);
(www.dsrtf.org)

Down Syndrome Research Foundation/Canada (DSRF) (604-444-3773;
888-464-DSRF—toll free in Canada; (www.dsrf.org)

National Association for Down Syndrome (NADS) (630-325-9112); (www.nads.org)

National Down Syndrome Congress (NDSC) (800-232-NDSC [6372]);
(www.ndsccenter.org)

National Down Syndrome Society (NDSS) (800-221-4602); (www.ndss.org)

Uno Mas! Down Syndrome Online (www.unomas21.com)

DYSCALCULIA

Terms used in this chapter: ADHD (attention-deficit/hyperactivity disorder); APD
(auditory processing disorder); DSM (*Diagnostic and Statistical Manual of Mental Disorders*);
ICD (*International Classification of Diseases*); IEP (individualized education program); LD
(learning disability); NCLD (National Center for Learning Disabilities)

Did you know?

LDs are lifelong afflictions, and dyscalculia is the LD involving math. The *ICD* classifies
it as acalculia, an arithmetical skills disorder, while the *DSM* assigns it to Gerstmann's, a
disorder that has a broader definition, beyond math.

Since LDs are often at the heart of Alphabet Disorders and they form a mix-and-
match menu, each LD could be affected by another. For instance, a child with a language
disability and a math disability will manifest symptoms differently than a child with a
writing disability and a math disability.

As with all LDs, one size does not fit all, and what is an inability for one child might
not be a problem for another.

Unlike those with more obvious reading LDs such as dyslexia, children with dyscalculia
are often not red-flagged in school, usually being labeled as just weak math students. By
the time the child is assessed with a disability, he or she might have fallen so behind that
catching up might seem impossible.

It is believed that about 6 percent of school-aged children suffer from a math LD. It is
as common as reading LDs among children who are classified with LDs.

Because Alphabet Disorders have fragile borders, parents should refer to other LD-
related chapters in this book, such as APD, DGS dysgraphia, dyslexia, and dyspraxia,
because a child with dyscalculia may have other(s) of these disorders.

Signs and symptoms

Children with dyscalculia have difficulty:

- comparing and contrasting using concepts like smaller/bigger, taller/shorter
- comprehending verbal instructions
- copying numbers or math calculation problems
- deconstructing pictorials, graphs, or other visual-spatial problems
- estimating number quantities
- figuring out how to apply knowledge and skills to solve math problems
- finding alternative ways to solve problems
- following multistep procedures
- identifying critical information needed to solve equations and more-complex problems
- learning days of the week, color, and shapes
- learning the meaning of numbers (number sense)
- learning to count
- measuring
- memorizing basic number facts
- moving on to more advanced math applications
- organizing objects in a logical way
- putting math facts down on paper in an organized way, even though the child understands them
- recognizing groups and patterns
- recognizing numbers and matching numbers with amounts
- remembering and retaining basic math facts (e.g., times tables)
- self-checking work
- solving basic problems using addition, subtraction, multiplication, and division
- sorting objects by shape, size, or color
- telling time
- understanding math vocabulary
- understanding writing on a board or in a textbook
- using money
- visualizing patterns and different parts of a math problem

Other signs include misreading information, working slowly, poor coordination, poor handwriting, reversing numbers, paying too little attention to details or focusing on them too much without results, transposing number sequences, and confusing arithmetic signs.

The NCLD offers these descriptions of a child as warning signs:

- good at speaking, reading, and writing, but slow to develop counting and math problem-solving skills
- good memory for printed words, but difficulty reading numbers or recalling numbers in sequence
- good with general math concepts, but frustrated when specific computation and organization skills are needed
- trouble with the concept of time: chronically late, difficulty remembering schedules, trouble approximating how long something takes
- poor sense of direction, easily disoriented and easily confused by routine changes
- poor long-term memory of concepts: can do math functions one day but cannot repeat them the next
- poor mental math ability: trouble estimating grocery costs or counting days until vacation
- difficulty playing strategy games like chess, bridge, or role-playing video games
- difficulty keeping score when playing board and card games

Cause

See the "LD: Learning Disability" chapter.

Diagnosis

In many cases, a child's other disabilities, such as reading, auditory and/or visual processing, and spatial and motor problems, take precedence over math concerns. But math problems could point to something more serious.

The child should first be evaluated with a full physical exam by a pediatrician to rule out any other medical condition, and then the doctor will suggest specialists to consult. These may include a pediatric neurologist, speech-language pathologist, audiologist, optometrist, ophthalmologist, occupational therapist, and/or a pediatric psychologist or psychiatrist.

Proper evaluation involves more than just testing math skills. Full psychoeducational testing should be administered. Due to the nature of LDs, evaluation needs to be more holistic, checking a child's ability to understand, memorize, problem-solve, organize, self-check, estimate, tell time, count money, and more. Besides checking basic math skills, the evaluator will check the child's ability to predict. A child might be able to add and subtract but not know *when* to add and subtract. A good evaluation will gauge skill levels against expected skill levels. The child's developmental milestones will be evaluated.

Treatment

After determining the child's strengths and weaknesses, a team of teachers, the parents, and school specialists will establish an IEP to aid the child while building math skills.

Beyond extra help in school, outside tutoring is highly recommended to help reinforce what is learned in school and help the child understand math concepts and "tricks" to compensate. The following are generally accepted recommendations on how to help a child with dyscalculia in his or her school work.

Children with dyscalculia might also have ADHD; even if they don't, their attention might wander because they are lost or confused by the lesson. Keeping their attention is imperative, so short study periods are suggested. Reinforcement activities prove helpful.

Children who have difficulty memorizing basic number facts should be allowed to use some aid to provide them with that fact, other than their fingers or broken pencil erasers they have collected. Calculators or fact charts should be allowed, to remove the pressure of memorizing facts, allowing the child to progress to other math applications and procedures as they memorize facts in the time their disability allows.

Games and music are effective alternate ways to teach math to kids with dyscalculia.

Another effective method uses turnarounds, switching math problems around: 3+2=5/2+3=5. The games should be kept fresh—after turnarounds, a teacher, parent, or therapist might implement doubles in calculations: 2+2+4 or other combinations. In addition, the problem's physical form should be changed: 3+2=5 as a horizontally presented problem and then as a vertically presented problem. Another option is to present a problem orally. A math worksheet should be printed out so that the child doesn't have to write out both problem and answer.

These techniques help kids who have trouble with concepts. What about those who understand concepts but can't compute? They *know* how to calculate difficult problems but lose track when actually doing it. These children need careful monitoring because they can be held back from participating in higher-level math classes, when, in fact, they can do better there than in the most elementary classes.

Then there are the kids with language, visual, and auditory-processing disabilities who have problems that seem unrelated to math but are. These children with visual-spatial motor problems might not understand a picture that seems obvious to another; the child with auditory problems doesn't hear the math question the same way it was verbalized. He or she doesn't understand the question when spoken or cannot properly comprehend the question or application when read. These kids often have a double or triple whammy of disabilities that further their inability to deal with math when, in fact, they might very well have that ability.

These children need many types of compensatory plans to help them succeed—from complementary materials like arithmetic flash cards and workbooks, to placement near the teacher in the front of the classroom. They often need a slowly spoken lesson.

These LD kids have many strengths, and particular strengths should be played up to. If they are visual learners, they need visual material for help. If they are auditory learners, that route should be emphasized. If they are neither, an IEP needs to be structured to support them.

But one thing is very important, no matter what type of learner the child is—*understanding* the material. Attempting to have them learn is one thing, but having them *understand* it is the key. It's not all about a teacher's rattling on; the student needs to repeat the lesson back so that the teacher knows the student "gets" it—it needs to make sense. Otherwise, it's just a garbled bunch of numbers and symbols to these kids.

The NCLD offers the following suggestions to help children with dyscalculia:

- Use graph paper for students who have difficulty organizing ideas on paper.
- Find different ways to approach math facts. For example, instead of just memorizing multiplication tables, explain that 8×2 = 16, so if 16 is doubled, 8×4=32.
- Practice estimating as a way to begin solving math problems.
- Introduce skills beginning with concrete examples, later moving to more abstract applications.
- For language difficulties, explain ideas and problems clearly and encourage students to ask questions.
- Provide a work place with few distractions, with pencils, erasers, and other tools on hand.
- Help students become aware of their strengths and weaknesses. Understanding how a person learns best is a big step in achieving academic success and confidence.

Prognosis

LDs are a lifelong problem. Through proper (and early) intervention, many aspects of dyscalculia can be overcome. Early detection is crucial. Do not simply write this off as a child who is not good in math.

Sources and resources

Dyscalculia Centre (www.dyscalculia.me.uk)
dyscalculiaforum.com (www.dyscalculiaforum.com)
Dyscalculia.org (www.dyscalculia.org)
Learning Disabilities Association of America (412-341-1515); (www.ldaamerica.org)
Learning Disabilities Worldwide (www.ldworldwide.org)
National Center for Learning Disabilities (212-545-7510; 888-575-7373); (www.ld.org)
National Joint Committee on Learning Disabilities (www.ldonline.org)
Schwab Learning Center (www.schwablearning.org)

See the "LD: Learning Disability" chapter and the individual LD and DGS chapters, as well as "General Resources," for more sources used in this chapter.

DYSGRAPHIA

D

Terms used in this chapter: IEP (individualized education program); LD (learning disability)

Sound familiar?

Mark is 16, but he cannot write a legible word. He cannot spell. He has been like this since he was little. When he sits at his desk, he looks as if he's in agony, as he writhes trying to get the words down. He has what some teachers call "the blank-page syndrome"—when he has to write something from scratch it is like asking him to climb a mountain. His eleventh-grade English teacher finds it hard to believe he has made it this far.

"His compensatory skills are truly unbelievable," she says. "It must be draining every other part of his brain to compensate for everything he's been compensating for his whole life."

She marvels at the lack of awareness for his disability as she skims through his school records. "No teachers 'got' him in his early years, and he really fell through the cracks," she remarks. "It wasn't until seventh grade, when he had a teacher who realized he was suffering from a learning disability, that he finally got help." He attended occupational therapy and got accommodations to use a computer for schoolwork.

If you look at one of his handwritten papers, she says, you would think a pre-schooler wrote it, or "an abstract artist." Fortunately, he now uses computers and is improving his memory and cognitive and organizational skills.

"He's such a smart boy," says his teacher, "but you'd never know it if you watched him try to write."

Mark has dysgraphia.

Did you know?

Dysgraphia is an LD that is a deficit in writing or fine motor skills.

Writing is an important skill—when done appropriately, it is an effective way to aid memory, process information, and organize thoughts. Dysgraphia affects a child's handwriting, spelling, and ability to express thoughts on paper. These children can learn, and they're not just lazy or purposefully sloppy—they simply do not have the ability to write properly. Just having poor handwriting does not make a child dysgraphic—dysgraphia is a processing problem.

Signs and symptoms

- abnormal wrist position when writing
- avoids writing or drawing tasks
- awkward body position when writing
- awkward paper position when writing
- copying is slow or labored
- difficulty organizing thoughts on paper
- difficulty previsualizing letter formation
- difficulty thinking and writing at the same time (taking notes, creative writing)
- difficulty with syntax structure and grammar
- gap between writing ability and expressive and receptive speech
- illegible printing and cursive writing
- inconsistent spacing between words and letters
- messy, unorganized papers
- omitted words
- pain in hand from writing
- poor fine motor skills
- poor spatial planning on paper
- poor spelling
- says words out loud when writing
- sloppy, seemingly careless written work
- tight, cramped, awkward pencil grip
- tires quickly when writing
- unfinished or omitted words or letters on paper
- unsure of right- or left-handedness
- writing inconsistencies: mixing print and cursive, upper and lower case, or irregular sizes, shapes, or slant of letters
- writing is slow or labored

Cause

See the "LD: Learning Disability" chapter.

Diagnosis

Many kids have bad handwriting. Dysgraphia is much more than that, and parents need to find a diagnostician who is familiar with LDs to get a proper diagnosis.

The specialist who can best help is the occupational therapist, but the child might also be referred to a pediatric neurologist, speech-language pathologist, audiologist, optometrist, and ophthalmologist and/or a pediatric psychologist or psychiatrist.

A proper evaluation involves more than just crossing the "Ts" with a straight line or making a proper "S." Due to the nature of LDs, the assessment needs to be holistic—a child's ability to understand, memorize, organize, and properly complete physical tasks all need to be checked. The assessment will gauge the child's skill levels against his or her expected skill levels. The child's developmental milestones will also be evaluated, so parents should be prepared to provide a family history.

Treatment

Many strategies can be used to help a dysgraphic child. Most involve school and are often completed with the teacher or occupational therapist. Numerous accommodations, modifications, and therapeutic remediations are available to dysgraphic children and to all children with LDs. The first step is to identify that disability.

Once dysgraphia is diagnosed, parents should consider getting the child a word processor. The child should be able to type work or present it in alternative forms such as a video presentation or a response on audio tape. Even with these alternatives, the child should always be encouraged to perfect his or her writing skills.

An IEP should be worked out in which the child is able to respond orally to some exams and be provided with notes or with a note-taker. The amount of writing the child should do should be minimized (handouts are helpful). A math worksheet should be printed out so that the child does not have to write out both problems and answers. Children should be allowed to tape lessons. When writing is necessary, these children should be allowed to use graph paper or paper with wide lines. There are also an assortment of writing aids, like pencil grips.

Demands on the rate, volume, and complexity of writing assignments need to be changed. The student should be allowed extra time on a project. If proper headings or other consistent aspects of homework are required, the child should be encouraged to have them ready in advance—or they shouldn't be made a requirement. As long as the child knows the content in the headings, the parent could do it.

Teachers have to give leeway when it comes to spelling and allow a dysgraphic child breathing room, such as the use of abbreviations. The child's "neatness" should never be judged, whether in the regular class or any specialty classes such as art. Many experts say that it is surprising how often a classified dysgraphic/LD child has come home with points taken off because of neatness, even with the teacher's having full knowledge of the child's disorder.

Parents should buy binder paper that is prereinforced. It is expensive, but well worth the investment.

Again, these accommodations are not made for kids who are lazy; they aid children who have serious problems with written work and skills requiring fine motor abilities. It is important that there is quality time within a child's learning environment and not just quantity time with the child struggling to write.

Here are tips from the National Joint Committee on Learning Disabilities that parents of dysgraphic children might want to pass on to their child's teachers:

- Break writing into stages and teach students to do the same. Teach the stages of the writing process (brainstorming, drafting, editing, proofreading, etc.). Consider grading stages on some "one-sitting" written exercises, awarding points on a short essay for brainstorming and a rough draft, as well as the final product. If writing is laborious, allow the student to make some editing marks rather than recopying the whole thing. On a computer, a student can make a rough draft, copy and revise it, so that both rough draft and final product can be evaluated without extra typing.
- Do not count spelling on rough drafts or one-sitting assignments.
- Encourage the student to use a spellchecker and to have someone proofread work, too. Speaking spellcheckers are recommended, especially if the student cannot recognize the correct word (headphones are usually included).
- Allow the student to use cursive or manuscript, whichever is most legible.
- Consider teaching cursive earlier than would be expected, as some find cursive easier to manage, and this will allow the student more time to learn it.
- Encourage primary students to use paper with raised lines, to keep writing on the line.
- Allow older students to use the line width of their choice. Remember that some students use small writing to disguise messiness or spelling, though.
- Allow the student to use different-colored paper or writing instruments.
- Allow the student to use graph paper for math, or turn lined paper sideways, to help with lining up columns of numbers.
- Allow the student to use the most comfortable writing instrument. Many students have difficulty writing with ballpoint pens, preferring pencils or pens that have more friction in contact with the paper. Mechanical pencils are very popular. Let the student find a favorite pen or pencil (and then get more like that).
- Have some fun grips available for everybody, no matter what the grade. Sometimes high-school kids enjoy the novelty of pencil grips or even big "primary pencils."
- Word processing should be an option. For many students, learning to use a word processor will be difficult for the same reasons that handwriting is difficult. Some keyboarding instructional programs address the needs of learning-disabled students. Features may include teaching the keys alphabetically (instead of the "home row" sequence) or sensors to change the feel of the "D" and "K" keys, so that the student can find the right position kinesthetically.
- Consider whether using speech recognition software will be helpful. As with word processing, the same issues that make writing difficult can make learning to use speech recognition software difficult, especially if the student has reading or speech challenges. However, if the student and teacher are willing to invest time

and effort in training the software to the student's voice and learning to use it, the student can be freed from the motor processes of writing or keyboarding.

- Reduce the copying elements of assignments and tests. For example, if students are expected to answer in complete sentences reflecting the question, have the student do this for three questions that you select, then answer the rest in phrases or words (or drawings). If students are expected to copy definitions, allow the student to shorten them or give the definitions and have them highlight the important phrases and words, or write an example or drawing of the word, instead of copying the definition.
- Reduce length requirements on written assignments—stress quality over quantity.
- Grade different assignments on individual parts of the writing process, so that for some assignments, spelling doesn't count, for others, grammar.
- Build handwriting instruction into the student's schedule.
- Teach alternative handwriting methods such as "Handwriting without Tears."

Prognosis

LDs are never cured, but they can be treated. Depending on the severity of the dysgraphia, how long it has gone untreated, and any other concurrent Alphabet Disorders, the prognosis can vary. In most cases, through treatment such as occupational therapy, a dysgraphic child can learn to compensate for his or her problems and lead a normal life.

Sources and resources

Learning Disabilities Association of America (412-341-1515); (www.ldaamerica.org)
Learning Disabilities Worldwide (www.ldworldwide.org)
National Center for Learning Disabilities (212-545-7510; 888-575-7373);
    (www.ld.org)
National Joint Committee on Learning Disabilities (www.ldonline.org)
Schwab Learning Center (www.schwablearning.org)

See the "LD: Learning Disability" chapter and the individual LD chapters, as well as "General Resources," for more sources used in this chapter.

DYSLEXIA

Terms used in this chapter: ADHD (attention-deficit/hyperactivity disorder); LD (learning disability); TS (Tourette syndrome)

Sound (and look!) familiar?

Hav ingdys lexiac anmake it hardtoread! Translation: Having dyslexia can make it hard to read! Writing that looks just fine to you might look like this to someone who has dyslexia:

Thew ord sare n otsp aced cor rect ly.

We spell wrds xatle az tha snd to us.

Sometimesallthelettersarepushedtogether

Aoccdrngig to rscheearch at an Elingsh uinervtisy, it deosn't mttaer in waht oredr the ltteers in a wrod are, olny taht the frist and lsat ltteres are at the rghit pcleas. The rset can be a toatle mses and you can sitll raed it wouthit a porbelm. This is bcuseae we do not raed ervey lterer by ilstef, but the wrod as a wlohe.

Did you know?

Dyslexia is a neurologically based LD that, according to the widely accepted definition, is characterized by difficulties with accurate and/or fluent word recognition and by poor spelling and decoding abilities. In effect, it is all about deviant reading. The popular notion of dyslexia is mixing up letters, but that isn't always the case, as involuntary cursing isn't always the case with TS.

Secondary consequences include problems in reading comprehension and reduced reading experience that can impede the growth of vocabulary and background knowledge.

LDs affect about 10 percent of children, according to the American Psychological Association. These children have normal intelligence and vision and, usually, normal speech—but because of dyslexia there are additional problems involved with writing and interpreting spoken language. Most schoolchildren receiving special-education services have deficits in reading, reports the Mayo Clinic, and dyslexia is the most common cause.

Dyslexia is a worldwide concern, but it manifests itself in different ways around the world. In Japan, for example, according to Yoichi Sakakihara, M.D., Research Center for Child and Adolescent Development and Education at Ochanomizu University, Tokyo, "The incidence of dyslexia is much lower … than with English-speaking children because of the different language system. The estimated incidence of dyslexia in Japan is less than 3 percent of the population. There are many studies describing the difference in the incidence of dyslexia among different languages. Dyslexia is mainly due to the dysfunction of phoneme [smallest unit of speech sound] awareness. The Japanese language does not have phonemes, but instead it has *mora* as the language unit. One Japanese character (*kana*) has only one *mora*. So these basic language differences could explain the low incidence of dyslexia in Japan."

Dyslexics' problems vary, even within one task. For example, a child might spell the word *automobile* five different ways in a short essay. Words can swirl, pages can strobe, letters can invert or transpose.

Up to 15 percent of the U.S. population has significant difficulty learning to read, according to the National Institutes of Health. People are born with dyslexia, and other family members often have the disability as well.

The International Dyslexia Association and other LD and health organizations provide the following facts on the disorder:

- Studies show that individuals with dyslexia process information in a different area of the brain than do nondyslexics.
- Many people who are dyslexic are of average to above-average intelligence.
- An individual can have more than one learning or behavioral disability. As many as 50 percent of those diagnosed with a learning or reading difference have been diagnosed with ADHD.
- Although disabilities may co-occur, one does not cause the other.
- From 15 to 20 percent of the population has a language-based LD.
- Of the students with specific LDs receiving special education services, 70-to-80 percent have deficits in reading.
- Dyslexia is the most common cause of reading, writing, and spelling difficulties.
- Dyslexia affects males and females nearly equally.
- If children who are dyslexic get effective phonological training in kindergarten and first grade, they will have significantly fewer problems in learning to read at grade level than children who are not identified or helped until third grade.
- At least 74 percent of children who are poor readers in third grade remain poor readers in the ninth grade. Often, they can't read well as adults, either.
- It is never too late for dyslexic individuals to learn to read, process, and express information more efficiently. Research shows that programs utilizing multisensory structured-language techniques can help children and adults learn to read.

Signs and symptoms

- adds new words slowly
- alienation
- behavioral problems such as aggression
- conceptual difficulties (now/then, up/down, etc.)
- delay in learning alphabet, nursery rhymes, colors, objects, etc.
- delayed speech

- delayed vocabulary acquisition
- difficulty comprehending rapid instructions
- difficulty following more than one command at a time
- difficulty remembering the sequence of things
- difficulty rhyming
- disorganization
- fails to hear and/or see similarities and differences in letters and words
- improper use of age-level grammar
- inability to recognize words and letters on a printed page
- inattention
- inconsistent spelling skills (sometimes good, sometimes bad)
- inversions of letters (m/w)
- low self-esteem
- may be unable to sound out the pronunciation of an unfamiliar word
- may not recognize the spacing that organizes letters into separate words
- poor reading comprehension
- problems with comprehending what is heard
- processing problems
- pronunciation problems
- reading ability level well below the expected level
- reads from right to left
- reversal of words (*lap* for *pal*)
- reversals of letters (b for d)
- sequencing problems when speaking
- substitutions (house/home)
- tendency to get overwhelmed
- transpositions (felt/left)
- withdrawal
- word retrieval problems

According to the Nemours Foundation, one of the largest health systems devoted to children's issues in the U.S., difficulty in any of these steps in reading can cause trouble for a dyslexic child:

- focusing on printed marks such as letters and words
- controlling eye movements across the page
- recognizing the way letters sound
- understanding words and grammar
- building images and ideas
- comparing new ideas to what is already known
- storing ideas in memory

Cause

Dyslexia is a neurobiological disorder (an illness of the nervous system caused by biological factors such as genetics or metabolic reasons). While there are other factors such as brain trauma or environmental causes such as lead poisoning, it is usually inherited, and the chance of a child's having it is increased if it runs in the family, which it often does. Dyslexia is an LD, and, like other LDs, creates a disparity between a child's ability and his or her performance. Even though most dyslexic children have average or above-average intelligence, their reading levels are much lower than they should be.

Treatment

There is no cure for dyslexia, but it can be treated. Once the child receives the correct diagnosis, early intervention is imperative. Remedial education is the treatment. Much hard work and educational services are needed for a child to improve his or her disability, but, with the right kind of home support and the correct school accommodations, there is reason to hope for a successful outcome.

A multisensory approach is the best way to treat dyslexic kids—through touch, sight, and sound. Reading to the child is of utmost importance, while pronouncing letters and spelling words. Children need to learn to read in a specific order—knowing that words are made up of certain sounds, associating sounds with written words, decoding words, and, finally, reading groups of words.

Prognosis

As with other LDs, dyslexia cannot be cured, but it can be treated, and the dyslexic child can lead a normal life. The earlier the detection and intervention, the better the prognosis.

Sources and resources

British Dyslexia Association (0118 966 2677); (www.bdadyslexia.org.uk)
Canadian Dyslexia Association (613-722-2699); (www.dyslexiaassociation.ca)
Davis Dyslexia Association International (www.dyslexia.com)
Dyslexia Teacher (www.dyslexia-teacher.com)
International Dyslexia Association (410-296-0232; 800-ABCD-123); (www.interdys.org)
Learning Disabilities Association of America (LDAA) (412-341-1515);
    (www.ldaamerica.org)
Mayo Clinic (www.mayoclinic.com)
National Center for Learning Disabilities (NCLD) (212-545-7510; 888-575-7373)
    (www.ld.org)

Nemours Foundation (www.nemours.org)
Recording for the Blind & Dyslexic (Audio Services) (212-557-5720);
    (www.rfbd.org/New_York.htm)
Schwab Learning (www.schwablearning.org)

See the "LD: Learning Disability" chapter and the individual LD chapters, as well as in the "General Resources," for more sources used in this chapter.

DYSTONIA

Terms used in this chapter: CP (cerebral palsy); DRD (dopa-responsive dystonia); NINDS (National Institute of Neurological Disorders and Stroke)

Sound familiar?

When Thomas first started getting cramps, his parents just thought they were growing pains. But it was much more than that. It seemed to get worse when he was under pressure or particularly agitated. When his whole body began to cramp and he started displaying involuntary movements, his mother, Jean, knew it was more serious than she first thought.

"That's when Tommy's nightmares started," the Houston office receptionist recalls. "He went from one doctor to the next, one needle prick to the next, one surgery to the next, one medication to the next. I can't even think of it in detail, it's so upsetting."

But Thomas, now 10 years old, two years after his first correct diagnosis, has begun to show great progress, and, although he still exhibits some unusual, twisted postures, he has some symptoms under control. "We're starting to see the light at the end of the tunnel," says Jean. "He seems happier, and that is all that counts."

Thomas has dystonia.

Did you know?

Almost everyone has had a case of writer's cramp. Now imagine that kind of cramping all over the body: that is dystonia. The movement disorder is manifested by involuntary muscle contractions that produce sometimes painful involuntary twisting, repetitive movements, and abnormal postures. These are caused by one muscle, a group of muscles, or all the muscles, which force part of the body or the entire body into an abnormal position or posture.

The disorder can be inherited and can also be acquired through another disease. There is no cure, but there are treatments.

The symptoms, ranging from mild to extreme, often occur in childhood between ages 5 and 16 and usually start in the foot or the hand. Progression to the limbs and torso can be rapid. The contractions often occur during voluntary movement or when the child is stressed or tired. Dystonia is not the same as involuntary, rhythmic tremors that have a back-and-forth movement.

The NINDS describes the different types of dystonia:

Generalized dystonia affects most or all of the body.

Focal dystonia is localized to a specific part of the body.

Multifocal dystonia involves two or more unrelated body parts.

Segmental dystonia affects two or more adjacent parts of the body.

Hemidystonia involves the arm and leg on the same side of the body.

Torsion dystonia, formerly called DMD (dystonia musculorum deformans), is a rare, generalized dystonia that may be inherited, usually begins in childhood, and becomes progressively worse. It can leave individuals seriously disabled and confined to a wheelchair. Genetic studies have revealed a mutation in a gene named DYT1.

Cervical dystonia, also called spasmodic torticollis, or torticollis, is the most common of the focal dystonias. In torticollis, the neck muscles that control the position of the head are affected, causing the head to twist and turn to one side.

Blepharospasm, the second most common focal dystonia, is the involuntary, forcible closure of the eyelids. The first symptoms may be uncontrollable blinking. Only one eye may be affected initially, but eventually both eyes are usually involved. The spasms may leave the eyelids completely closed, causing functional blindness, even though the eyes and vision are normal.

Cranial dystonia describes dystonia that affects the head, face, and neck muscles.

Oromandibular dystonia affects the jaw, lips, and tongue muscles. The jaw may be pulled open or shut, and speech and swallowing can be difficult.

Spasmodic dysphonia involves the throat muscles that control speech. Also called spastic dysphonia or laryngeal dystonia, it causes strained and difficult speaking or breathy and effortful speech. Meige's syndrome is the combination of blepharospasm and oromandibular dystonia and sometimes spasmodic dysphonia. Spasmodic torticollis can be classified as a type of cranial dystonia.

Writer's cramp is a dystonia that affects the muscles of the hand and sometimes the forearm, occurring only during handwriting.

DRD, of which Segawa's dystonia is an important variant, is successfully treated with drugs. Typically, DRD begins in childhood or adolescence with progressive difficulty in walking and, sometimes, spasticity. In Segawa's dystonia, the symptoms fluctuate during the day, from relative mobility in the morning to worsening disability in the afternoon and evening as well as after exercise. The diagnosis of DRD may be missed since it mimics many symptoms of CP.

Signs and symptoms

- all fingers extend when child tries to write
- body cramps
- dystonic movements occur during stress, fatigue, and voluntary movements
- elbow and wrist flexed with hand held near the body
- facial contortions
- fingers of hand are bent backward with wrist flexed
- foot cramps
- foot turns in at ankle, made worse when walking
- handwriting gets worse as it progresses
- jaw contortions
- neck contortions (torticollis)
- one foot drags
- one limb triggers dystonic movement in another limb
- rapid eye blinking
- tremors
- upward extension of large toe
- voice problems

Cause

It is thought that the basal ganglia—the area of the brain where muscle contractions are initiated—is the epicenter of the abnormal brain activity in dystonia, with a fault in the processing of neurotransmitters, which are chemical substances that carry impulses from one nerve cell to another. The disorder is inherited, spontaneous, primary or idiopathic (no known origin), or caused by a brain trauma before or after birth.

Diagnosis

When a child is being examined for dystonia, he or she will be clinically observed at rest, and then with the affected body part in action. The diagnostician will also attempt to distract the child, to aid in determining the child's triggers. The time of day the child's spasms and movements occur is also important in determining a diagnosis.

Tests that are used to diagnose dystonia include blood tests, electroencephalogram (EEG) to test brain activity, and an MRI scan to test for brain injury. Genetic testing might be performed, as well as a spinal tap.

Treatment

While there is no cure for dystonia, there are many treatments ranging from physical therapy and medication to surgery. According to the NINDS, the most frequent initial drug prescribed belongs to a group that reduces the level of the neurotransmitter acetylcholine—and Artane (Trihexyphenidyl) is the most common of those drugs. Also used are benztropine and procyclidine HCl. Other drug treatments include diazepam (Valium), clonazepam (Klonopin), valproate (Depakote), baclofen (Kemstro and Lioresal), carbamazepine (Tegretol), Reserpine, or tetrabenazine (Nitoman), which is not available in the U.S. Drugs that regulate the neurotransmitter Gamma-aminobutyric acid (GABA), such as the muscle relaxant Ativan, may be used in combination with these drugs or alone in patients with mild symptoms. Drugs that act on dopamine, a neurotransmitter that helps the brain fine-tune muscle movement, include levodopa/carbidopa (Sinemet) and bromocriptine (Parlodel). Remember that no drugs should be taken without a doctor's recommendation.

The NINDS reports that "DRD has been remarkably responsive to small doses of this dopamine-boosting treatment." But it has been indicated that dystonic patients also benefit from drugs that *decrease* dopamine, such as Reserpine or the investigational drug tetrabenazine. Anticonvulsants including Tegretol, usually prescribed to control epilepsy, have occasionally helped individuals with dystonia. Small amounts of Botulinum toxin (Botox) are effective when injected into affected muscles.

When medications don't work, surgery might be indicated. Some procedures, such as that performed in advanced dystonia, are extreme, destroying part of the thalamus deep within the brain, which controls movement. Some dystonias are aided by removing or cutting the nerve to the affected muscles or extending the tendons. The results of these extreme surgeries are not always permanent, and they carry many risks, as do many of the drugs prescribed.

Deep-brain stimulation implants are also used, especially for children with the genetic type of dystonia. An intrathecal baclofen therapy (ITB) pump brings the medication Baclofen directly to the spinal cord. Physical, occupational, and speech therapy are often beneficial, as are stress management and biofeedback.

Children with dystonia can sometimes use sensory tricks to decrease movement or spasms. We Move, an organization that advocates for those with movement disorders, suggests the following:

- Placing a hand on the side of the face, the chin, or the back of the head or touching these areas with one or more fingers may sometimes reduce neck contractions associated with cervical dystonia, abnormal movement, or postures of the neck and head.
- Applying pressure on the eyebrows or touching skin to the side of the eyes may improve involuntary contractions of eyelid muscles (blepharospasm).

- Touching the chin or the lips, applying pressure beneath the chin, or placing an object in the mouth, such as a toothpick, may reduce dystonia of the jaw, mouth, and lower face (oromandibular dystonia).
- Touching the affected hand with the other hand may help to alleviate writer's cramp.
- Leaning against the wall while standing, pressing on the hips, or applying pressure to the back of the neck may help to alleviate dystonia of the trunk (truncal dystonia).

Prognosis

Since dystonia has such a wide spectrum of disorders and symptoms, it is impossible to provide a general prognosis. But dystonia does not prevent its sufferers from having a fulfilling life. It's a matter of adjusting to the disorder. Most cases of dystonia will stabilize, usually within five years. But even with that stabilization, there are flare-ups and symptoms might return, especially under stressful conditions. Medications and surgery can help treat the symptoms, but there is no treatment that will stop the progression of dystonia.

As with so many other disorders, it is all about early detection and intervention and finding the proper treatments. If that is done, symptoms will improve as will the quality of life from education to recreation to marriage and having children.

Sources and resources

Bachmann-Strauss Dystonia & Parkinson Foundation (212-682-9900);
(www.dystonia-parkinsons.org)
Benign Essential Blepharospasm Research Foundation (409-832-0788);
(www.blepharospasm.org)
Dystonia Medical Research Foundation (800-377-DYST [3978]; in Canada:
800-361-8061); (www.dystonia-foundation.org)
National Institute of Neurological Disorders and Stroke (www.ninds.nih.gov)
National Spasmodic Torticollis Association (714-378-9837; 800-HURTFUL [487-8385]);
(www.torticollis.org)
Spasmodic Torticollis Dystonia/ST Dystonia (262-560-9534; 888-445-4588)
(www.spasmodictorticollis.org)
WE MOVE (Worldwide Education and Awareness for Movement Disorders)
(212-875-8312; 866-546-3136); (www.wemove.org)

E

ED (Eating Disorder)

EDS (Ehlers-Danlos Syndrome)

ERLD (Expressive-Receptive Language Disorder)

ED

Eating Disorder

Terms used in this chapter: AN (anorexia nervosa); BED (binge-eating disorder); BN (bulimia nervosa); ED (eating disorder); NIMH (National Institute of Mental Health); OCD (obsessive-compulsive disorder)

Did you know?

Although EDs are being diagnosed more and more in younger children, parents shouldn't get over-concerned. It is a good bet that if your 3- to 6-year-old is a picky eater, overeater, or even food phobic, he or she might simply be displaying normal behavior. However, unusual eating habits at a young age should be monitored.

Some studies, such as a U.S. Department of Health and Human Services Task Force report on EDs, have shown that 80 percent of girls have body image concerns by the sixth grade. The same percentage has dieted at least once by the age of 13.

It is no wonder that EDs have hit epidemic proportions: our children are inundated with images of skinny role models, society's preoccupation with dieting, and the convenience of fast food, while they lack family meals and proper eating supervision.

Most EDs are life-threatening and should be taken very seriously.

How it is manifested

There are four main types of EDs:

AN (anorexia nervosa) is characterized by very low body weight—less than 85 percent of expected weight—an abnormal fear of gaining weight, and a distorted view of body weight and body shape. *AN has the highest mortality rate of all mental and eating disorders!* Those with AN die from starvation and electrolyte imbalance. See the "AN: Anorexia Nervosa" chapter.

BED (binge-eating disorder) features uncontrolled intake of food, without any mitigating activities, such as purging or laxative abuse. See the "BED: Binge-Eating Disorder" chapter.

BN (bulimia nervosa) is manifested by binge eating and by mitigating activities—vomiting, laxatives. See the "BN: Bulimia Nervosa" chapter.

Pica is manifested by persistent eating of substances that have no nutritional value such as dirt or paint for at least one month. The *Handbook of Clinical Child Psychology* estimates pica prevalence rates from 4 percent to 26 percent among institutionalized children. Pica is an intentional activity not associated with any developmental disability or OCD. It is potentially life threatening because it can involve side effects such as lead poisoning, which can lead to developmental disabilities and even death. Other problems include non-nutritional eating; becoming ill from toxins, parasites, or bacteria found in eaten items; eating items that can't be digested, like rocks; and eating sharp items that can perforate the intestines. Pica usually is not long-term, lasting months rather than years.

Pica is best treated through behavioral therapy, as are all eating disorders. See the "Pica" chapter in this book.

By the numbers

According to Courtney E. Martin's book *Perfect Girls, Starving Daughters: The Frightening New Normalcy of Hating Your Body* (2007), EDs affect seven million females in the U.S. and up to seventy million people worldwide. In 1995, it was reported that 34 percent of American high school aged girls perceived themselves as overweight; that percentage has nearly tripled, a decade later.

The NIMH reports an estimated 5 to 15 percent of people with AN or BN, and approximately 35 percent of those with BED are male. But those numbers are increasing.

ANRED (Anorexia Nervosa and Related Eating Disorders, Inc.), an ED organization, cites an article published in 2001 in the *American Journal of Psychiatry*: "Twenty years ago it was thought that, for every ten to fifteen women with AN or BN, there was one man. Today, researchers find that, for every four females with AN, there is one male, and for every eight to eleven females with BN, there is one male."

BED, the most common ED, occurs almost equally in males and females. However, males might not consider it as great a problem as women do and might not seek help.

The generally accepted research shows that more than 90 percent of those who suffer from EDs are women between the ages of 12 and 25. However, increasing numbers of older women and men have these disorders. In addition, hundreds of thousands of boys are affected by these disorders.

In a February 2007 study, "The Prevalence and Correlates of Eating Disorders in the National Comorbidity Survey Replication," Harvard University Medical School researchers suggested that up to 25 percent of adults with EDs are male.

Signs and symptoms

See the chapters on specific eating disorders (AN, BED, BN, Pica) for the indications for each disorder.

Cause

There are many potential causes for EDs including genetic, sociocultural, neurochemical, and psychodevelopmental. Many Alphabet Disorders, such as OCD or various anxiety disorders and PDs (personality disorders), are comorbid, occurring with EDs. Comorbid mental disorders are exceedingly common, but the interrelationships are poorly understood.

There is not one cause of EDs, says ED expert, Sabine Naessén, M.D., Ph.D., a senior consulting doctor in obstetrics and gynecology at Karolinska University Hospital, Stockholm.

"It would be too easy to say that only one factor causes EDs," says Naessén. "The development of an ED is often attributed to our cultural environment, as exposed in mass media, which place a heavy emphasis on slimness. However, only a small percentage of all women who are exposed to these cultural mores develop eating disorders.

"The etiology of eating disorders [is] unknown. There are various contributory causes like biological, social, psychological, and genetic factors of eating disorders, and often several of these may act in combination. The personality traits which increase the risk of eating disorders are partly hereditary.

"There are several common comorbid problems in eating disorders. Addictive problems or affective disorders (depression, etc.) are more common among relatives.

"Eating disorders are more common in females than males, suggesting a possible role for female sex hormone signaling in the pathogenesis [the origin] of these diseases.

"We found a possible role of ERβ (estrogen receptor β gene) and/or neighboring genes in the etiology of disease in bulimic women. How the gene acts and the interaction with other factors we do not know.

"Hormonal changes seem to play a great role. Women with high androgen levels and polycystic ovary syndrome [POS] have a greater craving for sweets and tendency of binge-eating."

Treatment

The key to beating an ED is first admitting to it. And there are therapies that have helped.

EDs can be treated by psychotherapy, preferably cognitive behavioral therapy (CBT), which changes the child's negative behaviors and thoughts about those behaviors into more positive behaviors. EDs are also treated through pharmacotherapy. They can be separate treatments, but often need to be practiced in tandem. Psychotherapy will also be helpful in treating Alphabet Disorders that are usually comorbid with EDs.

SSRIs and other antidepressants are often used to help battle EDs. (See the "SSRIs" section in "What You Need to Know" for more information.)

The NIMH points to new findings that provide great hope. Scientists suspect that multiple genes may interact with environmental and other factors to increase the risk of developing EDs, so further research into these genes may turn up more effective treatment.

One area of research indicates that appetite and energy expenditure are regulated by a highly complex network of nerve cells and molecular messengers called neuropeptides. The NIMH states that further insight is likely to come from "studying the role of gonadal steroids whose relevance to eating disorders is suggested by the clear gender effect in the risk for these disorders, their emergence at puberty or soon after, and the increased risk for eating disorders among girls with early onset of menstruation."

Prognosis

People with EDs die from starvation, suicide, or electrolyte imbalance.

EDs can be effectively treated as long as the child wants help or, at the least, submits to help. With EDs, early intervention is crucial to stop the cycle before life-threatening or permanent symptoms occur. The ED relapse rate is high, so constant vigilance must be kept over the child's eating habits, even after they seem under control.

Sources and resources

Academy for Eating Disorders (AED) (847-498-4274); (www.aedweb.org)
Alliance for Eating Disorders Awareness (www.eatingdisorderinfo.org)
American Dietetic Association (www.eatright.org)
ANRED (Anorexia Nervosa and Related Eating Disorders, Inc.) (www.anred.com)
Asociacion Civil de Lucha Contra Desordenes Alimentarios
     (en español) (+54 627 22580/24290/24291 Int 211); (www.alda.org)
AWARE Foundation (www.awarefoundation.org)
Center for the Study of Anorexia and Bulimia (212-333-3444);
     (www.icpnyc.org/CenterForStudy.nxg)
Dads and Daughters (www.dadsanddaughters.org)
Eating Disorder Referral and Information Center (www.edreferral.com)
The Dressing Room Project (828-318-4438); (www.thedressingroomproject.org)
The Eating Disorders Action Group/Halifax, NS (902-443-9944)
Eating Disorders Anonymous (www.eatingdisordersanonymous.org)
Eating Disorders Association, Ireland (080 232 234914)
Eating Disorders Association (UK) (01603 621414); (www.b-eat.co.uk)
Eating Disorders Association of WA (Western Australia) (9221 0488)
Eating Disorders Clinic, New York State Psychiatric Institute and Columbia University
     Medical Center (212-543-5739); (www.eatingdisordersclinic.org)
Eating Disorders Coalition (202-543-9570) (www.eatingdisorderscoalition.org)

Eating Disorders Research Program, University of Minnesota (612-627-4494) (www.med.umn.edu/psychiatry/research/eatingdisorders/home)

The Elisa Project (214-369-5222); (www.theelisaproject.org)

The Handbook of Clinical Child Psychology, Wiley Series on Personality Processes, 3rd ed. (Hoboken, NJ: John Wiley and Sons, 2001).

Healing Connections, Inc. (www.healingconnections.org)

J. I. Hudson, E. Hiripi, H. G. Pope Jr., and R. C. Kessler, "The Prevalence and Correlates of Eating Disorders in the National Comorbidity Survey Replication," *Biological Psychiatry* 61, no. 3 (Feb. 2007): 348–58.

International Association of Eating Disorders Professionals (IAEDP) (www.iaedp.com)

Jessie's Wish (804-378-3032); (www.jessieswish.org)

Marino Therapy Centre, Dublin (353-1-8333126); (marinotherapycentre@gmail.com)

Multiservice Eating Disorders Association (MEDA) (617-558-1881); (www.medainc.org)

Courtney E. Martin, *Perfect Girls, Starving Daughters: The Frightening Normalcy of Hating Your Body* (New York: Free Press, 2007).

National Association of Anorexia Nervosa and Associated Disorders (ANAD) (847-831-3438); (www.anad.org)

National Eating Disorders Association (NEDA) (800-931-2237); (www.nationaleatingdisorders.org)

National Eating Disorders Screening Program (NEDSP) (www.mentalhealthscreening.org)

National Institute of Mental Health (www.nimh.nih.gov)

National Institute of Neurological Disorders and Stroke (www.ninds.nih.gov)

New York-Presbyterian Medical Center Psychiatric Center (www.nyppsychiatry.org)

Overeaters Anonymous (www.overeatersanonymous.org)

Somerset and Wessex Eating Disorders Association (01458-448600); (www.swedauk.org)

Something Fishy (www.something-fishy.org)

U.S. Department of Health & Human Services (www.hhs.gov)

Weight-control Information Network (877-946-4627); (www.win.niddk.nih.gov)

WINS (We Insist on Natural Shapes) (800-600-WINS)

D. B. Woodside, P. E. Garfinkel, E. Lin, et al., "Comparisons of Men With Full or Partial Eating Disorders, Men Without Eating Disorders, and Women With Eating Disorders in the Community," *American Journal of Psychiatry* 158 (April 2001): 570–74.

EDS

Ehlers-Danlos Syndrome

Terms used in this chapter: EDS (Ehlers-Danlos syndrome)

Sound familiar?

Nikki, from Dallas, Texas, is now 6-feet-1-inch tall, has blonde hair and blue eyes, and is a very happy, laid-back teenager. In seventh grade, she began playing basketball and had aspirations of playing college basketball. She had always been very healthy, but, after she started playing basketball, she began experiencing shin splints and pain in both hips.

One day during her freshman year in high school, Nikki passed out. The doctor said this was typical of teenaged girls and that she just needed salt in her diet. She fainted a few more times, but life went on. Nikki found that she needed to tape and brace her ankles to play basketball because she would turn them very easily. Once, she broke her arm at basketball practice and continued playing throughout the week. Her family realized that Nikki had a very high pain threshold. She didn't tell them how bad the broken wrist was until the bone completely broke in two pieces. X-rays showed it had likely been broken for a week.

During her sophomore year, Nikki started having back pain, describing it as "bone pain." The doctor thought she might have fractured her spine, but X-rays were inconclusive and a bone scan found no fracture. She attended physical therapy, but the pain got so bad that an MRI was ordered. It showed a fluid-filled cavity in her spine (spinal syrinx) at the site of her pain. The family decided to seek a second opinion.

The new doctor didn't initially check her spine; instead, he examined her joints, fingers, feet, wrists, and mouth. His diagnosis: a connective tissue disease. Because of Nikki's height and long arms, he thought that maybe it was Marfan syndrome, which affects connective tissue, but he suggested it could also be EDS (Ehlers-Danlos syndrome).

Nikki was then referred to a rheumatologist who said that her skin "wasn't stretchy enough" and that she "looked too healthy" for those other diseases; he diagnosed it as reactive arthritis. By this time, the spine pain was extreme, and Nikki was having severe pain in her ankles, elbows, and knees. The doctors repeated blood work, looking for lupus or JRA (juvenile rheumatoid arthritis), but all tests came back normal.

Michele, Nikki's mother, began researching and became increasingly convinced that Nikki did indeed have a connective tissue disease.

Through connections Nikki's basketball coach had, extensive records Michele kept and photos of Nikki's joint hypermobility were sent to a doctor who was familiar with EDS. A month later he saw Nikki and diagnosed her.

Michele says, "At the time I thought I had won the lottery."

In the process, Michele realized that her two sons had even more EDS physical characteristics than her daughter. In fact, she says, her oldest son, 16-year-old John, "looks like a rubber man." He suffered so many broken bones that doctors suspected low bone density. Her 11-year-old, Peter, has a lot of pain in his joints, primarily in his knee and shoulder. Peter has since been diagnosed as well, but John has been diagnosed with osteoporosis in his spine and has suffered a spontaneous pneumothorax (collapsed lung).

"Many children like my daughter don't begin to experience all of the problems associated with the disease until they finish growing. In fact, Dr. McDonnell at NIH doesn't even like to diagnose kids before puberty, because many young children are hypermobile," says Michele.

Now, at 17, Nikki has begun an entire new set of challenges, dealing with balance, vision, and more neurological problems. Because she has absolutely no gag reflex, the doctors learned that she has substantial craniocervical instability and that the connective tissue inside her head isn't holding her cerebellum in place as it should. Her cerebellar tonsils (brain stem) are lying low and, because her neck is so hypermobile, even simple movements put pressure on her brain stem.

Nikki was sent to the Chiari Institute in Great Neck, New York, where they learned that she has had POTS (postular orthostatic tachycardia syndrome). The disease had caused her blood vessels to be a little too elastic, so that, when she stands, the vessels don't constrict and pump blood up to her heart. Her blood pools in her legs, and her heart has to pump really fast to get the blood moving. This causes a lot of dysautonomia, a malfunction of the autonomic nervous system, and could be what contributed to her fainting.

Nikki and her brothers were also described as having Marfanoid habitus. "This is a relatively new concept," says Michele. "The researchers are seeing more and more 'crossover' issues. My children, especially my son, have many Marfan characteristics, but not enough to be diagnosed. And they don't have the genetic mutation for Marfan.

"The one thing that is vitally important in people with this disease," advises Michele, "is that they keep their muscles strong as a way to 'hold' their joints together. For many people, that proves to be very difficult. I can't say what will happen in five years or ten years, or even one year, to my daughter. But, today, she has had to give up basketball and all contact sports. With the craniocervical instability, one bad hit and it could be catastrophic. She has worked very hard to exercise, and it has been a lot of trial and error. She finds Pilates has been good in keeping her core strong. By doing this, she has really been doing well. She has good days and bad days and hasn't taken pain medication for many months." Nikki wants to pursue a nursing career.

Nikki and her brothers, Peter and John, have EDS—Ehlers-Danlos syndrome.

Did you know?

EDS is an inherited disorder that affects the body's connective tissue, which is supposed to support the skin, muscles, blood vessel and organ walls, and ligaments. Because of defective collagen—the fibrous protein that is the body's bonding agent, often called the glue that adds elasticity and strength—the child suffers from problems ranging from bruisable, tearable skin to unstable joints to ruptured arteries. The prevalence for EDS is one in five thousand. The severity can range simply from being "double-jointed" to the life-threatening vascular type.

The disease, which had been described as early as the fourth century BC, was first identified by two doctors—the 1901 work of Edward Ehlers, M.D., a Danish dermatologist, and the 1908 observations of Henri-Alexandre Danlos, M.D., a French physician who specialized in skin disorders, were eventually combined.

"EDS is an 'invisible' disease," says Michele Darwin, Nikki's mother. "On the outside, the kids look perfect. Inside is a different story."

There are many types of EDS, but recently they have been classified into six main types:

Types I and II

- extreme joint hypermobility
- fragile, smooth, velvety skin
- joint dislocations
- scoliosis
- skin hyperextensibility (laxity)
- skin tears and bruises easily
- sprains

Hypermobility Type (Type III)

- frequent joint dislocations
- joint hypermobility

Vascular Type (Type IV, arterial form)

- clubbed foot
- skin laxity
- spontaneous rupture of bowel
- spontaneous rupture of arteries
- veins visible through the skin

Kyphoscoliosis Type (Type VI)

- fragile globes of the eyes
- severe curvature of the spine (kyphoscoliosis)
- significant skin laxity
- significant joint laxity

Arthrochalasia Type (Type VIIB, arthrochalasis multiplex congenita); very rare

- joint dislocation
- joint laxity

- low muscle tone (hypotonia)
- possible skin laxity
- short stature

Dermatosparaxis Type (Type VIIC); very rare

- severely fragile skin
- skin that sags and folds
- soft, doughy skin

The other types, such as Type V, which is an extremely rare X-linked variant, are not included because they are not regarded as the "main types."

Signs and symptoms

- arterial fragility and rupture
- blood-clotting problems
- chronic diarrhea
- chronic, early onset, debilitating musculoskeletal pain
- early onset of osteoarthritis
- easy bruising
- fleshy, scarred lesions over pressure areas
- fragile, small blood vessels
- gum disease
- intestinal fragility and rupture
- joint pain
- lightheadedness due to low blood pressure
- loose joints (joint hypermobility)
- low muscle tone (hypotonia)
- mitral valve prolapse
- periodontal disease
- premature aging from skin exposure
- skin laxity
- slow and poor wound healing
- uterine fragility and rupture (in females)
- weakness of tissues

Cause

EDS is caused by a variety of genetic mutations that interfere with the production of collagen, which is the protein that is one of the key components of the body's connective tissue. These mutations affect different aspects of the collagen: its structure, production, or processing, which is what causes the different variations of EDS.

There are several ways the disorder is passed on. Autosomal dominant inheritance involves one copy of the altered gene in each cell. A child can inherit the mutated gene from one affected parent, in which case there is a 50 percent chance the child will have EDS.

Other children inherit the defective gene in an autosomal recessive pattern, which means two copies of the gene in each cell are mutated. The parents of a child with this pattern are carriers of one copy of the altered gene but do not show signs and symptoms of the disorder. And then there are new, sporadic genetic mutations that occur in people with no family history.

These are the genes that, when mutated, cause EDS: ADAMTS2, COLIA1, COLIA2, COL3A1, COL5A1, COL5A2, PLOD1, and TNXB. Most of these genes provide the body's protein-making map, and those proteins are used to put together the body's collagen.

Diagnosis

The doctor diagnosing your child will look for a family history and physical attributes such as extremely loose joints and fragile skin. The Mayo Clinic recommends that the following tests be performed:

Genetic tests: A few tests can detect collagen gene alterations through DNA analysis. These may help identify vascular and arthrochalasia types of EDS.

Urine test: This can help identify kyphoscoliosis type by measuring enzyme levels produced by the gene associated with kyphoscoliosis type. Abnormal levels typically indicate this form of EDS.

Skin biopsy: A small sample of skin is removed and examined under a microscope, which may reveal abnormalities in collagen fibers. Vascular-type EDS can be diagnosed by analyzing collagen produced by skin cells.

Heart ultrasound: To check for mitral valve prolapse, a heart condition that can occur with the classical and hypermobility EDS subtypes, your child's doctor may recommend a heart ultrasound (echocardiogram). This provides real-time images of the heart in motion. It can help identify heart muscle and valve abnormalities and find any fluid that may surround the heart.

Prenatal diagnostic tests: Prenatal diagnostic tests are indicated for certain types of EDS if a relative has the genetic mutation. Kyphoscoliosis type can be diagnosed through amniocentesis, a test that analyzes a sample of amniotic fluid surrounding the fetus, for levels of enzyme activity. Vascular-type EDS can be identified through genetic testing of amniotic fluid.

Treatment

There are several ways to help manage the symptoms of EDS. The main focus of care is to protect the joints and prevent injuries. Pain management through medication is an avenue often taken, and physical therapy is advised to help the child build his or her muscle strength and, in turn, help with joint problems. Exercise like weightlifting is not recommended for EDS children.

While surgery might be needed for EDS children to repair joints, it is recommended to remind the surgeon that the child has EDS, because stitches could tear out of the child's fragile skin. It is recommended that surgical glue or adhesive tape be used to close incisions. Elective surgery is not recommended for children with EDS.

Other treatments that are suggested include dieting to reduce weight and Vitamin C supplements, which has anecdotal success, but nothing officially documented.

Prognosis

There is no cure for EDS. What is important is managing the symptoms and learning techniques on how to protect the child from injuries.

According to the Ehlers-Danlos National Foundation, although life expectancy can be shortened with the vascular type of EDS due to the possibility of organ and vessel rupture, children with the other types of EDS have a normal life expectancy.

Sources and resources

Arthritis Foundation (www.arthritis.org)
Ehlers-Danlos National Foundation (www.ednf.org)
Ehlers-Danlos Support Group (www.ehlers-danlos.org)
Mayo Clinic, "Ehlers-Danlos Syndrome" (www.mayoclinic.com)

ERLD

Expressive-Receptive Language Disorder

Terms used in this chapter: ADHD (attention-deficit/hyperactivity disorder); APD (auditory processing disorder); ELD (expressive language disorder); ERLD (expressive-receptive language disorder); IEP (individualized education program); LD (learning disability); RLD (receptive language disorder)

Did you know?

ERLD is the diagnosis when children have difficulty with both their expressive (verbal expression) and receptive (comprehension) language skills. A child with ERLD has a communicative disorder, causing problems with understanding and expressing language.

It is believed that up to 5 percent of all children have an ELD, an RLD, or a combination of both, ERLD.

It is important to know the difference between speech and language. Problems dealing with speech involve the perception or articulation of speech sounds. Language problems involve communication and cognition.

ELD is a condition involving the ability to put words together to formulate thoughts, problems telling a coherent story, and difficulty naming objects. ELD is diagnosed when the child fits the diagnostic characteristics and tests lower on standardized tests for expressive language than on standardized measures of their receptive language and nonverbal intellectual ability. Children with ELD might have a limited vocabulary or have difficulty recalling words, difficulty producing sounds, make errors in tense, and have an inability to produce sentences that are age appropriate. ELD affects the child's academic and social performance.

RLD is simply a language disorder causing a child to have difficulty understanding what is said. Problems with the child's receptive skills begin before age 4, when he or she has difficulty understanding and using language. The ability to attend to, process, comprehend, retain, or integrate spoken language is impaired.

Signs and symptoms

- appears not to listen when spoken to
- articulation errors
- attention problems
- delayed speech
- difficulty acquiring rules of grammar
- difficulty naming objects
- difficulty responding appropriately to yes/no, either/or, who/what/where, when/why/how questions
- difficulty with word meaning (semantics)
- inability to follow directions or verbal instructions
- inability to start, hold, or maintain a conversation
- inability to understand complicated sentences
- lack of interest when being read to
- language skills below the expected age level
- misnaming items (mysnomia)
- not paying attention to spoken language
- problems relaying information
- problems retelling a story
- problems with verb tenses (morphology)
- repeats a question before responding to it (reauditorization)

- repeats words or phrases (echolalia)
- searches for the right word
- switches letters or syllables in words or phrases (spoonerisms)
- talks in circles
- tells rambling stories
- unintelligible speech
- uses "memorized" phrases and sentences
- uses short simple sentences
- uses wrong word in speech
- weak vocabulary
- word retrieval difficulties

Cause

The cause of ERLD is unknown, and pinpointing one is difficult because each child has a unique set of symptoms and etiologies. Various factors, some working in combination with each other, cause these disorders: the child's genetic susceptibility (it runs in the family); the child's exposure to language; the child's developmental abilities; environmental factors, ranging from toxins to vaccines; and trauma such as brain injury, disease, or a tumor.

The process of understanding spoken language is one of the human body's most complex processes. It involves hearing and visual cues; being able to attend and remember; the ability to distinguish sounds and employ grammar and vocabulary skills; and being capable of processing what is said.

Diagnosis

For a proper diagnosis, specialists including a speech-language pathologist, audiologist, pediatric neurologist, and someone who deals with pediatric developmental issues should be seen. Your pediatrician is the first stop, however; he or she will give the child a full medical examination to determine if there are any underlying medical issues.

Treatment

Children with ERLD are best supported by early detection and early intervention with several therapies, especially speech-language therapy. They can also benefit from occupational therapy to help them with social skills, as well as psychotherapy to prevent emotional or behavioral problems.

Educational interventions are aplenty and should be taken advantage of. A visit with an audiologist would be advised to make sure the child has no hearing problems or auditory processing difficulties. Many children with LDs including APD have related speech problems that are often missed and get worse if untreated.

A treatment program and IEP should be established with the specialists and teachers at school and adhered to strictly. Behavioral therapy and educational approaches, such as role modeling, reinforcement, sound shaping, and prompting, are also helpful for ERLD children. The child's being in an inclusion class with typical children is usually an extremely effective method and should be included in an IEP, which would include accommodations and therapies that are mandated by law. The ERLD child should be assessed for other comorbid disorders such as APD or ADHD and other LDs, which are commonly concurrent with ERLD. ERLD kids often have a long list of Alphabet Disorders.

Many standardized language tests are used to help diagnose these children, but parents should make sure they get the full results and have them assessed by a specialist in the field, especially someone not only expert in speech-language disorders, but processing disorders and LDs as well.

Prognosis

ELD, RLD, and ERLD cannot be cured, but they can be treated and modified. The child can have a productive academic and social life.

The most important thing to remember is that early detection and intervention can make all the difference in the world to your child, from academic success to social acceptance.

As was mentioned in the "APD: Auditory Processing Disorder" chapter, Priscilla L. Vail, M.A.T., author of the book *Words Fail Me: How Language Works and What Happens When It Doesn't*, describes in detail how the nuances of language can greatly affect a child's social status. "Popularity," she says, "hangs by a linguistic thread."

With a disorder such as ERLD, with so many potential causes, it is very important to get the proper diagnosis, which is often very difficult to come by and sometimes a torturous journey. These kids are at the heart of Alphabet Disorders, but, with the right kind of treatment, their futures can be very bright.

Sources and resources

American Speech-Language Hearing Association (ASHA) (www.asha.org)

See the "LD: Learning Disability" chapter and the "Autism" contacts and the mental-health contacts under "General Resources" for more sources used in this chapter.

F

FXS (Fragile X Syndrome)

FXS

Fragile X Syndrome

Terms used in this chapter: ADHD (attention-deficit/hyperactivity disorder); FXS (Fragile X syndrome); LD (learning disability); MR (mental retardation)

Sound familiar?

Arlene had many questions regarding her newborn twin son, Joshua: "Why is he spitting up his formula so much?" "Am I not holding him right?" "Why is he squirming so much when I change him?" "Am I not bonding correctly?" "His sister, Allison, seems so much more calm. Am I being impartial?"

The twins' birth was not an easy one. Arlene had difficulty getting pregnant, and prenatal tests showed that the twins were struggling. The first sign Arlene had that all was not right was when she saw her baby's nurse crying after the birth. When she asked why she was crying, the answer was, "He is so beautiful." It's the answer any parent would have loved to have heard, but Arlene didn't quite believe the response. And it took her five years to figure out what was wrong.

At the babies' six-month check-up, it was discovered that they had double ear infections—the first, Arlene says, of many. By the time they turned 1, they had each had ten ear infections. This, along with their lack of verbal skills and her son's poor eye contact, led the family to an ear, nose, and throat doctor, the first of many pediatric specialists they visited. They went through the standard hearing tests; everything checked out fine. The children just needed tiny tubes placed through their eardrums to equalize pressure on each side. Arlene's concerns were soothed for the time being. But soon she noticed that Josh was lagging behind his twin sister, Allison (Alli), in gross motor skills. At 1 year, he still was not crawling. The pediatrician, she says, "never gave my concerns much credence. She insisted that it all was because I was a first-time mother. 'He is a boy and a twin; he'll catch up,' the pediatrician said. My husband, Jeffrey, loved that answer, which only further fueled his displeasure with me for questioning that his son was not 'perfect.'"

Arlene continued urging the doctor to evaluate Josh further. She and Jeffrey were referred to the next specialist, a pediatric rehabilitation physician, or physiatrist, who found nothing obvious. And then, Josh started walking at 16 months. The situation was causing problems between Arlene and Jeffrey.

"By now, even the slightest suggestion that I still felt that something wasn't quite right was fodder for huge arguments with my husband," Arlene recalls, "but I insisted that we continue our quest for some answers."

Josh spoke fewer words than his twin and was showing no signs of improvement. So, they consulted a speech pathologist who found many areas to work on. They attended sessions twice a week, with Alli and Arlene biding time in the waiting room. After about a year, the speech pathologist commented about Alli's unique speech patterns and suggested that she could use some therapy, too. After a year of intensive speech therapy, Arlene's concerns were not alleviated.

F

"When I suggested more evaluations, I was again met with more opposition," she says.

"Next the pediatric psychologist evaluated my son and our parenting skills. As luck would have it, my husband was the stellar father, further fueling my feelings of inadequacy. He knew instinctively how to interact with my son, when I was struggling just to have him enjoy my touch."

There was promising news, though: this doctor felt there was a medical reason for Josh's delays.

"I finally had what I needed to combat our pediatrician and my husband," Arlene says.

They went to see the head of pediatric neurology at their local children's hospital. "This doctor was sure to find the answer," thought Arlene.

Josh went through a battery of tests including an MRI, EKG, and blood work. To Arlene's "great surprise," they found nothing.

Then, months later, the speech pathologist asked if they had ever tested for Fragile X. Arlene was sure they had ("The pediatric neurologist tested for everything under the sun"). Arlene rushed home and looked up Josh's test results and found that they hadn't done that test. When she checked with the doctor's office, he replied, "He's too high-functioning to have Fragile X," but said he'd run the test if Arlene brought Josh in. After having just put Josh through the battery of tests, Arlene declined. Six months later, the pediatrician, still trying to convince Arlene that everything was fine, suggested that they run the test.

"She was so sure it would find nothing," says Arlene. "They all knew better than me." ·

Josh was diagnosed with Fragile X syndrome in February 1994 at age 5. Shortly thereafter, Alli was also diagnosed with Fragile X.

"Not only did I learn that my children had Fragile X syndrome, the most common inherited cause of intellectual disabilities," Arlene says, "but I also learned that they inherited it from me."

"There were many dark days that followed," says Arlene, "but soon I realized that I could not let Fragile X defeat or define me or my children. My husband and I set out to learn as much as possible and to make a difference in their lives." Six months after the diagnosis, they attended the first of many international conferences sponsored by the National Fragile X Foundation. This set them on a path of not only educating themselves, but the rest of the world as well. They joined the foundation's board of directors and, Arlene says, "were motivated beyond belief to make the world embrace our children in spite of their differences. We went into their classrooms each year, educating teachers and students about [the disorder]. Speaking to their peers made a huge difference in their understanding of my children and themselves."

The thirteen years since their diagnosis have been "mind- and life-altering," Arlene says. "There are still those days when I say to myself 'if only.' But when I truly think about it, my life would not be as full and rewarding if not for going down this road. My kids are my compass and have a great deal to offer. In the end, it's about making the most of what you have and not about having the most.

"Now that Josh and Alli are 18, I can see where all this effort has gone and how much more needs to be done on their—and on my—road to independence."

Josh is a high-school senior and requires a full-time aide less and less. He goes to his classes completely unassisted and contributes in each, but still needs the regular curriculum to be modified. It is only now in his senior year that he has become truly comfortable in his role as a student, his mother says. Next year *he will be in a more skill-based program to help him learn an employable skill. For the first time, he will be in a segregated setting. "It will be interesting to see what that brings," says Arlene.*

Allison graduated from high school last year ("I do twins the hard way," jokes Arlene) and is in community college, driving, and working on weekends. It wasn't until last summer that Alli's IQ was tested as a requirement for a program she hoped to qualify for. That exam revealed that she has a normal IQ but also that she has a significant nonverbal learning disorder, which explains why she doesn't pick up social cues as others do. It also explains the fact that, while she reads at grade level, her comprehension is much lower. "But no one has a bigger heart or tries harder to succeed," says Arlene, "and it is that motivation which is sure to take her far."

Things have also worked out on the marital level.

"Jeffrey and I have accomplished much as a couple and as parents of these two wonderful young adults," says Arlene, "but what I think I'm most proud of is the attitude we have somehow been able to instill in them."

At a holiday party several years ago with members of their local Fragile X support group, Arlene was speaking with another mother about the prospect of finding a "cure" for the disorder. She was unaware that Alli was listening, but her daughter asked if she could join the conversation. Arlene said she could, "not having any idea where Alli was going with this," and Alli confidently stated, "If there was a cure, I would not take it." The other mother looked shocked and immediately asked why. Without missing a beat, Alli responded, "Because I'm happy with who I am."

"Raising any child who has that kind of positive self-image is truly the holy grail," says Arlene. "With any luck, the rest will take care of itself."

Joshua and Allison have FXS—Fragile X syndrome.

Did you know?

FXS is the most common inherited form of MR. Children with FXS can have intellectual impairment ranging from mild LD to profound MR and autism.

FXS is caused by a mutation of the FMR1 gene on the X chromosome. The mutation shuts down the gene responsible for producing FMRP, an essential protein for normal brain function. The disorder affects mostly males.

The delays and physical features associated with FXS are not seen at birth, but rather later in childhood, at around 8 to 10 months. In general, developmental delay is not diagnosed, usually, until around 24 months. In the case of FXS, it takes about another year for a diagnosis.

Boys are affected by FXS in a more severe way than girls because boys have one X chromosome, and girls have two. If a girl has a mutation in one, she still has another properly functioning chromosome to offset the bad one. Girls affected with FXS are usually not severely retarded and often manifest the disorder through LDs.

The mutation can be passed from either parent to a child, but the mutated gene can also be carried through generations without causing FXS through carrier status. It is a sex-linked genetic abnormality in which a mother has a 50/50 chance of transmitting the disorder to each son or daughter and in which a father will transmit the disorder to all of his daughters (who will only be carriers), but never to his sons. According to the Fragile X Association of Australia, "An average based on international statistics indicates that 1 in 360 males and 1 in 4,000 to 6,000 females are affected; 1 in 260 females and 1 in 800 males are carriers."

MR is a nonprogressive (does not get worse or degenerate with time) condition involving limitations and delays in many areas of development, including mental functioning, motor skills, communication, academics, social skills, and everyday life skills. These limitations cause the child to learn more slowly than his or her peers, but they will learn, for the most part, depending on the severity of the MR (MR is usually diagnosed when the child has an IQ test score below 70).

IQ test scores are read this way: the average score is 85–115; borderline, 70–84; mentally retarded (mild), 55–69; moderate, 40–54; severe, 25–39; and profound, lower than 25. It is very important to know that a child who does not have MR could score low on this test because of many reasons, ranging from LDs and attention deficits to behavioral problems. About 30 percent of girls with the full mutation score above 85 on an IQ test, with the other 70 percent placed mostly in the borderline or mild mental-retardation range.

These children do not usually regress. With the right therapies, they progress.

Signs and symptoms

- ADHD
- anxiety
- autistic behaviors
- broad forehead
- chest indentation
- chewing on clothes
- cognitive delays
- cross-eyed or wall-eyed (strabismus)
- developmental delays in sitting, talking, walking, and toilet training
- difficulties processing information
- difficulties understanding concepts
- dislikes being touched or held
- dislikes change in routine
- ear infections
- flat feet
- flexible finger joints
- fun-loving

- fussiness
- good copying skills
- good memory
- good mimicking skills
- good reading skills
- good sense of humor
- hand biting
- hand calluses
- hand flapping
- high palate
- hypersensitivity to stimuli
- impulsivity
- inability to cuddle
- interest in objects that spin
- large head
- large testicles develop in puberty (macroorchidism)
- LDs
- long face develops in puberty
- low muscle tone (hypotonia)
- math is a challenge (FXS girls)
- mitral valve prolapse
- mouthing objects
- MR
- poor abstract thinking
- poor socialization skills, but is social
- prominent ears
- prominent forehead
- repetition of phrases and activities (echolalia, perseveration)
- seizures
- sensitivity to noise, smell, touch
- sensory-motor problems
- short-lived eye contact
- shyness
- soft, fleshy skin
- squint
- strength in visual perception
- strong vocabulary skills
- tangential speech
- tantrums
- toe walking

- unstable moods
- vision problems
- weak fine motor skills
- weak gross motor skills

Diagnosis

Testing for FXS is carried out via a simple DNA blood test which is virtualy 100 percent accurate. Tests can be done on both parents to see if they are carriers and on the fetus as well.

Treatment

FXS has no cure, but physical, psychological, cognitive, speech-language, behavioral, and occupational therapies will all help your child. The earlier you get this help, the better, as with every Alphabet Disorder.

Although these children do not have many specific medical concerns associated with the syndrome, medications are suggested for the ear infections, seizures, and other concerns. They might also be treated for associated behavioral problems such as ADHD and aggression.

Prognosis

Children with FXS have a much better outlook with early detection and diagnosis than with later diagnosis. It is estimated that, if a child has a full fragile X mutation, about one-third of females and three-quarters of males have lifelong MR, often mild. FXS children can be expected to have a normal lifespan.

Sources and resources

Fragile X Association of Australia (www.Fragilex.org.au)
National Fragile X Foundation (USA) (1-800-688-8765); (www.fragilex.org)

G

GAD (General Anxiety Disorder)

GAD

General Anxiety Disorder

Terms used in this chapter: GAD (general anxiety disorder); OCD (obsessive-compulsive disorder)

Sound familiar?

Nora is a pretty 10-year-old girl with a smile that just lights up the room. She has a wild head of strawberry blonde hair, and the sweetest disposition you'd want in a child. She's funny and smart and likes watching Nickelodeon cartoons. She likes many things that her peers like—Girl Scouts, the Cartoon Network, Bratz dolls—but she also really hates some things.

She hates movie theaters, school, gymnastics, camp, and restaurants, and just about anything where her anxiety can act up. So, she is afraid of everything. She worries that she will get sick if someone touches her; she thinks she will throw up on the school bus; she worries about getting diarrhea at the movies; she wonders if saying a certain word will bring her bad luck. Will certain foods make her sick?

She constantly asks her parents for reassurance. Questions like: "If I drink that milk, will I throw up?" "If I see someone get hurt on TV, will I get hurt?" "Will the cat that lives ten blocks away be all right during the night?" And, of course, her closet light must be on at bedtime.

Most of the time, Nora reacts with avoidance and irritable bowel syndrome (IBS) symptoms—stomachaches, irregular bowel movements, nausea. She has begun exhibiting headaches and tics and is self-stimulating (stimming) by continuously licking her fingers. She does not want to go to school. She longed to have sleepovers but cancelled at the last minute, fearing getting sick at a friend's house or even her own.

One day, on the way to a gymnastics recital, Nora had her first full-fledged panic attack—at least the first her parents noticed. She complained of having "a heart attack" and was frozen with fear.

Nora was lucky. Because her mother had suffered from serious panic attacks for many years, she knew how to handle this episode and, for the long term, the importance of early intervention. For generations, Nora's matriarchal lineage had suffered from anxiety disorders, as did Nora's father and his matriarchal line, with OCD.

After the panic attack and the rapid appearance of physical tics that were appearing like OCD to Nora's parents, the young girl was quickly brought to a children's psychiatrist, who put her on Zoloft to cut the edge—and cut it, it did. Her most critical symptoms almost immediately disappeared, although she occasionally still needs reassurance that outside events will not harm her. Her parents say that, although they were afraid of putting her on medication, they knew it had to be done.

Nora suffers from, and will constantly fight, this family affliction. But her most intense symptoms have subsided, thanks to medication.

Nora has GAD—generalized anxiety disorder.

Did you know?

GAD is an illness characterized by chronic overworry and fear, occurring most days for a period of six months or more, that involves concern over a number of activities or events. The mean age for onset is around 8 years old.

The GAD child worries about a wide variety of topics—from past occurrences to events that have not yet occurred—even if there is nothing to provoke the fears. Unlike separation or social anxiety, which result from specific worries (a parent leaving, speaking in front of a classroom, etc.), children with GAD find an expansive, diverse assortment of subjects to make them anxious—"Will I get sick if a stranger sneezes near me?" "Will I have bad luck if I change my breakfast cereal?"

These children are not concerned only about their well-being, they worry about family, friends, and even incidents and conversations experienced the week before. They find concern with their academic and social abilities and just about anything else in the world. The fear persists even when the child is not being judged or is about a task they've always performed well.

Adolescents usually realize that their anxiety is at a higher level than normal, but young children do not have that ability. And considering how many adults don't seek help when they know something is wrong, children are often left to suffer in silence. As with Nora's story at the start of this chapter, children with this disorder are constantly requiring reassurance from those they trust.

While it is normal for children to worry and experience nervousness and anxiety, when these interfere with their daily routine, the parent should consider seeking help from a professional such as a pediatric psychiatrist or psychologist. No precautionary measures can prevent GAD in children, but, as with most Alphabet Disorders, early detection followed by early intervention can greatly enhance the child's well-being.

Signs and symptoms

- anticipatory anxiety
- attention problems
- breathing problems
- clinging behavior
- depression
- difficulty swallowing
- fear of natural disasters
- fearfulness
- feeling as though there is a lump in the throat
- feeling faint
- heart palpitations
- hot flashes

- inability to relax
- insomnia
- irritability
- lack of concentration
- mind goes blank
- nausea
- need for constant reassurance
- nervousness about participating in sporting events
- obsessive-compulsive symptoms
- overconcern about being late
- performance anxiety
- redoes tasks to make them perfect
- safety concerns for self, family, friends
- school aversion
- startles easily
- stomachaches
- sweating
- trembling
- twitching
- undue worry about academic performance
- vertigo

According to the Children's Hospital Boston, anxiety and worry are associated with at least three of the following symptoms: restlessness or feeling keyed up or on edge, being easily fatigued, difficulty concentrating, irritability, muscle tension, and sleep disturbance.

Cause

GAD, like all anxiety disorders, has several causes: biological, environmental, and family-based factors. It can be inherited, or it can be behavior learned from an anxious household. If a child's father openly fears dogs because one bit him when he was young, the child could pick up that fear. It can also be rooted in a real fear or traumatic event. Around the world, children who live in war-torn countries or areas prone to natural disasters can form these anxious behaviors. It is conventional wisdom that children whose parents have an anxiety disorder are more likely to have an anxiety disorder than those whose parents have no anxiety.

One thing we can be sure of: GAD is greatly influenced by an imbalance involving two brain chemicals (norepinephrine and serotonin).

Diagnosis

A mental-health professional is the best person to diagnose and work with your GAD child, but the child's pediatrician should first run tests to see if there is an underlying physical/medical problem. The mental-health professional will observe your child, speak with you and the child, and perform tests such as the Screen for Child Anxiety Related Emotional Disorders (SCARED) to determine a diagnosis.

Treatment

The good news is that anxiety disorders can be easily and effectively treated. Changing the disturbing, unwanted thoughts and relaxing are the main goals. Helping the child master and manage anxiety is achieved through cognitive behavioral therapy (CBT), which has proven successful in effectively helping to replace bad behaviors and thoughts with positive ones; antidepressant or anti-anxiety medication; or a combination of therapies. Family therapy and school participation are also strong approaches for effective treatment. Children need also to learn the physiological symptoms of their anxiety disorder, so they can learn to control it. A reward reinforcement program for positive behavior should also be established.

Relaxation and desensitization therapies should also be considered. But sometimes, medications are needed, as was the case with Nora. The deficiency of norepinephrine, serotonin, and Gamma-aminobutyric acid (GABA) greatly affect mood.

More natural aids such as L-glutamine, an amino acid that increases the amount of GABA, which sustains proper brain function and mental ability, have been found to be helpful, but some conditions do not tolerate L-glutamine—so, as with any type of medication or supplement, the parent must speak with a physician or expert in natural medicines before administering any to a child.

Long-acting, fast-working benzodiazepines (Ativan, Klonopin, Librium, Serax, and Valium) have been effective in helping the GAD child. But SSRIs are getting the most positive attention with their antidepressant and anti-anxiety abilities, although it takes longer for these to work effectively. (See the "SSRIs" section in "What You Need to Know" for more information.) Combination serotonin/norepinephrine agent drugs including Effexor, Remeron, and Serzone are also used to help GAD.

Other drugs range from more extreme tranquilizers to less powerful antihistamines. But, again, doctors should always be consulted before a child takes any drug, and it might be wise to get a second opinion whenever drugs are prescribed for a child.

There are also everyday habits that a parent can change for a child that will help minimize anxiety, including lessening stress, reducing the amount of stimulants such as caffeine, and regulating their amount of sleep. Asthma, cold, cough and nasal products, and other medications can bring on GAD.

The Children's Hospital Boston offers this advice: "Early detection and intervention can reduce the severity of symptoms, enhance the child's normal growth and development, and improve the quality of life experienced by children or adolescents with anxiety disorders."

Prognosis

With the proper treatment, especially with early intervention, GAD symptoms can be controlled and the child can lead a normal life.

Sources and resources

American Academy of Child and Adolescent Psychiatry (www.aacap.org)

American Psychiatric Association (www.psych.org)

American Psychological Association (www.apa.org)

The Children's Hospital Boston, "Generalized Anxiety Disorder" (www.childrenshospital.org)

DSM (*Diagnostic and Statistical Manual of Mental Disorders*)

National Institute of Mental Health (www.nimh.nih.gov)

Nemours Foundation (www.nemours.org)

See the mental-health contacts under "General Resources" for more sources used in this chapter.

H

HPD (Histrionic Personality Disorder)

HS (Hyperlexia Syndrome)

HTD (Hypothyroidism Disorder)

HPD

Histrionic Personality Disorder

Terms used in this chapter: HPD (histrionic personality disorder); PD (personality disorder)

Sound familiar?

Kalinda, 16, has tried to be the center of attention since she was 4, when her parents divorced. Her father, Karl, says she had a good role model in her mother, his ex-wife, whom he describes as a "diva, a crazy diva."

Kalinda lived with her mother and progressively worsened when it came to being overdramatic. She would tell her father incredible stories about her mother's friends and boyfriends, things so unbelievable that he knew they weren't true. She would tell him—and her friends and teachers (he later learned)—that she had met celebrities who became her close friends. She dressed in a dark, dramatic black-leather gothic style starting at age 11, which became more and more extreme—so much so that the school complained to Karl about inappropriate dress and behavior.

When Karl talked to Kalinda about her behavior, she would have an almost violent screaming tantrum. Then her mother would call with a similar tantrum, accusing Karl of being a "manipulative liar."

In school, with her peers, Kalinda's behavior got worse. She would bully, embarrass, and manipulate her friends in a very passive-aggressive manner, one minute saying that she was sad and suicidal and the next turning against them, for no reason. She started cutting herself in places on her body that were easily seen.

Kalinda acted as if she were the center of every social clique. She wasn't. She would yell, cry, feign fainting, and laugh inappropriately, making everyone around her uncomfortable. She would blurt out inappropriate statements in class. She rarely let anyone get a word in edgewise.

Starting at age 12, Kalinda began incessantly talking about sex and sexual encounters (which never happened). As she became older, the talk became actual flirting and seduction.

"She would be so intricate and detailed in what she was talking about, but there would be no real substance behind any of it," Karl recalls.

Kalinda was spiraling down so badly that Karl finally took action and regained custody. He brought her to a psychiatrist, and she was diagnosed for the first time in sixteen years with anxiety, mood and eating disorders, and one PD. Karl recently put her in therapy—which, he says, she likes because she's the focus of the session.

"I now know that her mother wasn't just obnoxious, she was sick," says Karl, "and I hope that Kalinda will now find the help she needs to change and have a good life."

Kalinda has HPD—histrionic personality disorder.

Did you know?

HPD is manifested by overdramatic behavior characterized by distorted self-image, expression of over-the-top emotions, and the intense need for attention and approval—in everyday terminology, the drama queen. HPD children—mostly teenagers—strive to be the center of attention in such an intense fashion that it interferes with their everyday life-functioning.

HPD children are not happy when not the focus of attention and will do anything to gain attention, from acting inappropriately to being seductive and provocative to fabricating tall, highly embellished tales. They will use all types of behavior to gain the attention they crave, from what they talk about to how they dress. Their emotions are as shallow as are their topics of discourse, which might sound flowery but usually lack detail. It's all for the "Wow!" factor.

Although more females than males are diagnosed with HPD, the schism is narrowing as social expectations change.

Signs and symptoms

- appears to lack sincerity
- attention seeker
- believes he or she is loved by everyone
- considers relationships more intense than they actually are
- dominates conversation
- dresses provocatively
- easily bored by routines
- easily suggestible
- emotions change rapidly
- exaggerates emotions
- exaggerates relationships
- exaggerates illnesses
- frustrated
- good social skills
- highly influenced by others
- inappropriate displays of emotion
- interrupts others
- jumps from project to project without finishing
- "life of the party"
- manipulative
- physical appearance draws attention
- rarely shows concern for others
- rash decision making

- seductive
- seeks constant praise
- self-dramatization
- theatrical
- threatens suicide
- uses grandiose language

Cause

As with so many PDs, the exact cause of HPD is not known, but it is believed that it results from both learned and genetic factors as well as physiological, developmental, cognitive, and social factors. HPD tends to run in families, but that could be the result of behaviors learned at home or an inherited trait. There are a slew of psychiatric theories, ranging from the child's not receiving enough parental attention to the child's receiving too much attention. Having free rein and not being criticized while growing up have also been cited as possible causes.

Diagnosis

The HPD diagnosis is made by a psychiatrist or psychologist and is determined by the child's history and information culled through clinical observation and interviews.

Treatment

While therapy is the proper treatment for HPD, it also creates a problem. Psychotherapy enables the HPD individual to find his or her ultimate audience. The therapist becomes captive, focusing all attention on the HPD patient, enabling the child to be, once again, the center of attention. The types of therapy used include psychotherapy, group and family therapy, and cognitive behavioral therapy (CBT), which helps the child identify his or her bad thoughts and impulses and work to change them. Medication is not recommended for HPD, unless it is to treat a concurrent disorder, such as antidepressants prescribed for depression. Since HPD children are likely to develop depression due to the clash between reality and their expectations, psychotherapy is highly recommended.

Prognosis

HPD characteristics are long-lasting and often lifelong. HPD affects social and family relationships, but it should not affect the child academically. The HPD child's future success depends on the success of therapy, but PDs, in general, are very hard to treat. Individuals with PDs, when left to their own devices as they age, often drop therapy. Some HPD children begin to lessen their symptoms as they mature.

Sources and resources

American Academy of Child and Adolescent Psychiatry (www.aacap.org)

DSM (Diagnostic and Statistical Manual of Mental Disorders)

Nemours Foundation (www.nemours.org)

psychologytoday.com

See the mental-health contacts under "General Resources" for more sources used in this chapter.

HS

Hyperlexia Syndrome

Terms used in this chapter: ADHD (attention-deficit/hyperactivity disorder); AS (Asperger syndrome); ASD (autism spectrum disorder); HS (hyperlexia syndrome); IEP (individualized education program); LD (learning disability); MR (mental retardation); NLD (nonverbal learning disorder); PDD (pervasive developmental disorder)

Sound familiar?

Jacob, who has had several developmental delays, just turned 4. He spoke early and then just stopped. He started walking only six months ago.

Melissa, Jacob's mother, had POS (polycystic ovary syndrome) and had to take a "fairly low dose" of Clomid, a fertility drug, to conceive Jacob. At birth, he had low muscle tone, hypotonia, and he was "floppy." Melissa was told that this resulted from blood-pressure medications she took during her pregnancy. She says she still has no idea how the Clomid might have affected her son.

Jacob was jaundiced soon after birth, had many ear infections during his first year, and took a lot of antibiotics. Many parents of Alphabet Kids cite those conditions in their child's history.

Throughout childhood, Jacob was inundated with therapies, interventions, and doctor visits, all seemingly useless. He had MRI scans, blood tests, and hearing tests, even a test for CF (cystic fibrosis). Melissa and her husband even went to a geneticist to find out what was wrong with their son. Jacob saw neurologists and therapists, but no one had an answer. The tests showed normal brain function. It would be years of incredible stress and feelings of guilt before Melissa would know the answer.

In fact, it was Jacob's neurologist, who had been testing him for a year, who matter-of-factly mentioned the diagnosis one day.

Melissa, a day-care worker in Alabama, was smart—and lucky. Even though she didn't know what was wrong with Jacob, she had him in early intervention programs since the age of 1.

"We had him evaluated by early intervention," Melissa recalls. "I was torn while waiting to see the results of their testing. He had to have a 30 percent delay in order for them to work with him. A part of me wanted him to not have that delay, but I knew he needed something to help. It turned out

he did have the delay in muscle development and motor skills, so he qualified. After the intervention began, he started sitting up more on his own, but couldn't for long periods of time.

"They say that early intervention has helped him a lot!" she says.

"I was exasperated as a parent, knowing there was something wrong. He lost speech at 18 months after being ahead," Melissa says of her only child. "He lost all of it overnight ... quit talking. I blamed myself ... blamed the hospital."

It was particularly shocking because Jacob had begun speaking at four months old, saying, "Mama." He had always been very alert and aware of his environment.

"At 18 months, I noticed that the words stopped," Melissa says. "He grunted and made noises but nothing that was understandable. When he went to checkups and therapy I pointed this out. No one seemed concerned. He started more speech therapy at this time. I got frustrated with the therapist. She saw him once a month and would seem irritated that he wouldn't cooperate. She pointed out that he didn't make eye contact with her. He became obsessed with lining toys up between his legs. If you moved something out of the lineup, he noticed it missing."

The therapist became upset with Jacob's focus on letters and shapes. Melissa was not happy with her. When Jacob stopped therapy with her around his third birthday, he began talking again.

Today, Jacob is obsessed with animals, letters, and numbers. Even before his first birthday he could count to ten. At five months, he began counting his fingers with a specific sound for each one.

After he turned 2, he became obsessed with the alphabet. He would draw the letters and within a week could write them all. When he entered a room, he gravitated toward letters. He'd identify them, taking his magnetic letters from the board and announcing what letters followed or preceded, identifying the alphabet forward and backward from any point.

"He did things that I couldn't do without thinking about it," says Melissa.

"He can read more than we know. He is big on spelling right now, and I am finding new words that he is spelling that we didn't know he knew. Yesterday he read the word 'Alabama.' He also knows shapes, colors, and, of course, how to spell and write the words for those shapes and colors."

Although Jacob was almost 2½ and couldn't walk, his written-language skills continued to grow. He would write words that he had seen on TV or in a book. He learned to write his first name, then his last name. Melissa says he couldn't say, "Mama, I am hungry," but could use letters in many complex ways.

Jacob flaps his arms when he is excited, moves his legs, and sometimes grinds his teeth. His need to line things up was one of the biggest red flags that his mother noticed. Melissa began to notice many autistic behaviors.

His eating habits, which had been normal, also began to change. Jacob hated getting dirty. He refused to let anyone feed him, lest they not be neat enough. He stopped eating "messy" foods like pasta. He refused to hold a spoon and, in fact, kept his hands behind his back, so they wouldn't get dirty when he ate. He wouldn't play with Play Doh and hated to paint. Jacob began collecting diagnoses, including ASD and ataxia, lack of coordination.

"I had carried so much of the blame," says Melissa. "If I had only slowed down during my

pregnancy ... if my blood pressure hadn't shot up. ... We had so many tests run and some therapist seemed to think I babied him or coddled him which I never did. We went to a geneticist who answered so many questions. When I asked my husband's family for their history, they said they had never had anyone with problems—must be from my side.

"After Jacob's diagnosis, I said something about us having a low percentage of having another child with the same disorder and my husband's grandmother suddenly remembered that her sister's daughter had two kids ... both autistic.

"I said, 'Aha!!!'"

Jacob is lucky. He is social and has a good attention span and a positive attitude. He started in a special-needs preschool and has come very far this past year.

Despite all his problems and obvious delays, Melissa had no idea what was wrong with Jacob until a year ago, when he was 3 and finally diagnosed. She looked up his diagnosis on the Internet and discovered that he was "a textbook case." Up until then, no doctor or therapist had made the proper diagnosis. "It was a shock to see how many other parents had children like mine," she says.

Jacob has HS—hyperlexia syndrome.

Did you know?

HS is characterized by a precocious ability to read words, but also by significant difficulty understanding and using verbal language, a significant NLD, and difficulty in reciprocal interaction.

Not officially recognized as a stand-alone disorder, HS, a condition thought to fall within the PDD diagnosis, is a tough syndrome to diagnose. It is usually comorbid or mimics other Alphabet Disorders such as ASD, ADHD, hearing impairment, giftedness, LDs, MR, or behavior, language, motor, and psychological disorders.

The syndrome's most obvious aspect is the child's precocious ability to read well beyond his or her chronological reading-level expectancy. These children are often intensely captivated with letters or numbers, but they could not care less about human interaction and have difficulty in reciprocal personal interactions. They manifest significant deficiencies in understanding verbal language and display a lack of social interaction skills and abilities.

While their auditory and visual memory is formidable, expressive language skills are often compromised and they usually exhibit echolalia (repeating words without comprehension) and reverse pronouns. They manifest many hypersensory symptoms.

Other characteristics found in HS children mimic autism or might be autistic in nature: the need for routine, problems with change and ritualistic behavior, self-stimulation (stimming), inability to initiate conversation, inability to respond to simple who/what/when/where/why questions, fearfulness, thinking literally, lack of subtlety, and selective listening.

Some people suggest that hyperlexia is a separate subgroup of children with PDD, a group of five disorders that includes ASD and AS, two conditions usually confused with hyperlexia. (See the "PDD: Pervasive Developmental Disorder" chapter.)

HS may coexist with autism, but it is different. While HS children have autistic qualities, many eventually emerge from those symptoms. Unlike with autism, hyperlexic children do not necessarily comprehend what they read.

Signs and symptoms

- appears to be deaf
- difficulty answering open-ended what, where, who, and why questions
- difficulty following verbal prompts
- difficulty with abstract concepts
- difficulty with transitions
- enjoys visual mechanical toys
- fascination with the printed word
- good fine motor skills
- intense need to keep routines
- learns quickly
- normal development until 18–24 months, then regression
- rarely initiates conversations
- repeating words or sentences (echolalia)
- reverses pronouns
- ritualistic behavior
- selective listening
- self-stimulatory behavior
- sensory hypersensitivity
- specific, unusual fears
- strong interest in brand logos
- strong interest in trains
- strong visual memory
- strong-willed
- superior motor coordination
- thinks in literal terms
- unusual interest in numbers and letters
- voice might be high-pitched and sing-songish

Cause

There is no known cause for HS, but ASD and LDs have been found in the previous generation of many HS children. As with similar disorders such as PDD and LDs, it is believed that there are genetic, biological, and environmental factors involved.

Diagnosis

After having a physical exam by a pediatrician to rule out other medical problems, the child should be brought to a pediatric neurologist and speech-language therapist, who are usually the specialists most familiar with HS. The doctor or therapist will give the child psychological tests focusing on the visual rather than the verbal if they suspect HS. One popular test is the Visual Decoding and Visual Association Sub-Tests of the Illinois Test of Psycholinguistic Abilities.

To obtain a diagnosis of HS, the child must be developmentally disabled; must have exhibited symptoms prior to five years of age; most likely taught him/herself to read, in a ritualistic and compulsive manner; and has an advanced ability to read words according to their age level.

Treatment

After assessment, the child will embark on a program to develop language skills, comprehension, and expression. The hope is that the diagnosis is made early, so intervention can start as soon as possible.

An IEP is very important, to set up the best modified academic plan. HS children need written and visual models in order to succeed. They need rules and patterned language. When being taught, they require concrete examples as opposed to more abstract explanations. Rote learning is the best way to teach them, but they also must learn how to cope with change, so teaching techniques should be switched around.

Behavioral therapy is also very helpful for these children.

Being around other children will help a hyperlexic child develop much-needed social skills, and as a complementary service, an occupational therapist or other professional should be utilized to build the child's social abilities.

Prognosis

The prognosis for HS children is good, with the proper early intervention. Since they do have advanced reading skills, they have an advantage. The HS child will often emerge from the autistic or autistic-like behaviors as they mature. They might always demonstrate a bit of shyness, aloofness, and remnants of other symptoms, but improvement is often significant. They sometimes become gifted students.

Sources and resources

American Hyperlexia Association (www.hyperlexia.org) **N.B.** This is not an active
  Web site (as of 8/6/04) but still offers valuable information and other contacts
  for this disorder.
American Speech-Language-Hearing Association (ASHA) (www.asha.org)
National Institutes of Health (www.nih.gov)

See "General Resources" for more sources used in this chapter.

HTD

Hypothyroidism Disorder

Terms used in this chapter: CHD (congenital hypothyroidism disorder); GD (Grave's
disease); HT (Hashimoto's thyroiditis); HTD (hypothyroidism disorder); LD (learning
diability); MR (mental retardation)

Did you know?

HTD is characterized by a deficit of thyroid hormone in the blood, due to an underactive
thyroid gland. In children, growth and development are delayed, causing varied symptoms
and inadequate organ stimulation. Hypothyroidism that is present at birth, known as
CHD, can be temporary or permanent. Hypothyroidism can also first appear later in
childhood or later in life.

At birth, delays might be obvious in several ways, from observing larger-than-normal
soft spots on the child's head to an infant's sleepiness and bowel problems. As the newborn
grows, short stature and MR might become dominant signs. Older children might suffer
from dry skin, inability to tolerate cold, and LDs.

A simple blood test will determine if the child has this disorder; a thyroid scan can
be done as well. Catching this problem early is the key to a good prognosis. While early
detection and early intervention are important in aiding developmental skills in other
Alphabet Disorders, with CHD and HTD, it is a matter of life and death—treatment
needs to begin immediately.

When blood testing detects low thyroid levels, the child will be put on daily doses
of synthetic thyroid hormone—easy and life-saving. But, if the hypothyroidism goes
unchecked for two months or longer of the newborn's life, it can lead to permanent
mental and physical developmental problems or even death. Most often it leads to a form
of MR called cretinism. If caught within the first month, however, treatment should be

effective, and symptoms should be reversible. Ninety percent of brain development occurs by the child's first few years, so the earlier parents can intervene with treatment, the better it is long-term for the child.

In the U.S. and other Western nations, newborns are routinely checked for thyroid problems. Other disorders such as DS (Down syndrome) can mask thyroid problems, so a thorough diagnostic exam is encouraged.

Some children will require hormone replacement therapy for the rest of their lives, while others appear to outgrow the disorder, often by age 3.

The thyroid, part of the hormone-secreting endocrine system, is a small, butterfly-shaped gland in the base of the neck, just under the Adam's apple, in front and at either side of the trachea. The hormone the thyroid secretes controls metabolism, the speed of the body's chemical functions. Iodine, the element that is essential to the thyroid, is found in foods such as salt, seafood, milk, yogurt, strawberries, vegetables, meat, eggs, and mozzarella cheese. The thyroid gland also produces the hormone calcitonin, believed to be part of bone metabolism. The bottom line is, if there's not enough thyroid hormone, the body slows down.

In the U.S., CHD occurs in about one in every four thousand newborns. In approximately 10 percent of those babies, the condition is temporary and resolves itself within months or even days.

Signs and symptoms

- anemia
- chronic physical fatigue
- constipation
- delayed bone age
- delayed puberty
- delayed tooth development
- discoloration of skin
- distended abdomen
- droopy eyelids
- dry skin
- elevated cholesterol
- enlarged tongue (macroglossia)
- feeding problems
- high carotene level
- hoarse cry
- inability to tolerate cold
- jaundice
- larger than normal soft spots on skull (fontanelles)
- LDs

- lethargy
- low muscle tone (hypotonia)
- mental fatigue
- puffy, swollen face
- sallow complexion
- short limbs
- slow heart rate
- slow speech
- umbilical hernia (protruding navel)
- weight gain

Cause

There are multiple possible causes for HTD.

About 95 percent of CHD cases are caused by a thyroid gland (or lack of) problem.

In less than 5 percent of cases, CHD is caused by abnormalities in the brain or the pituitary gland.

In 80 percent to 85 percent of cases, babies are born without a thyroid gland and with a gland that is not working properly.

In 10 percent to 15 percent of cases, HTD is caused by inheriting abnormal thyroid hormone production. While both parents have well-functioning thyroids, they are carriers with a one-in-four chance of having a CHD baby.

An abnormally formed or small thyroid might be the cause of later-onset HTD.

A poor-functioning thyroid might not produce enough hormones, despite appearing normal.

Having too little iodine in the body can be another cause.

Side effects of drugs such as Lithium or hyperthyroid medication can result in HTD. However, hypothyroidism caused by drugs is usually reversible.

Autoimmune diseases such as HT, where antibodies attack and wipe out thyroid cells, is another possible cause. HT occurs in up to 1.2 percent of the school-age population. GD in the mother can also set off an autoimmune attack on the thyroid, causing the cells to continuously produce thyroid hormone.

Hyperthyroidism, the opposite of hypothyroidism, appears in children, but very rarely. Hyperthyroidism is the overactivity of the thyroid and of the body's metabolism. In newborns, the most common cause of an overactive thyroid is neonatal GD, which can be life-threatening. It occurs when a mother who has or has had GD transmits her antibodies to the baby's thyroid gland. This is a serious, often fatal, condition for the baby. Signs and symptoms of hyperthyroidism include bulging eyes, diarrhea, difficulty breathing due to enlarged thyroid gland (goiter) pressing on windpipe, fast heartbeat (which can lead to heart failure), high blood pressure, hyperactivity, irritability, MR, nervousness, premature closing of bones in the skull (fontanelles), slowed growth, and vomiting.

Diagnosis

A simple blood test will determine HTD.

Treatment

The treatment for HTD is also simple: early detection, then daily doses of synthetic thyroid hormone.

Prognosis

If not diagnosed shortly after birth, HTD in newborns can be fatal, but with prompt treatment, babies usually recover completely within weeks. But parents should be aware that HD may recur during the first six months or year, before the thyroid is restored to a normal functioning level.

Sources and resources

American Thyroid Association (703-998-8890); (www.thyroid.org)
Thyroid Center of Santa Monica (www.thyroid.com)

L

LD (Learning Disability)

LKS (Landau-Kleffner Syndrome)

LNS (Lesch-Nyhan Syndrome)

LD

Learning Disability

Terms used in this chapter: ADHD (attention-deficit/hyperactivity disorder); IEP (individualized education program); LD (learning disability); LDA (Learning Disabilities Association of America); MR (mental retardation); NIH (National Institutes of Health); NIMH (National Institute of Mental Health)

Did you know?

An LD is a neurological disorder that affects processes in the brain that are involved with understanding spoken or written language, using spoken or written language, coordinating movements, directing attention, and the ability to learn, concentrate, listen, think, read, spell, write, or do math calculations. It's all about how the child's brain is wired—or miswired.

Larry B. Silver, M.D., is a child and adolescent psychiatrist, professor of psychiatry at Georgetown University Medical Center in Washington, D.C., and former acting director of NIMH. He is the author of *The Misunderstood Child*, a must-read for anyone who is interested in finding out about LDs, ADHD, and other Alphabet Disorders. Dr. Silver himself has LDs.

"With learning disabilities, the nervous system is wired a bit differently," he explains. "The brain is not damaged, defective, or retarded. The brain is just having trouble processing information. In some cases, it processes information in a different way than it is supposed to."

The brain wires itself differently in specific areas in the LD child, and in about 50 percent of children with LDs, Dr. Silver says, "the child's genetic code determines that different type of wiring." He says that genetic code is inherited.

Dr. Silver further explains, "There is a lot of research and information available to us, but there is no one real solid answer as to cause for the remaining 50 percent."

Knowledge of the brain, he reminds us, "is just 30 years old."

Fifteen percent of the U.S. population, or one in seven Americans, has some type of LD, according to the NIH.

"Learning disabilities by and large are not easily discernible; they are the hidden disease. And the repercussions are incredible," says Charles Giglio, president of the LDA. "[LDs] are lifelong disorders that are not curable, but they are manageable. The parents' job is to help the child to manage their disabilities and to be successful in their lives."

LDs are problems that affect the brain and its ability to receive, process, analyze, or store information. It can manifest itself in various ways, from how a child reads, speaks,

L

or does math calculations. It can be a spelling disorder or handwriting problem. It can interfere with a child's concentration or memory. It might even seem that the child is hearing- or vision-impaired.

Dr. Silver describes the learning process, the core of the problems LD children face. "First, it is about input. Information is input in the brain from the eyes and ears and other senses. Then, the brain needs to make sense out of this information when it arrives. That process is called integration. The information is then stored until it is later retrieved and used. That is the memory process. And, finally, the brain reacts through some action like talking or the child's using his or her muscles, and that is the output. That is the very basic set of processes that form the basis for disabilities."

Any miswiring or disruption in any aspect of those processes can cause a myriad of disabilities.

It might be said that no two learning disabled children are the same. There are numerous combinations of disorders, signs, and symptoms in LD children, and many children display manifestations that are unique to them. As Dr. Silver says, "There is no 'typical' child with learning disabilities."

But there is one constant: LDs do not have anything to do with a child's intelligence. Rather, they have more to do with how fast a child learns. Children with LDs usually show a deficiency in one area and good skills in another—the child may be a poor reader, but good in math computation, for example. Children with LDs usually have average or above-average intelligence.

"Children with learning disabilities have areas of strengths and areas of average ability along with the weaknesses," says Dr. Silver. "The distinguishing thing is that these children have larger areas of learning weaknesses than most other children. And each child with an LD exhibits their own patterns of those strengths and weaknesses."

Dr. Silver recommends that the child be looked at holistically—the weaknesses *and* the strengths—and not concentrate on just the weaknesses, as is often the case. "When you find the strengths, you can build upon them," he suggests.

"Learning disabilities is a neurologically based spectrum," explains LDA's Giglio. "People are all wired differently. My daughter, for example, is a really good speller, but not good at math. It also affects social skills, and management is needed in social situations. [LDs] have tremendous repercussions in school settings and later in job sites."

The Nemours Foundation, an organization concerned with children's health issues, warns about the impact of bullying on an LD child, reporting that social pressures can add to mental-health issues along with academic failure. LD kids have deficits that can be easily perceived by their peers: misinterpretation of facial expression, body language, or verbal cues that lead to awkward social interactions; impulsivity associated with ADHD; and poor social skills. LD children are more susceptible to teasing and bullying, which, in turn, may lead to alienation or social conflict.

Individuals of all ages with LDs and ADHD are subject to ridicule from peers and are often the objects of the kind of aggressive or mean-spirited behaviors that cause low self-esteem, a frequent byproduct of LDs.

With all the failures and roadblocks they face, LD children often think they are stupid—which they are not. It is important to remember that LD children are not mentally retarded and, in fact, often have impressive intellectual and creative abilities. Indeed, children with LDs who have a constant battle raging with frustration and low self-esteem might find solace in this list of well-known personalities who are all reported to have had or to have LDs: Prime Minister Winston Churchill, Leonardo da Vinci, Walt Disney, Albert Einstein, Whoopi Goldberg, Tommy Hilfiger, General George Patton, Vice President Nelson Rockefeller, and President Woodrow Wilson.

How it is manifested

The problems of an LD child are expansive and can be found in reading, comprehension, retention, writing, mechanics, handwriting, output of language, spelling, punctuation, capitalizations, organizing thoughts, and written language, math-remembering, or applications. It also affects quick-retrieval skills, higher-level problems, organization, writing papers, memory, and organizing thoughts. It affects the executive function of the brain that is involved with analyzing tasks, setting up a plan, and carrying it out in a timely way. That is why so many LD children are disorganized.

The following are the most common types of LDs, most of which are addressed in this volume. For more information, see the specific chapter on the individual LD:

- APD (auditory processing disorder): problems with comprehension, memory, attention, following directions, language, and reading
- Attention deficits, such as ADHD
- Dyscalculia: problems with arithmetic and math concepts
- Dysgraphia: writing disorder
- Dyslexia: a language and reading disability
- Dyspraxia: problems with motor coordination
- Language disorders (aphasia/dysphasia): trouble understanding spoken language; poor reading comprehension, auditory processing problems
- NLD (nonverbal learning disorder): trouble with nonverbal cues, e.g., misinterpreting body language and having poor coordination or being clumsy
- SID (sensory integration disorder): difficulty processing information from the five senses
- Visual Perceptual/Visual Motor Deficit: reverses letters; cannot copy accurately; eyes hurt and itch; loses place when reading; tracking problems when reading; struggles with cutting

L

Cause

There are several possible factors involved in why a child develops an LD, but genetics is a major player.

"About half of these learning disabled children have family members who have the same disability or disabilities," explains Dr. Silver. "The genetic code that they share is rewiring the brain." On the other hand, the fact that LDs run in families does not always point to genetics: the child could be modeling his or her behavior after that of a parent.

For the other half of LD children, it is believed that interference with neuroendocrines, the brain's chemical "messenger" system, might cause the miswiring.

Many factors that occur during pregnancy and involve the mother's illness, including her EDs (eating disorders), could cause LDs in a child. The mother's use of over-the-counter and prescription medications, alcohol, cigarettes, and drugs can affect the child's brain. Lack of prenatal care and premature birth can also contribute to LDs.

Other factors include viral, bacterial, and/or genetic injuries, chronic ear infections, and low birthweight.

Environmental factors include lead poisoning, vaccines, or poor nutrition, all of which can impact the child's brain in terms of LDs.

Diagnosis

Unfortunately, a child's LD might not be diagnosed until he or she begins school. It can be as late as fifth grade, Dr. Silver warns, because the child might not be required to use the weak skill until later grades. If it is missed, a child might develop compensatory skills, and it might go further undiagnosed through his or her teen years or even adulthood. And though adulthood is much later than what is preferred in terms of intervention, it is still important that the LD problem be addressed immediately upon diagnosis.

Complete psychoeducational testing should be administered to the child to determine the exact type and extent of the disabilities. There are many standardized tests as well as medical testing such as diagnostic imaging (e.g., MRIs) that are employed to determine a wide range of LDs. These scores along with clinical observation and family history are added together to provide a proper diagnosis. The types of professionals that usually need to be included in the diagnosis (and treatment) are a pediatrician, pediatric neuropsychiatrist or psychologist, LD-specialist teacher, audiologist (for hearing and auditory-processing problems), speech-language pathologist, occupational therapist, and pediatric neurologist. An optometrist and ophthalmologist should be seen so the child can be checked for vision and visual-processing problems, if these are suspected. Other specialists such as an otolaryngologist (ear, nose, and throat doctor) can be added if the need arises. Observation is important, especially in the youngest of children: how the child pays attention and organizes his or her thoughts; how the child gets a point across or expresses his or her needs, like asking for a toy or letting someone know that he or she wants to eat.

The Wechsler Intelligence Scale for Children (WISC) is often administered, but Dr. Silver warns of potential problems. He says the test, in isolation, "cannot be used, because the scores do not accurately measure the intelligence of a child with learning disabilities." He does say, however, that the subtest scores do help identify areas of weakness. He warns, "Never accept only an IQ score in determining how smart your child might be, especially the 'full-scale' IQ score on its own. You have to see the test in its entirety and look at the individual subtest scores."

According to Dr. Silver, 50 percent of LDs go undiagnosed altogether.

Treatment

There are many academic modifications that can be made to help a student with LDs, which is a recognized educational disability. Under the Individuals with Disabilities Education Act (IDEA), it is *required* that a learning disabled child receive services, and that should be reflected in the child's IEP. (Unfortunately, whether the school accepts the diagnosis is another story.)

The IEP might indicate placement in a special class for LD children or being put in an inclusion class, which is a regular classroom with an additional teacher who will help the LD child on a one-on-one level, as well as help any other child in the class who might need assistance. An LD child can benefit from working with an LD-trained tutor in the home environment or at school, and modifications might be set up for the child to have an extra set of books at home or a note-taker in school. Sometimes the IEP requires special equipment such as an audio amplifier, a tape recorder, calculator, computer, or books on tape.

Speech-language therapists and occupational therapists will help the child communicate in many ways, e.g., in improving vocabulary and the physical ability to speak and in learning conversational rules such as learning to listen and take turns.

Depending on the specific LD(s) the child has, a well-defined IEP should be prepared and dutifully followed. It rests on the shoulders of the already overburdened parent of an LD child to make sure that the modifications are in place and working. Those modifications might include a smaller teacher-to-student ratio in the classroom, the teacher's providing class notes, someone to whom the student can dictate essays, extended testing time with cueing, tests adapted to play to the student's strengths (multiple choice instead of open-ended questions), preferred seating (e.g., in the front of the classroom), the use of a resource room, and study-skills class, among other considerations. The parent should confer with the school district's director of special education because the school district might have services that can help the child that you haven't even thought of. Unfortunately, all this depends on if you have a cooperative special education department.

"Schools want to save money," Dr. Silver warns. "They'll find hundreds of reasons to find nothing wrong [with the child]."

L

Dr. Silver adds, "Now that we know more and more, kids are getting less and less help. [The] 'No Child Left Behind' [initiative] is draining money; money is taken from special education to train children to take tests. That's not the help they need; it's watered down.

"Schools use the 'Wait to Fail Model': they have to have at least two standard years deviated [in order to classify a child as having an LD]. They'll be years behind, and that means the child won't be diagnosed until third grade. They don't see school-based problems as medical problems. Parents have to be educated and be their own advocate."

What special education needs to address, says Dr. Silver, is "accommodation, teaching new strategies, treating it like a lifetime disability, and teaching the child how to adapt."

It is extremely important that the LD be detected early, treated early, and treated correctly. "What you need is habilitation," says Dr. Silver, "not rehabilitation" because it has never been addressed in the first place. It is a matter of learning how to live with the disability successfully.

Prognosis

Although LDs can be treated, and effectively so, they are never cured. They are life-long disorders, which can be compensated for in many ways. Early intervention can make a world of difference to a learning disabled child, but these disabilities are often missed until the child is already exhibiting problems in school. A child's being written off as a "late bloomer" can be the difference between years of suffering or years of success. Early intervention gives the LD child the potential to gain and maintain skills that would otherwise be lost. Citing an NIH study, the "Early Warning Signs of Learning Disabilities" report from the Coordinated Campaign for Learning Disabilities, a public awareness program of the LDA, states that 67 percent of young students who were at risk for reading difficulties became average or above-average readers after receiving help in the early grades.

Also, since LDs—perhaps, the heart of Alphabet Kids—are so intertwined with other disorders or so easily mistaken for other disorders, it is essential to get a proper diagnosis. Often LDs are comorbid or can mimic learning disorders, which are different from learning disabilities. Disorders are abnormal physical, psychological, or developmental conditions, such as MR or autism. Disabilities are the functional results of those conditions—an impairment, such as the inability to process certain sounds or a lack of balance caused by the disorder.

"There are now better and better scientifically based interventions," says Dr. Silver, "and better and better techniques to help these children. The earlier you intervene, the more chance there is of helping these children. When undiagnosed or misdiagnosed, the [child] does not do well socially, psychologically, does not pursue excellence."

Sources and resources

Coordinated Campaign for Learning Disabilities, "Early Warning Signs of Learning
   Disabilities" (1997) (www.readingrockets.org/article/226)
Learning Disabilities Association of America (LDA) (412-341-1515);
   (www.ldaamerica.org)
National Center for Learning Disabilities (888-575-7373); (www.ld.org)
The Nemours Foundation (www.nemours.org)
Schwab Foundation for Learning (800-230-0988); (www.schwablearning.org)
Larry B. Silver, M.D., *The Misunderstood Child: Understanding and Coping with Your Child's
   Learning Disabilities*, 4th ed. (New York: Three Rivers Press, 2006).

See individual LD chapters for more sources, information, and resources.

LKS

Landau-Kleffner Syndrome

Terms used in this chapter: LKS (Landau-Kleffner syndrome)

Did you know?

LKS, or better known in the U.K. as WDS (Worster-Drought syndrome) or acquired aphasia
with epilepsy, is a rare childhood neurological disorder characterized by the sudden or
gradual development of aphasia (the inability to understand or express language) and
abnormal brain activity as determined by an electroencephalogram (EEG). The syndrome
was first introduced in 1957 by William M. Landau, M.D., a neurologist, and Frank R.
Kleffner, Ph.D., a speech-and-language specialist.

   LKS is commonly confused with CDD (childhood disintegrative disorder) and is
considered by some experts to be synonymous with that disorder. LKS affects the parts
of the brain that control comprehension and speech. It is a rare form of epilepsy that only
affects children, causing them to lose their understanding of language. The main epileptic
activity happens during sleep and is usually not obvious to others. Seizures will appear
in the majority of these children within a few weeks of the first signs of the language
difficulty.

   Children with LKS usually develop typically, meeting normal milestones, but then
inexplicably they lose their language skills. (Some children may be aware of their loss
of abilities.) It is between the ages of 5 and 7 years when the disorder usually occurs.
While many of the affected children have seizures, some do not—about one-third of LKS
children will not have seizures.

The disorder is difficult to diagnose and may be misdiagnosed as other Alphabet Disorders such as ASD (autism spectrum disorder), PDD (pervasive developmental disorder), hearing impairment, learning disorders such as dyspraxia, APD (auditory processing disorder), ADHD (attention-deficit/hyperactivity disorder), MR (mental retardation), SM (selective mutism), CS (childhood schizophrenia), or emotional, conduct, and behavioral problems.

Another reason for misdiagnosis is the rarity of the syndrome (although it is believed the prevalence rates are actually higher than reported, because it is often misdiagnosed). In addition, because the child's physical aspect appears relatively normal except for slight movement and coordination problems, LKS slips through the diagnostic cracks.

Signs and symptoms

- aggressiveness
- autistic-type behavior
- behavioral problems
- complete loss of speech and language
- depression
- distress
- hyperactivity
- impaired motor skills
- irritability
- poor attention ability
- seizures while awake and asleep
- sensitivity to sound
- suddenly having difficulty putting thoughts into words (expressive dysphasia)
- suddenly having difficulty understanding what is said (receptive dysphasia)
- uncontrollable muscular movement (hyperkenisia)

Cause

There is no specific known cause for LKS. Some researchers believe it is brain damage due to an autoimmune or inflammatory disease. It is generally believed, however, that it is not inherited.

Diagnosis

An LKS diagnosis is made on clinical findings: doctor's observations, the child's history, and assessment. The core features are a history of normal early development followed by loss of language skills, often in association with mild seizures and behavioral changes. The only real test for LKS is the EEG.

Treatment

Treatment for LKS usually consists of medications, such as anticonvulsants and corticosteroids such as valproate (Depakote), levetiracetam (Keppra), and lamotrigine (Lamictal). Steroids and high doses of antihistamines like diazepam (Valium) given at bedtime have also provided positive responses. While it seems as if some anticonvulsants would make sense in treatment, it has also been shown that they often exacerbate the problem.

Steroids are the main treatment, but they are usually used short term because of the weight gain the child will experience.

Since language problems are the dominant concerns with LKS, speech-language therapy is required and should be started early.

Early intervention is crucial, and the child should be seen by his or her pediatrician, a neurologist, a speech-language pathologist, and a mental-health professional. It is important for the parent to keep accurate developmental and milestone records on the child and bring the child for consistent medical check-ups.

A relatively recent type of epilepsy surgery to prevent seizures—multiple subpial transection—is an often safe, but extreme, last resort in which the pathways of abnormal electrical brain activity are severed by cutting into the cerebral cortex, causing interruptions in fibers that connect neighboring parts of the brain. The operation does not cause any tangential long-term impairment.

Prognosis

The prognosis for children with LKS varies. Some affected children may have a permanent, severe language disorder, while others may regain much of their language abilities (although it may take months or years). In some cases, remission and relapse may occur. The prognosis is improved when the onset of the disorder occurs after age 6 and when speech therapy is started early. Seizures generally disappear by adulthood.

LKS is viewed by some as a spectrum disorder—one in which language is the prime skill affected, but with the impairment of an assorted number of skills. With all these variables, it is problematic to determine a prognosis—it depends on the age of onset, how language has regressed, how long the disorder has been active, and response to treatment.

The epileptic aspect of the disorder typically ends around adolescence, and it is believed that approximately 50 percent of LKS children make a satisfactory recovery. Twenty-five percent have a partial recovery, and an additional 25 percent remain impaired.

L

Sources and resources

American Speech-Language-Hearing Association (ASHA) (800-638-8255);
(www.asha.org)

Epilepsy Foundation (800-EFA-1000 [332-1000]); (www.epilepsyfoundation.org)

National Aphasia Association (800-922-4NAA [4622]); (www.aphasia.org)

National Institute on Deafness and Other Communication Disorders (800-241-1044);
(www.nidcd.nih.gov)

LNS

Lesch-Nyhan Syndrome

Terms used in this chapter: LNDR (Lesch-Nyhan Disease Registry); LNS (Lesch-Nyhan syndrome)

Sound familiar?

Philip Baker's is one of the most inspirational stories in this book. He tells his story in his own words:

I was born January 18, 1971. To my parents, I was just their first-born baby boy.

After coming home from the hospital, I started developing allergies from my formulas. I also started having breathing problems and rashes throughout my whole body. My parents started noticing I wasn't developing like a baby should. For example, I couldn't sit up or hold my head up. I was first diagnosed with cerebral palsy—until I started mutilating my fingers and my lips. I was unable to roll over or grasp anything like a normal child could do. After I started mutilating myself, the doctors sent me to New York Hospital, and I was diagnosed with Lesch-Nyhan syndrome. My parents needed to know more about the disorder, which then led them to meet with Dr. William Nyhan in California, who is a [co-discoverer] of the disease.

He experimented with several drugs which had no effect on me. My disease is an inborn error of purine metabolism in which there are devastating effects on the central nervous system, as well as an increased production of uric acid, which will eventually cause renal failure. I had to have numerous extractions of my baby teeth and adult teeth throughout the years to prevent me from biting my fingers, lips, tongue, and cheeks. I felt the pain, but I could not control my actions. I also bang my legs and my arms, if capable. My parents had to keep me restrained in my wheelchair so that I wouldn't hurt myself. They had to monitor me almost 24 hours a day, which is still going on today.

I had doctors mistreat me thinking that I was mentally retarded. Also, the doctors stitched me without Novocain when I was accidentally hurt, which caused me to scream in agony. The doctors told my mom that [I had] a very rare disease and life expectancy was about until 10 years old. I am now 37 years old and considered to be one of the oldest diagnosed with the disease. The doctors told my parents that I would end up only being retarded and that I would "Eat my body away."

My parents were told to leave me in [the] hospital and to forget about me as if I was never born. My parents paid no mind to this, and they took me home immediately. I understood everything that was going on around me and was hurt by the way people treated me.

Throughout my life, I attended numerous schools and had multiple therapies of which nothing physically helped. I lived in Matheny School and Hospital in New Jersey for five years before moving back home. While there, I created art work, songs, and poems—one of which is published.

Knowing that I am unable to physically take on tasks that I would like to do, I still mentally accomplish my goals. I love to watch most sports such as baseball, basketball, football, etc. I have created my own Web site with the help of my family so that I can share my experiences throughout the world. I have made numerous friends and have given much support to the families of younger children diagnosed with the disease.

I am an honorary fireman of Bayville Fire Company and Sea Cliff Fire Department [in New York]. My dad encouraged me to become who I am today because I wanted to follow in his footsteps. My dad has passed away recently; therefore, it is hard for my mom to do the things she does for me all by herself. I have friends and family who are a great help, and I appreciate what everybody does for me. I have a sister, Amy, and a brother-in-law, Don, who live in Virginia. Amy recently gave birth to their first child, Bella. I am excited about being a great uncle.

I cannot physically type, but I am able to speak, but my speech isn't up to par due to the fact I had all my teeth pulled so I couldn't harm myself. My muscles are not functioning well, but people are able to understand me very well. My mom or my cousin or my aunt type for me as I speak on the Internet. Through the State of New York, I am entitled to twelve hours a day of home care but, because of where we live in Bayville, Long Island, out of the way of everything, no one wants to travel here, so therefore I only get six hours and my mom does the rest, bless her soul.

I enjoy rap, hip-hop, and oldies music, and I love Billy Joel— he is one of my idols. My favorite shows on TV are ER, Deal or No Deal, House, and American Idol. I also watch the news for current affairs. My favorite movies are Forrest Gump, Die Hard, Top Gun, and Blue Lagoon. I love the Mets, Jets, Islanders, and Knicks. I am an all-around sports fan. I love sports! I've been to many, many Met games, hockey games, basketball games, etc.

Just because of my disability, nothing stops me from doing what I enjoy most. As I mentioned before, many people are misdiagnosed with this disease because everyone has different disorders; therefore, most are diagnosed as mentally retarded, which is not right. I will be speaking at local colleges about this disorder I have.

Throughout my life, I had dealt with a lot; and if you don't know me, then you will never know that I am a very successful, smart, and intelligent person. Through all of my challenges, I try to enjoy life as much as possible!

Philip Baker

Philip has LNS—Lesch-Nyman syndrome.

L

Did you know?

LNS is a disease that affects the body's basic genetic code. It is distinguished by neurological problems such as involuntary writhing and spastic movements, speech deficits, involuntary antisocial and aggressive behavior, and kidney problems. The syndrome was identified by Michael Lesch, M.D., and William Leo Nyhan, M.D., Ph.D.

One of the distinguishing symptoms of LNS is involuntary self-mutilation—especially lip and finger biting. If not contained, LNS children might chew off their fingertips and lips. Some children develop the self-injurious behavior as early as 2 years old, while some children might develop these problems later in life in their teenage years. Some don't develop them at all. It is believed that the earlier these behaviors manifest themselves, the more severe the future bad behavior will be.

According to the LNDR, at the New York University School of Medicine:

[LNS children] seem to be completely normal in many of the ways cognitive and intellectual abilities are measured. They have an excellent memory, their emotional life is appropriate, they have good concentration, they are capable of abstract reasoning, they have good self-awareness and are highly social. On the other hand, it is clear they are below expectation in traditional forms of academic ability. Most patients appear to have a specific LD in the areas of math and reading.

Cognitive and intellectual abilities are difficult to assess because of such things as uncoordinated movement, unintelligible speech, deliberate and misleading mistakes during testing, the difficulty of arranging appropriate schooling, monitoring of progress, feedback, etc. All of this has made intellectual measurement a contentious issue among researchers, teachers and parents.

The unusual aspect of the LNS child's self-injurious behavior, compulsive lying, and abuse of others—symptoms found in other diseases, especially PDs (personality disorders)—is that, in the case of LNS, the child is acting counter to what he really wants, according to the LNDR. The LNS child does not want to hurt himself; he does not want to say "no" when asked if he wants to watch his favorite TV show; he does not want to answer the test question incorrectly; he does not want to curse at his favorite caretaker. He is just compelled to do so. It is believed that the child is actually doing the opposite of what he really wants. (He loves ice cream, but says "no," when offered some.) Afterwards, the child feels guilty, sad, and out of control. Many experts, LNS advocates, and LNS patients themselves call this behavior inexplicable.

Because stress often makes all of the LNS behaviors worse, stress-reduction therapy is usually a great benefit to those with LNS.

What further compounds the condition of LNS children is that they are often very social and caring, with good senses of humor and a good ability to assess a social situation, but they are caught up in a body they can't control and, as Philip mentioned, are often viewed as mentally retarded when they are not.

LNS is a disease of boys. Girls are carriers of the gene. They are often asymptomatic, but they do have an increase in uric acid excretion, and some girls may develop symptoms of hyperuricemia, which is high levels of uric acid in the blood and is a cause of gout, a condition that they might manifest when they get older. It's important to detect LNS in asymptomatic girls so they are aware of their condition when they are older and thinking about having children of their own.

How it is manifested

Most LNS children start exhibiting symptoms between 3 and 12 months. Those early symptoms are involved with delayed motor development, most commonly by low muscle tone (hypotonia), involuntary movements, delayed growth, and the child's failure to reach normal milestones for motor skills. Symptoms, especially involuntary movements, become more extreme between 6 and 18 months.

One of the first signs of LNS (as well as other Alphabet Disorders) is that the baby is limp (due to the hypotonia) and unable to raise his head. At 6 months, the child might have an arching of his back. At 9 months, the child is unable to pull himself into a standing position and does not crawl. The LNS child does not walk by 12 months, which is the typical developmental milestone, and by 18 months, the LNS child begins to have involuntary "jerky" and twisting twitches and unusual posturing of the body and limbs.

Some children have symptoms that are related to the overproduction of uric acid, where it seems that there is "orange sand" in the baby's diaper.

Signs and symptoms

- absent or delayed puberty
- aggressiveness, such as hitting and spitting
- biting, gouging, self-injuring body tissue
- central nervous system problems
- compulsion to hurt others
- compulsion to lie
- delayed growth
- facial grimacing
- gout-like arthritis
- head banging
- impaired cognitive function
- impulsiveness
- involuntary cursing (coprolalia)

- involuntary movements of intermediate speeds (choreoathetosis)
- involuntary obscene gestures (copropraxia)
- kidney problems, such as stones
- low muscle tone (hypotonia)
- megaloblastic anemia
- overactive or overresponsive reflexes (hyperreflexia)
- repetitive movements of the arms and legs
- spasticity
- speech that is difficult to understand
- swollen joints
- testicular atrophy
- twisting, writhing, and repetitive movements of body, arms, and legs (dystonia)
- violent movement of the limbs (ballismus)

Cause

LNS is an X-linked recessive, inherited disorder caused by a deficiency of hypoxanthine-guanine phosphoribosyltransferase (HPRT), the enzyme involved with purine (units in RNA and DNA that make up the body's genetic blueprint) metabolism. The LNS gene is passed on to the son by his mother and is present at birth. (There are only two documented cases of a girl having LNS.) In one-third of cases, it occurs by a spontaneous genetic mutation.

LNS is characterized by three major elements: overproduction of uric acid, neurological disabilities, and behavioral problems. LNS affects how the body builds and breaks down purines.

The lack of HPRT causes a build-up of uric acid in all body fluids. This deficiency can result in gout, muscle-control loss, and moderate retardation, which manifest in the child's first year. The high uric levels lead to kidney, central nervous system, and joint problems.

Diagnosis

The definitive diagnosis of LNS is made by analyzing HPRT levels in red blood cells or cultured fibroblasts (a cell that synthesizes and maintains the structural integrity of connective tissue). Other diagnostic tests include serum chemistry, urine chemistry, and skin biopsy (to check for fibroblasts, which would show deficient HGP enzyme).

Genetic testing is suggested for those who might be carriers or those who have LNS in their family history. If a mother is a carrier, there is a 50/50 chance that her son will have the disease and a 50/50 chance that her daughters will be carriers. The disease can be identified prior to birth by culturing amniotic fluid fibroblasts. According to the LNDR, "the disease does not usually stay in families much longer than one or two or perhaps three generations."

Treatment

There is no cure for LNS, but the symptoms can be treated by medications. Allopurinol is considered a required medication in very effectively aiding the renal problems of LNS, because it controls the excessive amounts of uric acid. It is believed that the death rate for LNS has been lowered because of use of this drug. Kidney stones may be treated with surgery or lithotripsy, a procedure where sound waves are used to break up the stones. Valium is one of the most common drugs given to those with LNS because it relaxes the muscles as well as the mental state of the person. The neuroleptic drug Haloperidol has also been used to control some of the behavioral symptoms. Gabapentin, an anticonvulsant drug, and the atypical antipsychotic Risperdal are also used to alleviate LNS symptoms. Sometimes all it takes is some Benadryl at night time, to help the child sleep. Other drugs used to help the neurological symptoms include Carbidopa, Levodopa, and Phenobarbital. After a full-spectrum analysis of your child, your physician will be able to determine what drugs are best.

If the LNS child has severe self-injurious problems with biting, as awful as it sounds, tooth extraction is the accepted treatment, in order to protect the child from further injuring himself, as in Philip Baker's case.

Restraints are an important aspect of LNS care. The best restraint, of course, is one that keeps the LNS child both safe and comfortable. In many cases, the child will inform the caretaker when he feels self-injurious behavior or violent movements will occur and will request the restraints.

Behavior modifications and stress-reduction therapies are also employed for children with LNS.

Prognosis

The National Institute of Neurological Disorders and Stroke reports that the prognosis for those with LNS is "poor," that death is usually due to renal failure in the first or second decade of life, and that living past 40 is rare. But the LNS registry has a somewhat more optimistic take stating that the average lifespan "has a considerable range. With good medical and psychological care the patients can live to be much older."

LNS advocates say the answer to a good life for these children lies in the right caretaker. They suggest that the caretaker should be very familiar with LNS behavior and know that, when a child gives one response, he might really mean the opposite. The caretakers of LNS children need extra patience and physical strength.

L

Sources and resources

Children Living with Inherited Metabolic Diseases (CLIMB) (0800-652-3181; 0845-241-2172); (www.climb.org.uk)

Lesch-Nyhan Disease Registry, New York University School of Medicine (www.lndinfo.org)

National Information Centre for Metabolic Diseases, United Kingdom (climb.org.uk)

The National Institute of Neurological Disorders and Stroke (www.ninds.nih.gov)

Purine Research Society (email: purine@erols.com); (www.purineresearchsociety.org)

M

MCSS (Multiple-Chemical Sensitivities Syndrome)

MD (Muscular Dystrophy)

MR (Mental Retardation)

MSDD (Multisystem Developmental Disorder)

MCSS

Multiple-Chemical Sensitivities Syndrome

Terms used in this chapter: MCSS (multiple-chemical sensitivities syndrome)

Sound familiar?

Peter, 9, and Helen, 7, were typical, healthy children until a deadly mold invaded their California home sixteen months ago. Their mother, Grace, described them prior to their exposure as "healthy, happy, smiling, good color in their faces—typical California surfer kids."

Today they are pale, sickly, and, she says, "lucky to be alive."

In May 2006, the family's washing machine overflowed, and for up to eight hours, their house filled with three inches of water. The company that was hired to fix their home did not do it properly, and the house didn't properly dry. Without the family's knowledge, mold began to grow: Aspergillus, Penicillium, Chaetomium, Stachybotrys, Cladosporium, Alternaria, and Aspergillus versicolor, which is highly carcinogenic. Grace, the children—who were home-schooled—and their seven pets, including dogs and cats, remained in the house not knowing there was a deadly menace growing behind their walls. Grace's husband spent most of his day outside the house at work and was not affected as badly as the rest of the family.

Fans were installed to help dry the house, but instead, the mold was spread throughout by the circulating air. The family suffered a few short, intense blasts as well as long-term, six-week exposure.

"There's a reason people wear HAZMAT suits when they handle this stuff," says Grace. The family did not have such suits.

The first signs that there was serious trouble were frightening. One by one, the family pets began to die. The children began suffering sore throats, were becoming pale, had dark circles under their eyes, and no longer tanned in the sun.

Peter, who was a straight-A student, began to stare into space, losing his attention and focus.

"He was acting autistic," says Grace.

Both children were feeling depressed and stopped wanting to play.

Helen was becoming hypersensitive to light and sounds, especially repetitive ones.

"Something was zapping the zest out of the kids," Grace says.

A remediation team came to the house to investigate and cut the wall open while Grace and the kids stood by watching. They should not have been there—and it should have been contained, which it wasn't.

A few days later, Grace says, "We all had burning chests and were all down for the count."

Helen began losing her voice, which became dry and raspy. "She started sounding like Demi Moore," Grace now jokes. But it is no joke; the child's chronic laryngitis is a symptom of real physical damage.

Within six weeks, the pets died in similar ways to each other, with blood coming out of their mouths.

"I began thinking," Grace recalls. "If this was happening to our pets, what is happening to my 39-pound daughter?"

The family finally moved to a hotel, but even there they had problems. The initial exposure has caused the family to be hypersensitive to everything, and there was mold in the hotel.

"We were diagnosed with reactive airway disease and neurological problems. Peter didn't even have enough strength to blow his nose. The exposure began to affect his brain, and he started losing some functions."

Grace had to learn, on her own, how to detox him.

People began to doubt the family's sanity. "It's common to be mocked when you're suffering like this," says Grace. But she didn't care. Saving her family was more important.

"The worst was that we were just being treated for allergies," Grace says. "That's what they did at the beginning for us."

This has turned into a sixteen-month ordeal. The family is just now hoping that their latest move (their sixteenth) to a dry, arid area in the western U.S. will prove beneficial.

"Listening to doctors almost killed us," says Grace, "by them adding more toxins and mold to our compromised bodies by giving us antibiotics."

Realizing pulmonary doctors and allergists weren't the answer, the family finally began finding help when they visited a neurotoxicologist who noticed little bumps on Peter's hand, which to him indicated mold toxicity. The specialist explained that mold toxins get stored in fatty tissue of the palms.

Grace says that when Peter almost died last Christmas, the family visited Vincent Marinkovich, M.D., a mold exposure pioneer in Redwood City, California. He put them on the road to proper treatment—which was crucial at that point considering that they had found Agent Orange in Peter's urine, according to Grace.

"Most doctors treat you orally," she explains, "but what you need for mold exposure is to be treated internasally, and then [with] oral antifungals."

Now out of money, with absolutely no possessions, they are starting a new life.

"It's sad," says Grace, "because the end result is that the children are not doing great. Any new exposure is setting them back."

Peter and Helen have MCSS—multiple-chemical sensitivities syndrome.

Did you know?

MCSS is a common but only newly discussed condition that is caused by the combination of toxins found in everyday health, cleaning, and household products. These toxins bring on disorders of the nervous system, allergies, asthma, and chemical sensitivities.

The National Institute of Environmental Health Sciences (NIEHS) defines MCSS as a "chronic, recurring disease caused by a person's inability to tolerate an environmental chemical or class of foreign chemicals." The onset of this syndrome can range from gradual environmental intolerance to sensitivity to one traumatic toxic exposure. Although the current popular name for this disorder is MCSS, it is also known in the medical world as

IEI (idiopathic environmental intolerance). MCSS, unfortunately, is becoming more and more widely diagnosed.

Signs and symptoms

- abdominal cramping
- aching joints
- anxiety
- arthritis
- asthma
- balance problems
- burning sensation in chest
- burning throat
- candidiasis
- CFS (chronic fatigue syndrome)
- choking
- coordination problems
- cough
- chronic bronchitis
- chronic low blood sugar (hypoglycemia)
- chronic pelvic pain
- dental amalgam disease
- depression
- diabetes mellitus
- diarrhea
- difficulty concentrating
- discomfort
- dizziness
- dust mite sensitivity
- earache
- fatigue
- fibromyalgia
- food coloring
- headache
- heart palpitations
- heat intolerance
- heightened sensitivity to odors
- hepatitis
- hoarseness (dysphonia)
- IBS (irritable bowel syndrome)

- increased sensory sensitivity: odors, loud noises, bright lights, touch, extremes of heat and cold, and electromagnetic fields
- itchy eyes
- loss of memory
- lung inflammation
- malaise
- mental confusion
- migraine headache
- mucous membrane irritation
- nausea
- numbness
- painful and irregular menstrual cycle
- panic attacks
- pneumonia
- runny nose
- scalp pain
- scratchy throat
- seizures
- sleepiness
- swollen glands
- tingling
- twitching
- upset stomach
- weakness

Cause

The specific cause of MCSS is unknown, although it is believed that it is a gene–environment interaction. What is known is that it is set off by a specific environmental event—the smell or touch of a chemical that affects an organ or multiple organ systems. The response can then be exaggerated or worsened in future encounters with those same stimuli, even if it is presented in much lower doses or by chemical triggers that are unrelated to the initial one.

MCSS ranges from mild discomfort to severe disability and, as some claim, even death. Parts of the scientific and medical communities continue to debate the legitimacy of a MCSS diagnosis, but there is a growing number of scientists, researchers, medical experts, environmentalists, and public-health advocates supported by increased public concern who swear by its validity. In 1995, several U.S. federal agencies formed the Interagency Workgroup on Multiple Chemical Sensitivity to help come up with policy on this growing and controversial disorder.

Diagnosis

MCSS is extremely under- and misdiagnosed because it mimics so many other allergic, physical, and mental disorders. This is a very controversial disorder but one that is attaining more and more respect as the world turns "green," as parents become more attuned to environmental issues that affect our children, and as more holistic and environmental-awareness issues are absorbed by mainstream medicine. As with numerous other Alphabet Disorders, popular advocacy is in the shadow of conventional medicine, which is becoming more sensitive to protecting our children from environmental toxins, especially those found in everyday household items, auto fuels, exhaust fumes, and food additives.

Although there is not a specific official diagnosis for MCSS, there is a consensus on the criteria for a diagnosis, which includes reproducible symptoms with repeated (chemical) exposures; the condition is chronic; low levels of exposure (lower than previously or commonly tolerated) result in manifestations of the syndrome (i.e., increased sensitivity); the symptoms improve or resolve completely when the triggering chemicals are removed; responses often occur to multiple chemically unrelated substances; and symptoms affect multiple organs.

Some items that cause MCSS are aerosols, after-shave lotion, air fresheners, asphalt pavement, carpeting, chalk, cigar and cigarette smoke, cleaning products, clothes from the cleaners, cologne, cosmetics, deodorant, diesel exhaust and fuel, dry-cleaning fluid, floor cleaner, furniture polish, gasoline exhaust, glue, hair products, hairspray, household cleaners, insect repellant, lacquer, laundry detergent, make-up, mold, nail polish and remover, paint, paint thinner, perfumes in health and beauty aids, pesticides, preservatives in food, shampoos, shellac, soap, tar fumes, varnish, and water-proofing products. These items are used in many settings as are other toxins that are often used in schools and playgrounds. The non-profit organization Grassroots Environmental Education is a valuable resource for information on this topic.

Treatment

Getting the proper diagnosis and singling out the exact causes for the MCSS attack is the best way to begin an effective treatment. Parents should start the diagnosis process with the child's pediatrician who will rule out other medical conditions. The pediatrician will refer you to an allergist, preferably an environmental allergist—one who is familiar with MCSS. Many conventional doctors might miss the MCSS diagnosis and, therefore, not know how to properly treat the MCSS symptoms, but a natural or holistic doctor or a doctor who specializes in environmental illnesses might best provide the child with the proper therapies. On the other hand, parents should be careful that a holistic or MCSS-friendly doctor doesn't diagnose MCSS when there are other underlying problems.

Eliminating many of these potential stressors and toxins is not a bad idea, even if your child doesn't have MCSS, and many parents attest to a remarkable lifesaving change in their child once the problem is eliminated from the environment, so there is great hope.

Prognosis

The outlook for children with MCSS is difficult to gauge because of all the sensitivities the child develops. If the case is serious enough, it can be life-threatening; but, in many cases, removing the stressor and "greening up" the child's environment will be sufficient.

Sources and resources

Chemical Injury Information Network (CIIN) (www.ciin.org)

Grassroots Environmental Education (516-883-0887); (www.grassrootsinfo.org)

The Interagency Workgroup on Multiple Chemical Sensitivity, "A Report on Multiple Chemical Sensitivity," predecisional draft, August 24, 1998 (http://health.gov/environment/mcs/index.htm)

MCS America (www.mcs-america.org)

MCS International (www.mcs-international.org)

MCS Survivors (www.mcsurvivors.com)

The National Institute of Environmental Health Sciences (NIEHS) (www.niehs.nih.gov)

The Toxic Times (www.toxic-times.com)

MD

Muscular Dystrophy

Terms used in this chapter: BMD (Becker muscular dystrophy); DMD (Duchenne muscular dystrophy); FMD (facioscapulohumeral muscular dystrophy); LD (learning disability); LGMD (limb-girdle muscular dystrophy); MD (muscular dystrophy); MMD (myotonic muscular dystrophy)

Did you know?

What is commonly called MD is actually a group of more than thirty genetic diseases—actually muscular *dystrophies*—characterized by the progressive weakness and degeneration of the skeletal muscles that control movement. It primarily affects voluntary muscles, and most forms of MD affect the heart muscle. In MD's later stages, fat and connective tissue often replace muscle fibers, as in the case of enlarged calf muscles found in MD children.

The most common types of MD appear to be due to a genetic deficiency, and there is a wide range of onset, types of muscles affected, severity of the disease, and the ways in which it is inherited.

A large number of children with MD have normal milestones in their first few years, but there are telltale signs when MD begins to go into effect. A parent will notice the child is beginning to have difficulty walking—the child may fall, exhibit an unusual gait, toe-walk, and have difficulty walking stairs. A child's failed attempt to push things like a wagon or to sit up might also prove to be signs of impending MD.

How it is manifested

These are the most common forms of MD:

DMD is the most common of all the muscular dystrophies. Mostly affecting boys, it is caused by the lack of dystrophin, a protein involved in preserving the well-being of muscles. The onset age is between 3 and 5 years old with a rapid progression. By age 12, the boys cannot walk and are most likely in wheelchairs; they are soon unable to breathe on their own, requiring a respirator. Girls have a 50 percent chance of being born carriers, with no symptoms. DMD is found in one in 3,500 boys.

BMD is very similar to DMD, but BMD children do have dystrophin—just not enough or it is defective. This form of MD affects approximately one in 30,000 boys. Symptoms usually manifest during the teen years and then follow the DMD pattern. Muscle weakness first begins in the pelvic muscles and then moves into the shoulders, back, and arms. Many BMD children lead fairly normal and active lives.

MMD, also known as SD (Steinert's disease), is known as the "adult" form; but, in reality, in 50 percent of cases, it is diagnosed in children under 20. The symptoms include myotonia (in which the muscles have trouble relaxing once they contract), muscle weakness, and muscle shrinkage. Cataracts and heart problems are also associated with MMD.

FMD does not affect the child until the teenage years. The muscles of the face, arms, legs, shoulders, and chest begin to get progressively weaker. The child can have a mild case or can be fully disabled by FMD. The child with FMD is unable to close his eyes, whistle, or puff out his cheeks. The shoulder and back muscles gradually become weak, and those who are affected have difficulty lifting objects or raising their hands overhead. Over time, the legs and pelvic muscles also may lose strength.

LGMD affects boys and girls equally. Typically, symptoms begin when the child is between 8 and 15 years old. This form of MD progresses slowly, affecting the pelvic, shoulder, and back muscles. The severity of muscle weakness varies from child to child. Some kids develop only mild weakness, while others develop severe disabilities. As adults, LGMD sufferers need a wheelchair to get around.

Signs and symptoms

- cardiac arrhythmias
- cataracts
- cognitive impairment
- constipation
- curvature of the spine (scoliosis)
- diarrhea
- difficulty breathing in infancy
- difficulty rising from a lying or sitting position
- difficulty running
- difficulty sucking and swallowing in infancy
- dizziness
- drooping eyelids (oculopharyngeal muscular dystrophy)
- enlarged calf muscles and calf pain
- fainting
- fatigue
- frequent falls
- gonadal atrophy
- inability to push items such as a wagon
- inability to relax muscles at will (myotonia)
- joint deformities
- lack of concentration
- mild diabetes
- mild MR, in some cases
- muscular weakness in shoulders, back, arms, and legs
- often have normal intelligence, but, in DMD, one-third have LDs
- respiratory problems
- sleep problems
- stiffness of the spine
- stumbling
- toe walking
- waddles when walking

Diagnosis

A doctor might first suspect MD because of muscular weakness. Tests can be administered to determine if the child has MD and what type of MD the child has. The child will be checked for genetic abnormalities, and his or her blood will be checked for certain enzymes. One such blood test measures the levels of serum creatine kinase, an enzyme that is released when muscle fibers deteriorate.

A muscle biopsy might be performed to determine the level of dystrophin and to determine the extent of muscle deterioration.

Other tests include electromyography (EMG), in which a thin-needle electrode is inserted through the child's skin into the muscle to measure electrical activity as the child relaxes and tightens his or her muscles; and the noninvasive ultrasonography, or ultrasound, in which high-frequency sound waves produce images of the inner body.

Treatment

There is no known treatment that cures or reverses MD. There are treatments, however, that help address the symptoms. Those treatments include respiratory, physical, occupational, and speech-language therapy, and assistive orthopedic appliances. There are pharmaceutical therapies, including corticosteroids that help slow the progression of muscle degeneration; immunosuppressants and antibiotics that help to combat respiratory infections; and anticonvulsants to help with seizures. Surgery is also used to correct orthopedic abnormalities, such as tendon-release surgery and spinal fusion to correct severe scoliosis. Respirators are used to help ease breathing difficulties, and pacemakers are inserted for heart problems. The use of hot baths (hydrotherapy) can help maintain range of motion in joints.

If your child is diagnosed with MD, a team of medical specialists will work with you and your family. That team may include a pediatric neurologist, orthopedist, pulmonologist, physical therapist, occupational therapist, pediatric cardiologist, registered dietician or nutritionist, and perhaps a social worker.

MD is often degenerative, so children may pass through different stages as the disease progresses and require different kinds of treatment. During the early stages, physical therapy and bracing of the joints (and the steroid prednisone in the case of DMD) are the usual courses of action. In the case of prednisone, parents should discuss its use in depth with all of the child's doctors because this drug has some serious side effects, along with the positive effects it might provide. During the later stages of MD, doctors may add assistive devices such as ventilators to help the child breathe and wheelchairs and robotics to help with daily activities. For MMD, the drugs of choice are Mexitil, Dilantin, Phenytek, Tegretol, Carbatrol, quinine, Procanbid, and Pronestyl. They are all used to treat the delayed muscle relaxation that occurs in this form of MD. Discuss all medications with your doctor before administering them to your child.

The physical therapist is a necessity for an MD child. Through exercise, the therapist helps maintain the child's joint flexibility and muscle strength. It is believed that the right kind of bracing can lengthen the period that an MD child can walk independently.

There is a bright light in terms of treating DMD, and that is the use of tamoxifen, the drug best known for fighting breast cancer. In tests, the use of the drug has shown increased muscle strength in mice. This research is hopeful because it is the first that indicates that the biochemistry of MD children might be corrected, improving survival and prognosis.

Prognosis

The outcome of MD depends on the severity and type of the disorder. Some MD children die in infancy, while others live well through adulthood with very few problems; there are many different manifestations of symptoms in between. Sometimes the progress of the disease is slow, while, at other times, there is a rapid progression toward muscle degeneration and inability to walk or function. The good news is that there is a vast amount of research going on in this field.

Sources and resources

Facioscapulohumeral Muscular Dystrophy (FSHD) Society (781-860-0501);
   (www.fshsociety.org)
Federation to Eradicate Duchenne (703-683-7500); (www.duchennemd.org)
International Myotonic Dystrophy Organization (866-679-7954);
   (www.myotonicdystrophy.org)
Muscular Dystrophy Association (800-344-4863); (www.mda.org)
Muscular Dystrophy Canada (866-MUSCLE8); (www.muscle.ca)
Muscular Dystrophy Family Foundation (800-544-1213); (www.mdff.org)
Parent Project Muscular Dystrophy (PPMD); (800-714-KIDS [5437]);
   (www.parentprojectmd.org)

MR

Mental Retardation

Terms used in this chapter: CHT (congenital hypothyroidism); IEP (individualized education program); IFSP (individualized family services plan); MR (mental retardation); NIH (National Institutes of Health); PKU (phenylketonuria)

Did you know?

MR, the most common developmental disorder, is diagnosed when a child has limits in mental functioning that causes him or her to learn and develop more slowly than normal. Please see the introduction for an explanation of terminology between the U.S. and U.K.—in the U.K., MR is known as "learning disability." The general term used in this book will be MR.

Mentally retarded children have impairment of communication skills, social skills, and the ability to take care of themselves. The MR child will take longer to develop developmental milestones such as walking, talking, eating, dressing, grooming, and toileting skills. The child's cognitive skills will also be impaired. These children will learn and develop most of the skills, but there will be a delay.

There is a wide spectrum in MR. In some children, delays might not even be obvious, and there will never be an MR diagnosis. In other children, the disability is profound.

These children do not usually regress, but instead, with the right therapies, they progress.

According to The Arc, an organization of and for people with intellectual and developmental disabilities, as many as three out of every one hundred people in the U.S. have some level of MR.

Onset of MR can occur before birth, at birth, or during childhood years, anytime before the age of 18. It can be caused by a genetic defect, problem in the brain, an illness, or an injury; but, in all but 25 percent of cases, the cause is not known, according to the NIH.

Signs and symptoms

- decreased learning ability
- delays with crawling
- delays with sitting up
- difficulty comprehending social rules
- difficulty solving problems
- difficulty with concepts like making change and telling time
- does not comprehend consequences
- failure to meet intellectual developmental markers
- gullibility
- inability to meet demands of school
- infantile behavior
- jaundice
- lack of curiosity
- language and speech delays
- poor memory
- poor motor skills
- poor pragmatic skills
- poor self-help skills such as personal grooming and hygiene
- problems with logical thinking
- quiet disposition
- walks later than peers do

Cause

There are several causes of MR. These are the main ones:

- **unexplained:** largest percentage of cases
- **trauma before and after birth:** intracranial hemorrhage before or after birth; lack of oxygen to the brain before, during, or after birth; severe head injury; SBS (shaken baby syndrome)
- **infections present at birth or occurring after birth:** congenital rubella, meningitis, congenital CMV (cytomegalovirus), encephalitis, congenital toxoplasmosis, listeriosis, HIV infection
- **chromosomal abnormalities:** errors of chromosome numbers as in DS (Down syndrome); defects in the chromosome or chromosomal inheritance as in FXS (fragile X syndrome), AS (Angelman syndrome), and PWS (Prader-Willi syndrome); chromosomal translocations; chromosome deletions as in CDCS (cri du chat syndrome)
- **genetic abnormalities and inherited metabolic disorders:** galactosemia caused by lack of liver enzyme, TSD (Tay-Sachs disease), PKU, HS (Hunter syndrome), HS (Hurler syndrome), SFS (Sanfilippo syndrome), ZS (Zellweger syndrome), MCLD (metachromatic leukodystrophy), ALD (adrenoleukodystrophy), LNS (Lesch-Nyhan syndrome), RS (Rett's syndrome), and tuberous sclerosis
- **metabolic abnormalities:** Reye's syndrome, CHT, hypoglycemia, poorly regulated diabetes mellitus
- **toxic abnormalities:** intrauterine exposure to alcohol, cocaine, amphetamines, and other drugs; methylmercury poisoning; lead poisoning
- **nutritional problems:** malnutrition
- **environmental problems:** poverty, low socioeconomic status, deprivation syndrome

Jaundice can be another comorbid condition with MR. Many newborns display a yellow pigment (bilirubin), which can be normal; but if there is a build-up of that pigment, the baby's brain can be damaged, causing kernicterus.

Diagnosis

There are two main facets of an MR diagnosis: the child's cognitive abilities, which is his or her intellectual functioning ability to cope with everyday life (from the ability to gather knowledge to understanding and working out problems with that knowledge), and their adaptive skills, how they take care of themselves and respond to the world around them. MR is often diagnosed when the child does not reach his or her milestones.

MR is usually diagnosed when the child has an IQ test score below 70.

IQ test scores are read this way: the average IQ score is 85–115; borderline, 70–84; mild mental retardation, 55–69; moderate MR, 40–54; severe MR, 25–39; and profound, lower than 25. It is extremely important to know that a child who is not MR could score low on an IQ test for many reasons, ranging from LDs (learning disabilities) to ADHD (attention-deficit/hyperactivity disorder) to behavioral disorders.

A simple blood test can determine many of the problems that cause MR. If the child is treated early enough, as in the case of CHT, he or she has a good chance of being spared MR. There are also developmental screening and adaptive skills tests.

Treatment

Early intervention does not necessarily mean starting therapy after the child's birth—a lot can be done prenatally. Women with PKU, for example, should follow a special diet while pregnant. Of course, expectant mothers should refrain from alcohol or other substance abuse while pregnant.

There is no cure for MR, but there are many therapies and treatments that can help build up skills. Early intervention programs are available for children 3 years old and younger. An IFSP covers the ages of birth through 3 years, in order to obtain needed services. When the child attends school, an IEP will be created to service the child's needs in an academic setting. There are many educational and social services for mentally retarded children, and there is much information available from organizations that service these children and for the individual disorders that might be associated with MR.

Depending on the severity of the retardation, a child can be provided with a wide array of accommodations, ranging from slight accommodations and services in school to placement in a residential program.

Parents should become familiar with the numerous organizations dedicated to issues surrounding MR and speak with a developmental pediatrician to determine the best course of therapy and the best academic setting for their child. Therapies that can help include speech-language, physical, occupational, social skills, music, psychological, behavioral, sensory integration, and cognitive-skills-building therapy.

Prognosis

The largest percentage of people with MR (87 percent, according to The Arc) have a mild version of the disorder. Indeed, some might not ever know they have the condition since they might never have been diagnosed with the disorder due to their slight symptoms. Children with mild MR can be successful in school and in social situations; and with the proper encouragement and therapies, as adults, they can often live independent lives. For these children, there are many programs in school, for which the state in which the child lives is responsible.

For those with more severe MR, the remaining 13 percent with IQs lower than 50, there is hope as well, as new types of therapies are incorporated into more modern and progressive group homes and institutions.

Sources and resources

American Association on Intellectual and Developmental Disabilities (formerly the American Association on Mental Retardation, AAMR) (800-424-3688); (www.aaidd.org)

The Arc of the United States (800-433-5255); (www.thearc.org)

Division on Developmental Disabilities, The Council for Exceptional Children (888-232-7733); (www.dddcec.org)

National Center on Birth Defects and Developmental Disabilities/CDC (www.cdc.gov/ncbddd)

MSDD

Multisystem Developmental Disorder

Terms used in this chapter: ADHD (attention-deficit/hyperactivity disorder); APD (auditory processing disorder); AS (Asperger syndrome); ASD (autism spectrum disorder); LD (learning disability); MSDD (multisystem developmental disorder); NLD (nonverbal learning disorder); PDD (pervasive developmental disorder); PDD–NOS (pervasive developmental disorder–not otherwise specified); SID (sensory integration disorder)

Sound familiar?

Bruce is 11 years old. He has all the distinctive traits of Asperger syndrome (on the high functioning end of the autism spectrum)—he's a little professor who will lecture anyone on sharks or bugs—and he has taught several adult experts a thing or two about the subjects with which he is obsessed.

But that's not all Bruce has to deal with. He also has many social problems, not knowing how to interact properly with others. Along with his autism-spectrum-disorder symptoms and a diagnosed nonverbal learning disorder, he is also labeled with social anxiety, dyscalculia (math learning disability), dyslexia (reading learning disability), severe visual-motor perception problems, and gross motor dysfunction. He takes occupational, speech, and physical therapy for these and other disorders including dysgraphia (writing learning disability), stuttering, sensory integration disorder, general anxiety disorder, insomnia, attention-deficit/hyperactivity disorder, auditory processing disorder, multiple phobias, and possibly as-of-yet undiagnosed Tourette syndrome, considering the tics he has. According to a simple count, that would be AS, ASD, NLD, SAD, LDs, VPD, GMD, SID, GAD, ADHD, APD, and possibly TS—talk about an Alphabet Kid.

Is Bruce overdiagnosed, or is he the perfect example of how all these Alphabet Disorders are comorbid and part of a spectrum?

Bruce's mother, Michelle, who blogs about her son's condition, thinks that he will ultimately be diagnosed with "very high-functioning Asperger's."

Going from doctor to doctor for diagnoses over the years has been frustrating for Michelle, but recently Bruce was diagnosed at his local autism center. Michelle felt that the very cold and detached evaluation she received there was just a catch-all diagnosis, one given without much thought, He was diagnosed with MSDD, which is what it sounds like after listening to Bruce's shopping list of diagnoses he has collected over the years.

Michelle says that the combination of comorbid disorders that Bruce has, MSDD, "will one day be considered a subset population of the PDD–NOS diagnosis. Currently it's a 'we're-not-sure-what-exactly-is-going-on' waste-pail diagnosis for kids with 'autistic tendencies' who do not meet full criteria for the other spectrum diagnoses."

Bruce's younger brother, Jack, has been diagnosed with an autoimmune disorder called Hyper IgE syndrome or Job's Syndrome (JS). He has some of the same personality/learning traits as Bruce as well.

"I am of the belief that there is a strong genetic component to both of these syndromes and that both appear to some degree in me and in the rest of my family, as well," says Michelle. "Doctors, thus far, have been reluctant to link the two, however."

Michelle is one of those mothers who says she'll talk about her child's disorder to anyone and everyone, from the moms in school to "the grumpy lady on line" to whom she feels she must explain away Bruce's behavior, which can range, she says, from "belligerent to pedantic." Michelle will admit that she is "obsessed" with Bruce's concurrent conditions, and it has become the center of all her attention. Some people might think she's overdoing it, but those are probably parents with typically developing children, she says.

All Michelle wants is for her children to lead successful, happy lives. And to help them on that road, she has begun home-schooling them.

For the time being, Bruce has been diagnosed with MSDD—multisystem developmental disorder.

Did you know?

The *Diagnostic Classification of Mental Health and Developmental Disorders of Infancy and Early Childhood* introduced the diagnostic category of MSDD (multisystem developmental disorder) to classify and describe children who were suffering from a variety of Alphabet Disorders—children who manifested a wide variety of communication, social, and sensory-processing symptoms that were previously misdiagnosed or thrown into some disorder's NOS (not otherwise specified) classification, especially PDDs. For a long time, many doctors diagnosed MSDD when they suspected CBPD (childhood borderline personality disorder) or, as in more recent cases, when they were not ready to diagnose autism or PDD. But now, because of the surge of prevalence of interconnected Alphabet-Disorder symptoms, that old diagnosis of MSDD is enjoying a resurgence and many children classified with other disorders, such as PDD–NOS, are now receiving the MSDD diagnosis.

Sometimes MSDD and PDD/autism are confused, but they are different disorders. One of the aspects that differentiates the two is good news for MSDD children—they have a better prognosis for being successfully treated. They have less severe and long-lasting cognitive developmental delays than autistic children who demonstrate more ritualistic and repetitive behaviors than MSDD children. That said, the two disorders appear very similar because they share so many characteristics, as MSDD also shares with APD, OCD (obsessive-compulsive disorder), NLD, and LDs.

Signs and symptoms

- abnormal sensory responses: smells, sounds, tastes, textures, noise, movement, temperature, and other bodily sensations
- attention problems
- autistic characteristics, especially very-high functioning Asperger's traits
- aversion to touch
- clumsiness
- communication-development impairment
- coordination problems
- disinterest in social interaction
- emotional outbursts
- focus on narrow interests (perseveration)
- food issues—obsessions and refusals
- LDs
- obsessions and rituals
- organizational problems
- pragmatic speech problems
- receptive speech problems
- self-stimulation (stimming), such as spinning, hand flapping, etc.
- sleep disturbances
- tantrums
- toe walking

Cause

Considering the multisystem aspect of MSDD, there is no known cause, although it is believed, as with most other Alphabet Disorders, that it is a combination of genetic, biological, and environmental factors that can affect a predisposed child.

Diagnosis

The child should first see his or her pediatrician to rule out any undiagnosed medical conditions, after which the doctor may send the child to a pediatric neurologist for further testing. There is no one diagnostic test for MSDD, but standardized developmental and psychological tests can help provide answers, along with a detailed account of the child's history. Depending on the symptoms, the child might then be referred to other specialists including an audiologist, ophthalmologist, occupational therapist, and/or speech-language pathologist. Often autism centers have specialists on board who are familiar with MSDD.

Treatment

As with its sister disorders autism, SID, and PDD, there are many similar types of therapies that are employed for the MSDD child.

Sensory-integration therapy is one of the most common and effective therapies for MSDD. Since so many of the MSDD issues are related to sensory disturbances, activities are employed to sensitize or desensitize the child by such techniques as brushing, massage, and trampolining or swinging.

Behavioral therapy—or, more specifically, cognitive behavioral therapy (CBT)—is important in helping to replace unwanted behaviors with more positive ones. Speech and language therapy is also essential. Occupational therapy helps the child with his or her everyday skills and with social and pragmatic issues. An audiologist should be able to help the child with auditory processing concerns.

Children with symptoms of several Alphabet Disorders that have no distinct borders are the ones who need the most parental vigilance. The parents of MSDD children must remain aggressive advocates in their children's health care and social and academic life. These are the parents, like Michelle, who, as she says, can easily become overwhelmed and single-mindedly obsessed with their multisymptomed children.

You know your child, and you will develop a gut feeling of what makes sense regarding your child and what doesn't. These types of disorders (MSDD and PDD–NOS, and even LDs) are often misdiagnosed or not diagnosed at all. Multiply the various symptoms that can be present in MSDD and note how many of them mirror other disorders, and you'll see how difficult the MSDD diagnosis is—or how simple.

Parents of MSDD children should become involved with an advocacy group for moral support to fight for the proper medical, therapeutic, and academic services for their child. It is well to keep in mind that, when many of the other, now-established disabilities were not officially recognized, the children with those disorders fell through the cracks. ADHD and autism were once discounted, but they are now official diagnoses and ones that school districts often address.

Many parents are being forced to go along with an incorrect diagnosis just to get their child needed services. So, while medical experts are still debating PDD–NOS, APD, and MSDD, and as those "umbrella" disorders are becoming more clearly defined (MSDD is now being taught in early-childhood special-education courses), parents need to determine what their child needs and get the child the services that are required for a full, rich, successful, and productive life.

Sources and resources

Diagnostic Classification of Mental Health and Developmental Disorders of Infancy and Early Childhood (Washington, D.C.: 1999)

See the "ASD: Autism Spectrum Disorder," "LD: Learning Disability," and "PDD: Pervasive Developmental Disorder" chapters, as well as "General Resources," for more sources used in this chapter.

N

NLD (Nonverbal Learning Disorder)

NLD

Nonverbal Learning Disorder

Terms used in this chapter: AS (Asperger syndrome); *DSM* (*Diagnostic and Statistical Manual of Mental Disorders*); *ICD* (*International Classification of Diseases*); LD (learning disability); NLD (nonverbal learning disorder); PDD (pervasive developmental disorder)

Sound familiar?

Pia Savage is a successful, popular blogger ("Courting Destiny"), who lives in Manhattan. This is her story:

My breathing was shallow. I couldn't catch my breath. I couldn't stop moving, playing with my hair or tearing it out. I was 17 and in the grip of a panic attack. I was used to them. I had my first one in second grade when I waited in line during notebook inspection day. The long wait ended with my teacher laughingly making a public example of my notebook, which was filled with illegible chicken scratch and was completely disorganized.

Laughing, they were always laughing. My teacher laughed when he threw me out of driver's education and told everybody I came to school stoned. It wasn't true. I was humiliated. I was just ... different, I couldn't write legibly, stay organized, walk straight, and I couldn't learn the simple ten-two hands-on-steering-wheel position. Those were my failures.

In fourth grade I was unable to learn many subjects despite having a very high IQ. I was physically awkward. I couldn't run. I began acting out. NYU Medical Center gave me every test. The tests were hell and there wasn't a diagnosis. Doctors and teachers said that I was lazy: nobody could be so bright yet so stupid. I became used to teachers sighing and telling the class how I didn't try when I had been up for nights working. By 12, I felt like I deserved nothing. There was something off about me. I was cold. I looked at the world from a sea of hair, and looked nobody in the eye. Everybody had to hate me. I was the most unpopular girl in the world. Even my dentist told me I was odd—he couldn't believe I was unable to floss.

When I was a teenager, a psychiatrist put me on Thorazine. I spent the entire week fending off sleep. He had no idea what was wrong with me but insisted I needed this drug. I took myself off it. I would rather be my awkward self—clumsy, constantly playing with my hair or pulling it out, and "acting weird"—than be a zombie. My body was always in motion; I looked nervous, twitchy. I bumped into things and tripped. I still put shoes on the wrong foot. I felt physically anxious, and that made me mentally anxious. It affected the way I spoke; there were times I couldn't get words out, let alone give a whole speech in front of a class. I did begin to walk and talk at a very early age. It was all downhill from there. At 13 months I had pneumonia. Maybe that's what did it.

I tried explaining to doctors I couldn't see space properly. I have no spatial perception. That translated into "You are spacey." I stopped trying to explain.

Teachers constantly told me to try harder, and they made fun of me. Some would encourage kids to continue making fun. I would never fight back or defend myself in any manner. I didn't know how to react properly, so I didn't react at all. I thought they had the right to tell lies about me. The only real difference is that I'm an instinctive learner. If it weren't for that, I would have failed junior and senior high school, since I didn't learn anything in school.

Angry, I was always angry. The only people I felt comfortable yelling at were my parents. They never laughed at me.

I was doomed to a life of being laughed at and misunderstood by teachers, doctors, and kids. But then I grew up and weird became cool.

Pia has NLD—nonverbal learning disorder.

Did you know?

It is believed that more than 65 percent of all communication is conveyed nonverbally.

NLD (sometimes referred to as nonverbal learning disability) is a neurophysiological condition that results in both deficits and strengths in a child's development in regard to cognition, intuitive thinking, organization skills, processing, and visual-spatial skills.

There are four main types of nonverbal learning disorder:

- motor: poor coordination, balance, and fine motor skills
- sensory: auditory, tactile, etc.
- social: inability to comprehend nonverbal communication, difficulty with change or new situations, poor social interactions and skills
- visual-spatial-organizational: poor spatial perceptions, relations, and visual recall

NLD, a subtype of LDs, can be debilitating, but it is not always recognized or understood by some school districts and medical professionals to be a separate and distinct disorder. This can be frustrating to a parent whose child exhibits the distinct signs of this problem but does not fit the criteria of other disorders such as ASD (autism spectrum disorder), PDD, and AS, to which NLD symptoms are often ascribed. NLD children often show strong auditory retention and sometimes display above-average intelligence or great knowledge in one particular subject, similar to the "little professor" syndrome characterized by AS.

On their own, school districts might not accept NLD as a diagnosis that will allow the child to receive the services he or she needs; but when there is an obvious discrepancy between IQ and performance, the child should receive those services. The question is how to provide services to the children with NLD who fall between the cracks. The answer, unfortunately, is that some parents turn to incorrect officially accepted diagnoses such as ADHD or PDD to gain those services. Whatever the case, parents of an NLD child will have to adopt an advocacy role and fight for every service they can get, whether they themselves take on the school district or they bring aboard an advocacy lawyer. The bottom line is that, no matter what it is called or when the *DSM* or *ICD* will officially recognize NLD, these children need services and should not be left untreated.

Byron P. Rourke, Ph.D., FRSC, of the Department of Psychology, University of Windsor, Ontario, Canada, is an internationally respected expert in the field of NLDs. He has proposed his own *ICD* definition of NLD. He refers those interested in NLDs to his Web site, www.nld-bprourke.ca, where this description can be found:

The syndrome of Nonverbal Learning Disabilities [NLD] is characterized by significant primary deficits in some dimensions of tactile perception, visual perception, and complex psychomotor skills, and in dealing with novel circumstances. These primary deficits lead to secondary deficits in tactile and visual attention and to significant limitations in exploratory behavior. In turn, there are tertiary deficits in tactile and visual memory and in concept-formation, problem-solving, and hypothesis-testing skills. Finally, these deficits lead to significant difficulties in the content (meaning) and function (pragmatics) dimensions of language.

In contrast, neuropsychological assets are evident in most areas of auditory perception, auditory attention, and auditory memory, especially for verbal material. Simple motor skills are most often well developed, as are rote verbal memory, language form, amount of verbal associations, and language output.

This mix of neuropsychological assets and deficits eventuates in some formal learning (e.g., academic) assets, such as single-word reading and spelling. It also increases the likelihood of significant difficulties in other aspects of formal learning (e.g., arithmetic, science) and informal learning (e.g., as transpires during play and other social situations). Psychosocial deficits, primarily of the externalized variety, often are evident early in development; psychosocial disturbances, primarily of the internalized variety, are usually evident by late childhood and adolescence and into adulthood.

Signs and symptoms

NLD is often characterized by both deficits and strengths.

- anxiety
- better auditory processing skills than visual processing skills
- depression
- difficulty interpreting facial expressions, body language, tone of voice, and other nonverbal communication
- difficulty making and keeping friends
- difficulty understanding language subtleties and nuances
- difficulty with abstract thinking

- difficulty with math, especially word problems
- difficulty with spatial relationships
- dislikes new situations
- early language development
- excellent vocabulary and verbal expression
- focuses on details
- gets upset when routine is changed
- good memory, especially when information is verbalized
- gross motor skills impaired: has trouble riding bikes, playing catch, running, hopping, skipping, jumping, kicking
- hyperactivity as a younger child
- hypoactive as an older child and adolescent
- IQ is average to above-average, especially verbal IQ, but low performance scores
- lack of common sense
- not good at team sports or activities
- poor balance
- poor conversational skills
- poor handwriting
- poor motor skills
- poor social skills
- rote verbal, expressive, and receptive language skills are good
- takes things literally
- unable to see the "big picture"
- weak conceptual skills
- weak problem-solving skills
- weak visual-spatial-organizational skills
- weaker physically on left side of body
- withdrawn

Cause

There is no known specific cause for NLD, but it is believed that somehow the brain is miswired. Contributing factors can range from genetics to environmental issues. There are some medical causes for it as well, ranging from fluid on the brain to disease.

Diagnosis

Your child's pediatrician, if he or she suspects NLD, should refer you to a pediatric neuropsychiastrist or psychologist, specialists who can assess your child for NLD as well as any other comorbid psychological problems that are accompanying or caused by the disorder. They will test your child's cognitive, sensory, and motor skills, as well as his or her ability to process both auditory and visual-spatial information. A speech therapist will be brought in to determine language and speech concerns.

One of the problems in diagnosing NLD is that the child's abilities and deficits can be easily overlooked, as the focus shines on one particular strength or weakness. As children grow, their NLD problem will probably manifest in new and more obvious ways—in other words, worsen, especially if some of the symptoms have gone untreated.

These children have a very deceiving condition. For example, your child can appear to be a precocious reader, decoding the words on the page, but he or she will not get the nuances or full comprehension of the story being read. The same goes with math. The child might be able to calculate as if he or she were a human computer, but when it comes to writing the problems on the page … disaster!

Socially, these children usually have a terrible time, especially as they grow older and they don't "get" their peers' jokes or even their simple conversation. NLD kids are often the brunt of bullies' verbal and physical attacks, but even children who are well behaved might find it difficult to interact with an NLD child.

Treatment

Working with NLD involves a wide-ranging group of medical professionals, including a pediatrician, pediatric neuropsychiatrist/psychologist, mental-health professionals, speech-language pathologists and therapists, occupational and physical therapists, sensory integration therapists, and social-skill therapists and groups.

Prognosis

Depending on the severity and when treatment was begun, NLD children can have a wide spectrum of prognoses. Many of the symptoms of the disorder are treatable and respond well to the prescribed treatment. But early detection and early intervention are essential for the best outcome. NLD cannot be cured.

Sources and resources

NLD Online (831-624-3542); (www.nldline.com)
Nonverbal Learning Disorders Association (860-658-5522); (www.nlda.org)
Dr. Byron P. Rourke (www.nld-bprourke.ca)

O

OCD (Obsessive-Compulsive Disorder)

ODD (Oppositional Defiant Disorder)

OCD

Obsessive-Compulsive Disorder

Terms used in this chapter: ADHD (attention-deficit/hyperactivity disorder); CBT (cognitive behavioral therapy); *DSM* (*Diagnostic and Statistical Manual of Mental Disorders*); ERPT (exposure and response prevention therapy); NIMH (National Institute of Mental Health); OCD (obsessive-compulsive disorder); OCF (Obsessive-Compulsive Foundation)

Sound familiar?

Richard Downing is a 21-year-old tough-looking guy from Oceanside, New York, with a close-cropped beard, glint in his eye, and tattoos. But the minute he opens his mouth, he turns out to be an articulate, deep-thinking young man who is being ripped apart by his disorder—OCD.

"I didn't know what was going on with me," he says of his lifelong ordeal, which has brought him to numerous frightening emergency-room visits. "I was just diagnosed four months ago."

He realized at age 11 that something was wrong ("I always had the urge to keep things neat and in order"), and by 13, he was performing rituals.

"I was obsessively closing the door. I never felt it was closed all the way. I broke a couple of door knobs [because] I would be closing them so much.

"I didn't know what was going on with me. I was so embarrassed."

A year ago, Richard saw a TV show that changed his life: MTV's True Life: I Have OCD.

"The things these kids were doing related to me substantially. This is what I have!

"I was worried. How do I approach anyone to get help? I was always a hypochondriac as a kid, I always cried wolf. No one believed me.

"Everything went terribly wrong. I began self-medicating. I fell into drugs. I was so afraid. I didn't know what was going on. Before you get diagnosed, you feel all alone. You feel like you're losing your mind. You feel like you're going crazy. You feel so abnormal, and you think they're gonna lock you up in a mental institution in a straitjacket."

Richard's rituals have become more intense. He has started a hand-washing routine. If he thinks the door is not closed properly, he will sweat profusely and break out into a full-scale panic attack. He now has to perform activities for an even number of times—two, four, and now eight. He is also obsessed with microscopic dust. "I bang out my towel, fold it, bang it out again. I'm afraid of lint. Even if I don't see it, I'll feel it."

Richard spends an inordinate amount of time checking and rechecking the air-conditioning settings and plug in his basement apartment (he lives with his grandmother, who attends support-group meetings with him).

An animal lover, he recently lost his job in a pet shop because his rituals were interfering with his work. He has been to "ten to twelve shrinks."

Richard describes his most recent terrifying experience: "I was running ragged in my room, pacing, I couldn't hear, my brain was running like an overheated engine. I couldn't sleep. I knew I needed help." But he has no health insurance. The only thing to do was go to the emergency room, where he sat for eight hours, "freaking out."

He says he has forty-eight rituals, which include washing; setting/resetting his air-conditioner; cleaning dust from clothes, sheets, towels, shoes ("That's a big one")—he taps them out eight times; tapping out imagined water in his ears ("That's a big one"), which stopped him from taking showers ("I had to shake my ear twenty-eight times"); blowing "contaminated" air out of his mouth; rinsing his mouth with water; pushing plugs into outlets; washing his face eight times in a row and then washing his neck; preparing his bed by getting rid of all wrinkles in his sheets, and sometimes sleeping on a bare mattress; shaking out his blanket eight times on each of the four sides; making sure each side of his sheet is even on the bed—throughout the night. He'd perform these rituals in a number system, two times, twelve times, forty-eight times ("I'd never go more than forty-eight"). He'd get up in the middle of the night to do these things. Even at work he had to hold his breath when he swept the floors, and shake his head numerous times to free it from dust. These rituals took hours out of his life each day.

"I keep saying to myself, 'I know this is ridiculous. I need to stop.' But I can't."

But Richard has found help, after several very frightening and nonproductive visits to emergency rooms and clinics. Now that he has the OCD diagnosis, he doesn't feel so all alone. In fact, he feels compelled to go public and get the word out to others who are suffering in silence.

He is on medication ($220 worth out-of-pocket every month) and attends therapy. He finds his OCD support group very helpful and practices the ERP therapy at home.

"I had no hope," Richard says. "I needed to be on suicide watch. Now I have so much hope."

Richard has OCD—obsessive-compulsive disorder.

Did you know?

At first glance, they look like they came out of central casting for a sitcom: there is Richard, the 21-year-old tattooed punk, and his grandma; the statuesque young blonde; the 76-year-old army veteran; the bearded baby-boomer; and the well-tanned mother of three. But this turns out to be no joke.

They are meeting as members of a local OCD support group, and although the media—the hit television series *Monk* is a perfect example—portrays those afflicted with OCD in comical ways, this is a debilitating disorder.

These OCD sufferers meet at the Long Island OCD Support Network's (LIOCDSN) free support group every other week at a Mental Health Association office. The gatherings are run by Warren Barlowe, a former special-education teacher and behavioral coach who has OCD. Serious-looking, Barlowe enters the meeting with two briefcases. For at least five minutes, he searches futilely through them, looking through hundreds of papers for a printout of an article on SAD (seasonal affective disorder) for a new member. It is ironic to note that this OCD expert's rituals revolve around organization, a subtype of OCD.

"I was born with OCD," says Barlowe. "I inherited it. I see it in my parents." His father was an inventor and "collector," and his mother was a "neat freak" who always asked and re-asked questions for reassurance, a typical OCD activity. Barlowe is saddled with several incapacitating manifestations of the disorder, including constant checking and rechecking, resulting in past employment problems. But now he has the condition under control, and he has found the perfect job—as a counselor to those suffering with the illness.

When Barlowe was younger, his obsessions and compulsions greatly interfered with school and, later, work. The condition resulted, he says, in dismissal from "twenty to thirty jobs." He would keep returning home to check his lights, his doors, the oven, all the while "knowing nothing was wrong—but something forced me to come back."

"It was a paralyzing fear," he recalls, "until I convinced myself it was OK. You think you're going crazy."

Now Barlowe, who has his OCD under control through therapy and medication, devotes his life to helping others, both as leader of the support group and as a counselor who visits patients in their homes. Those who attend meetings say he is very comforting, and it is easy to see how, through his own experience, research, and behavioral therapy, especially ERP therapy, he is making a difference in people's lives.

"Through ERP therapy, the problem goes from scary to boring to funny," explains Barlowe.

This behavioral therapy, he strongly suggests, should be paired with antidepressant medications like Prozac and Zoloft.

Barlowe sits patiently as the members of his group start pouring their hearts out. Nikki, a tall blonde, is a 33-year-old who admits that she's a bit obsessed with support groups—she belongs to Overeaters Anonymous (she's as thin as a rail); Co-Dependents Anonymous (CoDa), for those in an addictive relationship; the OCD support group; and Recovery, Inc., for anxiety. Her issues initially seem slight, until she goes into detail. She constantly prays, constantly eats, and constantly exercises—but she has such an intricate routine for these activities that it's hard to believe she has time for anything else. And that's the point: she doesn't—that's why her actions are unhealthy. She was also a registered nurse but quit, afraid that she might do someone unintentional harm, a very common fear among OCD sufferers. A lot of her problems fall into the religious scrupulosity subtype and revolve around prayer and "trying to please God." And while she has faith in Barlowe's counseling, she says, "Warren is going to help me. But God is above Warren."

Bob is 76, and he, too, has the fear of doing harm. He provides one heartbreaking example, which actually involved him *helping* someone, but to Bob, it was harming that person. His ritual consists of constantly trying to prove his innocence—that is, to himself.

He has been hospitalized seven times.

But he has hope. "When you're 76, you don't want to look forward to a future of suffering," he says.

Peter, 41, has what most people recognize as classic OCD. He became a hand-washer at the age of 8. Fortunately, his supportive family realized that he had a problem and sought help for him. This was before OCD was officially recognized, so he was diagnosed with "phobias" and told there was little treatment. Meanwhile, his behavior became so intrusive that he quit school when he was 12.

It's not germs he fears—it's being "unclean." When someone of "questionable hygiene" would pass him in a public place, he would find the need to clean himself. Today, through years of medication and effective and ineffective therapies, he has overcome the cleanliness ritual and considers himself in remission.

"Therapists," Peter laughs. "I've seen more than Woody Allen. I always had a great wanting to be like everyone else."

Tracey was new to the session and remained quiet for the majority of its two-hour duration. But when she opened up, it was as if a dam had burst. She has suffered from OCD since she was a child. She has multiple rituals and comorbid conditions, including depression. The worst part, however, is that her husband is not the least bit understanding, and she worries that their fighting will affect their kids.

Fred Penzel, Ph.D., a Long Island behavioral psychologist specializing in OCD, says that unsupportive family members can stress out the OCD patient even further and make the condition worse. He says that people have to know that OCD "is not just a bad habit. People just can't stop their behavior. They need to take medication to take care of the biological aspect of it. And they need to complement it with therapy."

And then there's Richard and his forty-eight manifestations of OCD.

OCD is one of seven categories of anxiety disorders listed in the *DSM-IV-TR*, the most current version of the bible used by most mental-health professionals. The others are PD (panic disorder), GAD (generalized anxiety disorder), phobias, anxiety disorders from physical causes, stress disorders such as PTSD (post-traumatic stress disorder), and anxiety disorder not-otherwise-specified. All of these can be comorbid, or exist simultaneously and independently, with ADHD, ASD (autism spectrum disorder), depression, SID (sensory integration disorder), or CS (childhood schizophrenia).

How it is manifested

OCD is caused by a person's brain getting stuck on a thought. The disorder is transferred into severe worry, doubt, or superstition. Next, rituals are performed to alleviate the anxiety brought on by these symptoms. Of course, everyone has some quirk, so when do rituals or superstitions become harmful?

"When they start interfering with your daily routine," says Richard Schloss, M.D., a psychiatrist who shares a practice with Penzel and specializes in OCD.

The essential features of OCD are recurrent obsessions (intrusive thoughts) and compulsions (repeated behaviors) that are time-consuming and cause significant impairment in daily functioning.

Obsessions are persistent ideas, thoughts, impulses, or images that are experienced as intrusive and inappropriate and cause marked anxiety or distress. Most common obsessions are repeated thoughts about contamination, doubting oneself, needing to have things in a particular order, or aggressive impulses. Usually, the child with obsessions tries to neutralize these disturbing thoughts with some other thought or action (a compulsion). Compulsions are repetitive behaviors or mental acts (e.g., hand washing, ordering objects, checking, praying, counting, repeating words silently), the goal of which is to prevent or reduce anxiety or distress, not to provide pleasure. In most cases, the person feels driven to perform the compulsion to reduce the feelings of distress that accompanies an obsession or to prevent some event from occurring.

There's a difference between a healthy routine and OCD. For example, a person might feel compelled to say "God bless you" every time someone sneezes, out of habit or social politeness. But if that person feels panic because she thinks the sneezer will die if she doesn't say "God bless you," then she may have OCD.

Other warning signs include the ritual's taking more than an hour and the person's being compelled to perform rituals but not finding relief by performing them. Most adults suffering from the disorder realize that what they are doing is senseless, but many children and some adults do not know why they are performing the rituals.

As discussed in numerous studies and reported in publications such as the *British Journal of Psychiatry Supplement* and the *American Journal of Psychiatry*, untreated and misdiagnosed or undiagnosed OCD sufferers may self-medicate, turning to drugs or alcohol.

"You never get cured," warns Dr. Penzel. "It's a chronic condition." The most common symptoms he sees in practice are morbid thinking (fear of deliberate self-harm or harming others), religious scrupulosity (fear of doing moral wrong), fear of being homosexual or being viewed as homosexual, germ and dirt contamination, and checking and rechecking.

Ian Osborn, M.D., a psychiatrist at Penn State University and author of *Tormenting Thoughts and Secret Rituals: The Hidden Epidemic of Obsessive-Compulsive Disorder*, says that it's easy to see the difference between normal and OCD behavior. He offers the example of a person's getting up out of bed at night to check that the front door is locked. "[Someone without OCD] will find it locked, and the thought of an unlocked door is automatically gone," he explains. But the OCD sufferer, he explains, will get up, "check the door, see that it's fine, return to bed, and the fear remains."

"OCD is all about persistent doubt," says Dr. Penzel. His colleague Dr. Schloss refers to it as "the doubting disease." The ritual is supposed to work to put right the obsession, although it doesn't always succeed.

"The fearful thought sticks too much with people who have OCD," explains Dr. Osborn. "The automatic mechanism that dismisses bad thoughts does not work."

What separates the behavior of a person afflicted with OCD from someone with a psychosis or another serious disorder?

"The person, as a rule, knows [their OCD behavior] is not rational," explains Dr. Osborn. "They know it's stupid."

Dr. Penzel agrees. "People know it's a little crazy. But people who have it need a sense of humor about it."

There's apparently a lot to have a sense of humor about.

Patricia Perkins, cofounder and executive director of the OCF in New Haven, Connecticut, says that OCD, like autism, involves a spectrum of disorders: hypochondria, body dysmorphia (preoccupation with how a body part looks), trichotillomania (hair pulling), hoarding, scrupulosity (over-conscientiousness, religious obsessions), and more.

Fugen Neziroglu, Ph.D., the clinical director of the Bio-Behavioral Institute in Great Neck, New York, explains, "The OCD spectrum involves obsessions and/or compulsions, and there's a high probability that if you have one condition, you may have at some point in time one of the other disorders."

In their 1983 book *Obsessive-Compulsive Disorder Spectrum: Pathogenesis, Diagnosis and Treatment*, Dr. Neziroglu and her husband Jose Yaryura-Tobias, M.D., even went so far as to add EDs (eating disorders), HD (Huntington's chorea), and TS (Tourette syndrome) as part of the OCD spectrum, the latter being a very controversial stance. They found a chromosomal link between OCD and TS and strongly believed that the urge to "tic"— the rapid repeated movements or sounds that those with the syndrome make—was a compulsion. Dr. Neziroglu is of the school of thought that, because OCD is a spectrum, a disorder can be either a compulsion or obsession, not necessarily both.

By the numbers

This chapter deals with children *and* adults, because OCD is so highly inherited that adults reading this chapter might recognize a problem of their own and be more sensitive to the possibility of their child having OCD as well.

It is estimated that between 1 and 3 percent of Americans—at least 2.2 million, according to an article in the 2005 *Archives of General Psychiatry*, to 7 million, according to the OCF—suffer from the disorder. And some experts say that number is much higher, because it often goes misdiagnosed, undiagnosed, or kept secret by the sufferer.

Nemours, the nationwide children's health foundation, estimates that 2 percent of kids suffer from OCD, although Dr. Schloss and other experts feel it could be as high as 5 percent, and perhaps even higher, because, as with adults with OCD, children with symptoms often keep the condition secret from their family and friends. Schloss says that children often manifest OCD through touching and tapping a prescribed amount of times or thinking that a certain word or number is bad. OCD kids are often involved in "magical thinking," such as saying, "If I do or think action 'A,' then the result will be 'B' and it will prevent something bad."

According to OCF's Perkins, OCD kids usually do well in school academically, so there aren't as many red flags as with adults.

"But they are rule players," she says, "so sometimes they might get caught up [in] some action by being a perfectionist and not getting anything done because they do too much preparatory work, or they are so busy making things look good that they erase so much they smudge the paper."

Dr. Osborn cites an important study by NIMH, conducted in the early 1980s, which randomly chose 20,000 subjects in a door-to-door survey. The survey found that 2 to 3 percent of the respondents had OCD. But, says Osborn (who suffers from OCD), the survey only counted those who were under a doctor's care or on medications, and not the large group of subclinical sufferers who could bring that number up to "as high as 8 percent of the population."

Dr. Penzel, the behavioral psychologist who specializes in OCD, says the disorder is found in one out of 40 people.

"It's more common than asthma," Dr. Penzel says. Unfortunately, although people are born with OCD, it may take eight years from the time they realize they have the disorder to get the help they need, says Barlowe. Dr. Schloss says that one-third of adults with OCD had it as children, but Perkins, of the OCF, estimates that as many as one-half of adults with OCD developed symptoms as children. Research from many sources, including the NIMH Genetics Workgroup, indicates that the disorder is hereditary. Most people with OCD have relatives with the disorder. Osborn believes that there is "a strong genetic component" that may be as high as 50 percent.

"The same as high blood pressure," Dr. Osborn says.

OCD can affect people differently. It can even ease up and go away, in a sort of remission. It often gets worse, though, when it is unchecked, and renders a person unable to work or function in everyday life.

Although there are researchers who estimate that approximately one in two hundred women may suffer from OCD while pregnant or after giving birth, most researchers say that the illness affects both men and women equally.

Signs and symptoms

OCD is an organic, medical brain disorder, driven by fear (and anxiety), which is subdivided into two subcategories—obsessions and compulsions. These rituals include hand washing, counting, checking and rechecking, praying, arranging, needing symmetry, and odd physical activities (like always walking right foot first). But practicing these repetitions results in only temporary relief of the obsession. If the rituals are not completed or are done "wrong," the anxiety level will increase.

Both symptoms—severe obsessions and mental compulsions—are required for the classic diagnosis of OCD to be made, says Dr. Osborn. Other experts, however, believe OCD is a spectrum of disorders that may include only one of the symptoms.

Primary symptoms

Typically, the obsessions and compulsions cause marked distress, are time-consuming, and may significantly interfere with the child's functioning at home, school, or in social activities. Also, because obsessive intrusions can be distracting, kids may show poor performance at tasks that would require concentration, such as schoolwork. In addition, many kids may avoid objects or situations that provoke obsessions and compulsions.

According to Dr. Penzel, warning signs of OCD in children include their display of any unusual fears—strange things that most people are not usually afraid of, such as moving or changing things in the child's room. He notes that it is more difficult to spot these reactions in children because they are "mental events" and therefore harder to notice.

Other primary symptoms include the following:

- checking and rechecking things such as a backpack
- asking many repetitive questions
- asking for a lot of reassurance ("Are you sure?" "How do you know?")
- avoiding socializing and school and sports activities
- exhibiting uncommon superstitions ("If I don't turn around six times when I see a cat, something very bad will happen")
- being concerned that harm will come to parents, especially the mother, which might result in separation anxiety and a lot of "Do you love me?" questions

Subtypes of OCD in adults and children

1 aggressive obsession: for example, seeing a sharp object and having the fear of harming someone with it; doing something embarrassing or dangerous. Aggressive obsession includes horrific thoughts such as driving off a bridge or killing someone. Those suffering with it believe that, because they thought a specific thought, they can carry out the action ("If I think about killing my teacher, then I might kill him"). OCD sufferers would generally never act on these negative thoughts, but they can't dismiss the thoughts. OCF's Perkins suggests that John Mark Karr, who falsely confessed to killing JonBenet Ramsey, might suffer from this.

2 checking … and rechecking: "Did I turn off the lights?" "Did I shut off the gas?" "Did I run someone over?" (All three are common obsessions.)

3 cleaning and washing (the compulsion)

4 contamination (the obsession): afraid they will contaminate others or afraid they will be contaminated or get sick from others

5 counting

6 hoarding and saving

7   magical and superstitious thoughts: "If I shut my eyes and count to [pick any number], then my dog won't die"

8   need to know and remember: "When did I eat my last hamburger?" "When did the last red car pass?"

9   ordering and arranging: rectilinearity, or lining things up, keeping things symmetrical or in order

10 repeating rituals: continuously going back and forth through a doorway

11 scrupulosity: all about right and wrong and perceived hurt feelings: "I took Jim's pen and have to get it back to him." "Did I hurt your feelings?" "I talked too fast, and I will continue to call back to tell you I'm so sorry; will you forgive me?" (a) religious scrupulosity: thinking that one is possessed by the devil, or having blasphemous thoughts, or needing perfect prayer

12 sexual obsession: staring at people's genitals; fear of being or being considered gay (a common obsession seen by experts)

13 somatic: excessive concern with illness—counting breaths, constantly taking one's pulse

Cause

The human brain is affected by serotonin, a hormone that acts as a chemical messenger between nerve cells, affecting mood, attention, emotions, and sleep. In the brains of those with OCD, there may not be enough serotonin, researchers have discovered.

Dr. Schloss believes that the connections in the brain's frontal lobes and basal ganglia (clusters of nerve cells), where OCD is located, become overactive, so the brain doesn't receive what the eyes are seeing. He adds that, because of the brain's serotonin deficit, "thoughts get caught in a loop." Perkins theorizes that, since the basal ganglia is that primitive part of the brain that helped early civilizations in basic survival, OCD may be some sort of protection device. The current focus of OCD research, Perkins says, is on serotonin and genetics.

Dr. Schloss also believes that childhood OCD follows strep infections, a growing theory behind many pediatric autoimmune neuropsychiatric disorders associated with streptococcus infection (PANDAS).

Most importantly, one usually needs a biological disposition, or the genetic factor, to get OCD.

Treatment

An early medication that proved successful in treating those with OCD, and one that is still used, is the antidepressant clomipramine (Anafranil). Currently, medications called SSRIs have proven very effective.

Support-group facilitator Barlowe suggests that not enough serotonin gets reabsorbed into the system of OCD sufferers. Drugs such as SSRIs correct this, he says, by blocking the "leak" in the nerve cell. These don't change the person's mood, Barlowe says, but instead make it easier for the individual to resist the compulsion.

He demonstrates this by moving his hand toward a switch to turn it off. But his hand keeps returning, illustrating how a person with OCD does not have the message transmitted or does not receive the message that the switch has been turned off—so the hand has the need to keep returning.

Experts agree that medication must be complemented with cognitive behavioral therapy (CBT)—specifically, ERP therapy—in which the patient confronts the negative thought and is encouraged not to ritualize. ERP desensitizes the patient, and, according to Dr. Schloss, is "pretty fast and focused, and can make a significant difference within three months."

In 1972, Dr. Neziroglu and her colleagues were frustrated that there was very little information about OCD in medical texts ("three pages," she scoffs). So she and her husband, psychiatrist Dr. Yaryura-Tobias, conducted a double-blind study (an experiment in which neither the patients nor the doctors know which patient is receiving which treatment) using Anafranil. In 1977, her team published "Obsessive-Compulsive Disorder: A Serotonergic Hypothesis," a paper demonstrating that individuals with OCD had lower serotonin levels than people in the control group.

The following year, the two formed the Obsessive-Compulsive Society, a group of OCD sufferers, based at a local library. The participants, she says, became the first patients in the country to go on Anafranil, which became the breakthrough drug for OCD.

But then Novartis, Anafranil's manufacturer, stopped producing it, believing there were not enough potential users (OCD was not very well-known then). So Dr. Neziroglu and her group continued getting the medication from other countries such as Canada and Mexico. The patent was eventually extended so that Novartis resumed production, and on Long Island Dr. Neziroglu started the nation's first intensive CBT treatment program.

Thanks in part to Dr. Neziroglu and Dr. Yaryura-Tobias, and their work with CBT and serotonin research in the 1970s, OCD became generally recognized around 1990. At that time, the very effective drug Anafranil was finally approved by the FDA for treating OCD, and the OCF was formed out of a Yale research project, generating a lot of media.

In 1989, Dr. Neziroglu published another paper indicating that OCD patients could get the same serotonin changes through CBT only, and no medication. But without medication, the changes are temporary, she says.

Dr. Neziroglu says that both therapy and medication are indicated only in resistant OCD. "Cognitive therapy is more long lasting," she explains. "With medications alone, when [they] are discontinued there is a 90 to 99 percent chance of symptoms returning. That does not occur with therapy." She maintains that the first line of treatment is always CBT and that medications should always be used in conjunction with therapy—never alone.

Treatment strategies commonly used to treat OCD in children include ERPT, in which they are taught to face the fear that triggers the obsessive thoughts or anxiety. By facing the feared situation, anxiety is triggered, and through repeated exposure over repeated trials, the anxiety decreases or "habituates." The principle of "response prevention" means that children are taught to stop the performance of the ritual that decreases their anxiety (e.g., washing hands to feel less anxious, checking the door, etc.). Early in treatment, this may involve partial prevention (i.e., washing the hands ten times rather than twenty times) or altering ritualistic behaviors. Particularly during this phase, allies such as parents need to be included to assist children in carrying out this treatment effectively. As treatment progresses, complete response prevention is introduced. Other strategies employed include teaching children to challenge and change their obsessive thinking and to learn new adaptive ways of coping with anxiety. Further, rewards are often included to praise children for their successes. Because children's OCD symptoms have been found to have a significant impact on the family, many clinicians incorporate family therapy into their treatment protocol.

Prognosis

OCD is not an easy disorder to live with, but it can be helped. Perkins says, "OCD is a tricky disease, because it constantly throws impediments up in front of people who are trying to get better."

And Dr. Schloss reminds us, "You're never cured, but you can be treated." There is hope.

"People who suffer with OCD can look forward to living normal lives," says Dr. Schloss. "With therapy and medications, they go into a sort of 'remission,' where OCD is a dim noise."

As Peter, an OCD sufferer who attends Barlowe's support group, says, "If life never got any better than [that], I could live with it."

Sources and resources

Awareness Foundation for OCD and Related Disorders (www.ocdawareness.com)
Warren Barlowe, OCD behavioral therapist, Long Island OCD Support Network
(516-681-7861); (www.ocd.hereweb.com)
Bio-Behavioral Institute (516-487-7116); (www.bio-behavioral.com)
Madison Institute of Medicine, Obsessive-Compulsive Information Center
(608-827-2470); (www.miminc.org)
National Institute of Mental Health (www.nimh.nih.gov)
Nemours Foundation (www.nemours.org)
Fugen Nezirogulu and Jose Yaryura-Tobias, *Obsessive-Compulsive Disorder Spectrum: Pathogenesis, Diagnosis and Treatment* (Washington, DC: American Psychiatric Press, 1997).

Obsessive Compulsive Foundation (617-973-5801); (www.ocfoundation.org)
OCD Action (0870-360-OCDA [6232]); (www.ocdaction.org.uk)
OCD Hotline (www.ocdhotline.com)
Ian Osborn, *Tormenting Thoughts and Secret Rituals: The Hidden Epidemic of Obsessive-Compulsive Disorder* (New York: Dell, 1999).

ODD

Oppositional Defiant Disorder

Terms used in this chapter: ADHD (attention-deficit/hyperactivity disorder); LD (learning disability); ODD (oppositional defiant disorder)

Sound familiar?

Annette has always given her parents a hard time. Whether it was just slight acts of bad behavior around the house or moments of lapsed attention in school, it was always just considered as "part of her personality," her mother, Laura, a Minnesota state employee recalls. Annette's two older brothers also had "strong personalities," says Laura, but they always did extremely well academically in school, so her parents wrote off their oppositional behavior at home as "boys being boys."

But Annette was always different from her brothers. Although her IQ was actually higher than her siblings', she did very poorly in school, and that was the red flag—for Laura at least, who wanted Annette psychologically tested. Annette's father, George, who Laura describes as "stoic and jaded," was against it. That is, until Annette entered high school and, at 14, began acting out in much more serious ways than not clearing her plates from the table and having very public tantrums at family events.

She started failing most of her subjects, and she hooked up with a crowd of known troublemakers. She had a boyfriend with whom she became sexually involved, and she began smoking cigarettes and marijuana and abusing alcohol.

Annette fights with her parents constantly and sneaks out of her house, usually her bedroom window, blatantly defying her parents' warnings and punishments. She cuts classes and lies about it, even when she is confronted with indisputable proof. And then she'll do it again. She talks back to the school principal and any other authority figure who intervenes.

"She does things that are obvious," says Laura. "Almost like she wants to be caught."

Recently, during a prolonged period of being suspended from school and grounded at home, Annette had begun to lose her temper and has cursed and physically lashed out at her parents.

"Annette spends more time grounded than unpunished," says Laura, who is currently at her wit's end. "I know she's a good girl basically, and we have moments of peace and joy with her, but right now she is mostly hell on earth."

Not being able to deal with this any longer, Laura, George, and Annette have agreed that psychological therapy was overdue, and Annette has finally been diagnosed. She is in her first month of therapy.

Annette has ODD—oppositional defiant disorder.

Did you know?

CDs (conduct disorders) are behavioral and emotional problems exhibited in children who display a high difficulty following socially acceptable rules, and ODD is a psychiatric disorder that is one of the more controversial of all the Alphabet Disorders and one of the more mild conduct disorders.

ODD is a persistent disruptive behavior that is characterized by antisocial behavior that is directed more toward family and other adults or authority figures known to the child than by destructive illegal behaviors such as assault or thievery, which would fit more under the ASBD (antisocial behavior disorder) category. The child exhibits disobedience, defiance, and hostility. These children deliberately break rules and don't comply with requests.

There are many experts who argue that ODD is just bad behavior—or, for that matter, normal behavior. And the fact is it is in most cases. But when the uncooperative, defiant, or hostile behavior begins to become worse than the norm for a child's age and seriously interferes with and negatively impacts the child's daily functioning, whether at home, in school, or with peers, it becomes a classifiable disorder. That's when the behavior needs intervention.

All children between the ages of 2 and 3 (you've heard of the "terrible twos") and during adolescence display defiant behavior. They may rebel, resist, confront, challenge, disobey, dare, disregard, ignore, talk back, and sometimes treat others with contempt. They fight their parents, their teachers, their older relatives, and acquaintances. It's their job. It's what they're programmed to do. But when it starts to exceed the limits set by universally accepted standards in terms of duration and intensity, parents should seek help.

The American Academy of Child and Adolescent Psychiatry (AACAP) reports that 5 to 15 percent of all school-age children have ODD.

Disruptive behaviors are often comorbid. Many of these oppositional behaviors are found in children who also have ADHD.

Signs and symptoms

- argumentative with adults
- blames others for his or her mistakes or misbehavior
- bullies others
- defiant

- deliberately attempts to annoy or upset people
- difficulty being soothed
- easily annoyed
- frequent anger
- frequent fighting
- frequent temper tantrums
- hostile behavior
- hypermotor activity
- intimidating
- loses temper
- low frustration tolerance
- mean and hateful speech when upset
- negative behavior
- often being "touchy" or easily annoyed by others
- refusal to comply with adult requests and rules
- resentful
- sensitive
- spiteful
- vindictive

Cause

While the specific cause of ODD is not known, it is believed that there are several possible causes for it that include psychological, genetic, biological, and environmental factors—social deprivation such as family discord, inconsistent child care, or lax, inconsistent, unpredictable, or nonexistent parenting; neurological damage, low birthweight, ADHD, and/or LDs.

And, unfortunately, it could very well be just your child's innate temperament.

Diagnosis

Children who display ODD characteristics should first be brought to their pediatrician to check to see if there are any underlying medical conditions that might be causing the behavior. If everything checks out fine in that respect, the child will be referred to a pediatric psychologist or psychiatrist who will use standardized personality testing, assessments of school testing and evaluations, and their own clinical observations to determine the diagnosis of ODD.

Treatment

Early intervention is very important in helping to prevent the early signs of ODD from turning into a lifelong problem. A child who exhibits these early ODD signs can be and should be tested as soon as possible to see if his or her aggressive behaviors require any sort of treatment.

It should be determined what other disorders are at play: ADHD, LDs, anxiety, and mood disorders. If the comorbid disorder remains after the ODD is treated, the condition can still worsen into other conduct or psychological disorders.

Parents are crucial in the treatment process, and they can learn many techniques on how to deal with and remodel their ODD child's behaviors. Positive reinforcement is a key treatment mode along with reinforcing the parent–child relationship. Also important is modeling behaviors such as "time-outs." If a parent and ODD child are at odds, the *parent* should take a time-out. The child will learn that he or she, too, needs a breather when acting out. Parents should pick their battles, and consequences should be reasonable and always consistently enforced. Parents should also offer choices to the child; it provides the ODD child with a sense of power.

Cognitive behavioral therapy (CBT) is an effective therapy in which negative behaviors are modified and through which the child can learn problem-solving techniques. The child should also be taking social-skills training (SST) to learn the best way to deal with social interactions.

Drugs have not been proven consistently effective in helping to treat ODD.

Prognosis

With the proper treatment, ODD can be modified; if left untreated, it can progress into other serious behavioral and personality disorders.

Sources and resources

American Academy of Child and Adolescent Psychiatry (AACAP) (202-966-7300); (www.aacap.org)
American Psychiatric Association (www.psych.org)
American Psychological Association (ww.apa.org)
National Institute of Mental Health (www.nimh.nih.gov)

See the mental-health contacts under "General Resources" for more sources used in this chapter.

P

PAPD (Passive-Aggressive Personality Disorder)

PD (Panic Disorder)

PD (Personality Disorder)

PDD (Pervasive Developmental Disorder)

PDD–NOS (Pervasive Developmental Disorder–
Not Otherwise Specified)

Phobias

Pica

PKU (Phenylketonuria)

PPD (Paranoid Personality Disorder)

PWS (Prader-Willi Syndrome)

PAPD

Passive-Aggressive Personality Disorder

Terms used in this chapter: *DSM* (*Diagnostic and Statistical Manual of Mental Disorders*); PAPD (passive-aggressive personality disorder); PD (personality disorder)

Did you know?

PAPD or negativistic disorder is a chronic PD in which a child responds with passive compliance to the requests and needs of others, giving in to the requests. However, in turn, the child resents those requests or needs, so hostility and anger start building within the child when these demands are expected. The PAPD child will perform inefficiently on purpose, passively resisting the job or actions at hand. Being passive-aggressive is an oftentimes common behavior, but when it becomes a pervasive pessimism that is disabling, it is regarded as a disorder.

A PAPD child would agree to complete a timely chore, for example, but then procrastinate and miss the deadline for the chore or do the chore so badly that the child believes he or she will never be asked to perform it again.

There is a generation of kids whose motto is a dismissive "whatever." It is for the most part typical youthful behavior and jargon and, for some children, the mildest end of passive-aggressiveness. But when that "whatever" turns to an overall negativity and begins to disable the child socially and academically, then it is time to consider it as a possible disorder that needs immediate attention.

Signs and symptoms

- ambiguity
- argumentativeness
- blaming problems on others
- complaining frequently
- deliberate inefficiency
- disliking other people's ideas, even if they are good
- disliking people who are in charge
- fear of competition
- feeling underappreciated
- feigned forgetfulness
- irritability
- lying

- making excuses
- manipulation
- minimal insight
- procrastination
- putting blame on those more meek
- sarcasm
- stubbornness
- sullenness
- trying to come off as a hero
- unreasonable criticism of authority figures

Cause

The cause of PAPD is unknown, but it is thought to be both inherited and the result of the child's environment, ranging from factors as common as modeling after PAPD parents or to the more extreme of child abuse and maternal substance abuse during pregnancy.

Diagnosis

The disorder is controversial, and many psychiatrists no longer diagnose it, especially since it was moved to the *DSM-IV*'s Appendix B category (the section for disorders that need further study) from an Axis II personality disorder in the *DSM-III*. There are, however, many who continue to use the diagnosis when the symptoms stick closely to the original official diagnosis criteria.

Treatment

As with other PDs, psychotherapy is the best course of action. But as with PDs in general, treatment of PAPD can be problematic due to the very nature of a PD—patients are not inclined to trust a therapist or the results of the therapy, often misleading or manipulating the therapist. Passive-aggressiveness is a difficult concept to get across to any patient, especially a child, and the therapist is often met with resistance.

Prognosis

For treatment to be effective, the PAPD child must stick with treatment, despite his or her tendency to be resistant to the therapy. If the child has the proper treatment, the prognosis is good. If the child grows into a passive-aggressive adult, then he or she is in for future problems with relationships and at work.

Sources and resources

American Academy of Child and Adolescent Psychiatry (www.aacap.org)
American Psychiatric Association (www.psych.org)
American Psychological Association (www.apa.org)
DSM (Diagnostic and Statistical Manual of Mental Disorders)
Mayo Clinic (www.mayoclinic.com)
National Institute of Mental Health (www.nimh.nih.gov)

See the "PD: Personality Disorder" chapter and the mental-health contacts in "General Resources" for more sources used in this chapter.

PD

Panic Disorder

Terms used in this chapter: APA (American Psychological Association); CBT (cognitive behavioral therapy); NIMH (National Institute of Mental Health); PD (panic disorder)

Sound familiar?

Carl's mother, Barbara, and a large part of her side of the family suffer from depression, anxiety, and panic attacks; and it is the same on Carl's father's side of the family. Barbara herself suffered from panic attacks, which she's had under control for about fifteen years. Carl suffered from intense SAD (separation anxiety disorder) through fourth grade. In fact, it was so bad that his parents could not get Carl to go to school many days. But then it suddenly ended, and Carl, according to his mother, became an active, social, normal child.

Now Carl is 19. He is in his sophomore year at a top college in an intense science program; and when he's not in school, he's at work. At night, he hangs out with his friends until past midnight. He doesn't eat that well, and he's tired all the time.

A few months ago, Carl needed a blood test. As his blood was being drawn, he fainted. Since that incident, he has never been the same. At work, he became fearful of fainting. One day he got lightheaded, and his heart began to race because he thought he was having a heart attack. He thought he was dying.

Fortunately, Barbara knew what was wrong and immediately called the doctor who suggested that Carl was having an intense anxiety attack and that he should take a Xanax. Without exaggeration, his mother says, the minute he put that pill in his mouth, his labored breathing, the pins and needles in his extremities (a sign that he was hyperventilating), and pounding heart all subsided.

P

"It was just a time bomb waiting to happen," says his mother. "Although I did think at some point that he was safe from this." Carl's younger sister suffers from an anxiety disorder as well.

The next day Carl went to his doctor and to a psychologist where he was diagnosed. "Welcome to the world of late-adolescent boys," his doctor said. Carl was prescribed Xanax, which he takes occasionally when he feels an attack coming on, and he attends therapy weekly. He has changed his eating habits (he eats more healthily) and takes vitamins, niacinamide, and Omega 3, among other supplements. He visited a naturopathic osteopath who administered a complete blood screening (which was finally completed in Carl's car, after three aborted attempts in the doctor's office), and has determined that, among other things, Carl's adrenaline level was low. The doctor put Carl on a very restrictive diet. Carl's panic attacks stopped for several months, but have since returned.

He has not gotten over the fear of having these attacks, and is terrified of the thought of having to give blood.

Carl has PD—panic disorder.

Did you know?

PD seems to strike out of nowhere. It is a common and very treatable condition that affects children and adolescents without warning with repeated intense periods of fear, anxiety, or dread, accompanied by specific physical sensations. It is accompanied often by other symptoms such as a racing heart, feeling faint, feeling like throwing up, or shortness of breath. The panic periods can last a short or an extended period of time. A diagnostic sign of anxiety or panic attack is a tingling in the fingers and legs/feet, which is almost exclusively caused by hyperventilation.

The panicked child is overwhelmed by irrational fear.

PD usually is paired with stressful life transitions, but often there is a genetic predisposition. It often begins during adolescence, although it may start during childhood, and sometimes runs in families.

One month of ongoing anxiety after a panic attack is usually the criterion for an official PD diagnosis, which is sometimes comorbid with depression and other anxiety disorders.

Early intervention is important for helping PD because it is so easily treated. If left untreated, it can affect all aspects of a child's life from social interaction to mood to academic achievement. Children do not necessarily have to have panic attacks to be considered panic disordered—often the PD child is constantly anxious without having an attack. It is easy for a PD child to develop other psychological disorders such as SAD (separation anxiety disorder) or CA (childhood agoraphobia), which is anxiety about being someplace or in some situation where there is no escape, if one was perceived to be needed. These situations include being in a store, driving on a bridge, attending a concert, standing in a line, or being in a classroom. People with CA refrain from leaving the perceived safety of their homes. PD children can also develop depression, which can lead them to self-medication such as drugs or alcohol.

A panic attack occurs suddenly, with an out-of-control fear that is disproportionate to the situation. The attack itself might last minutes, but anxiety might remain for a much longer period. The fear then takes on a life of its own, and the child is afraid of having another attack, more so than being afraid of a specific stressor. A panic attack can occur in a stressful place or time or can occur in a calm, tranquil place or time.

By the numbers

According to the NIMH, more than 3 million Americans will experience panic disorder during their lifetime. Donna Pincus, a therapist at Boston University's Center for Anxiety and Related Disorders, states that 10 percent of those under 18 have anxiety disorders. The APA reports that one in seventy-five people might experience PD. It is believed that twice as many females as males have PD, but that can be deceiving because that statistic could be representing just those who seek help.

Signs and symptoms

- abdominal distress
- chest pain
- chills
- dizziness
- fear of being in a public setting (agoraphobia)
- fear of dying
- fear of fainting
- fear of having a heart attack
- fear of losing control
- feeling detached
- feeling of choking or being smothered
- feeling that something terrible is going to happen
- headache
- heart palpitations
- hot flashes
- hyperventilation
- inability to breathe easily
- lightheadedness
- nausea
- numbness
- paralyzing terror

- pounding or racing heartbeat
- sense of unreality
- shaking
- shortness of breath
- stomachache
- sweating
- tingling in extremities (parasthesia)
- trembling
- tremors

Cause

There are many theories on the cause of panic attacks. One theory says that there is a biological malfunction such as a mild heart anomaly that causes the disorder. Another theory is that it is genetic and passed from parent to child. Stress is often cited as a cause, as is diet. As with Carl, noted above, it could be a biological cause such as a low level of adrenaline. Pharmaceuticals such as asthma medications can also bring on an attack.

Besides occurring through genetics, a parent can pass down a fear to a child through his or her behavior that turns from a fear to anxiety to panic in the child. For example, if the parent gets visibly anxious every time he or she sees a dog and the child observes this behavior, the child can model that fear. Stressful life transitions such as starting high school or college, marriage, divorce, or illness can initiate an attack.

Some experts believe that panic attacks are caused by an abnormality in the part of the brain that involves relaying information about how much carbon dioxide (CO_2) is in the blood. When the brain is being told that there is too much CO_2, the body thinks that it is not breathing fast enough; or the body senses that there is too much CO_2 in the air (panic attacks often occur in stuffy rooms), and it sends messages to increase respiration and increases input of adrenaline—a primal reaction that would help if there were some real imminent danger. In the case of a panic attack, the message is being sent incorrectly: the body senses danger when there is none.

Diagnosis

Unless there is reason to believe the child is suffering from PD, such as family history, the disorder is often untreated and sometimes difficult to diagnose. Some children are afraid or too embarrassed to tell their parents of a panic attack, although it is not hard to miss when observing one. Some parents and doctors might just write it off as nervousness or another psychological disorder. But since the disorder runs in families, as each generation learns more and more about the disorder, it is often observed and treated earlier and earlier.

A pediatrician can diagnose the problem after observing the child and his or her symptoms and obtaining a family history. In most cases, the child will be referred to a mental-health specialist to start one of many effective and often short-term treatments.

A child suspected of having PD should have a thorough medical screening. PD can be caused by many physical ailments, ranging from thyroid problems to fatigue to a bad diet. The pediatrician needs to rule those medical conditions out. Caffeine can trigger the attack, and although the child might no longer ingest caffeine, he or she is still susceptible to the anxiety endured when suffering the first attack.

Treatment

There are several types of effective treatments for PD. According to the APA, most specialists agree that a combination of cognitive and behavioral therapies is the best treatment for PD. Medication might also be appropriate in some cases.

Psychotherapy may teach the child ways to cope with attacks. CBT is the psychological treatment of choice. It helps the child learn ways to change his or her behaviors to be able to control anxiety or panic attacks. A combination of medications and CBT is often the route taken.

As with so many of these Alphabet Disorders, early intervention is the key. With early intervention, many complications that are associated with PD—agoraphobia, depression, OCD (obsessive-compulsive disorder), EDs (eating disorders), substance abuse, etc.—are prevented.

Exposure and response prevention (ERP) therapy is encouraged for those children who develop specific phobias or fears. The child is exposed to the fear and desensitized to that fear by actually performing the task that causes the anxiety. Carl, for example, would be reintroduced to a syringe or a blood lab several times in a nonthreatening situation.

The APA says that it often takes between ten to twenty weekly sessions of therapy to help the PD patient, and the patient should be well on his or her way to a normal life within a year.

Anti-anxiety drugs such as Xanax, Buspar, Valium, and Librium are prescribed as are the antidepressant medications, SSRIs such as Celexa, Prozac, Zoloft, Paxil, and Lexapro, some of the more popular antidepressants used. (See the "SSRIs" section in "What You Need to Know" for more information.) SSRIs improve the reabsorption of the important neurotransmitter serotonin, which helps regulate mood and fear. Sometimes lower doses of SSRIs are more effective than higher doses, so parents should always have a thorough discussion with the child's doctor when considering medications.

While drugs are always a last resort, it is believed that a combination of drugs and psychotherapy is the most effective method to combat PD. Sometimes it is important to cut the edge of the attacks for the child by putting him or her on a brief initial regimen of a drug like Xanax, while determining the future course of treatment.

Medications such as Xanax might help cut the edge, but they can become addictive. Some parents find a change in diet and the use of vitamins and supplements beneficial. Some parents have turned to wheat-free, gluten-free diets or have given their child multivitamins or supplements such as chelated calcium, magnesium, Taurine, and Coenzyme Q10.

Relaxation therapy, deep breathing, meditation, and yoga are also helpful alternative therapies.

The PD child should be taught to stay in the present and realize that what is happening to him or her is an exaggeration of a bodily function that can be controlled.

PD is not a disorder children can cure by themselves, but those suffering from PD should be encouraged that there is a way to control the attacks and that they are not going to lose control or die, as they often fear.

Prognosis

The course of PDs is chronic, but it is highly treatable. In some cases, the child does not have a reoccurrence, while in most cases, there are mild reoccurrences. Children with PD can grow up to lead normal lives.

Sources and resources

Academy of Cognitive Therapy (610-664-1273); (www.academyofct.org)
American Psychological Association (www.apa.org)
Anxiety Disorders Association of America (240-485-1001); (www.adaa.org)
Boston University Center for Anxiety and Related Disorders (www.bu.edu/card)
The Freedom from Fear (718-351-1717); (www.freedomfromfear.org)
NIMH (800-64-PANIC); (www.nimh.nih.gov)
Panic Anxiety Disorder Association/Australia (08-8227-1044);
(www.panicanxietydisorder.org.au)

See the mental-health contacts under "General Resources" for more sources used in this chapter.

PD

Personality Disorder

Terms used in this chapter: *DSM* (*Diagnostic and Statistical Manual of Mental Disorders*); PD (personality disorder); PD–NOS (personality disorder–not otherwise specified)

Did you know?

PDs are mental illnesses that are characterized by the chronic use of inappropriate, stereotyped, and maladaptive manners of coping. PDs are long-term, rigid, and distressing disorders that are manifested in most, if not all, aspects of the child's life. The areas where these problems are seen are in the child's thoughts and the way they perceive themselves and others; how they function and interact in their relationships; the appropriateness, intensity, and range of their emotional functioning; and impulse control.

The *Psychology Today* diagnostic dictionary offers a quick lesson on personality:

The word personality *describes deeply ingrained patterns of behavior and the manner in which individuals perceive, relate to, and think about themselves and their world. Personality traits are conspicuous features of personality and are not necessarily pathological, although certain styles of personality may cause interpersonal problems.*

Personality disorders, though, are rigid, inflexible and maladaptive, causing impairment in functioning or internal distress.

A personality disorder is an enduring pattern of inner experience and behavior that deviates markedly from the expectations of the individual's culture, is pervasive and inflexible, has an onset in adolescence or early adulthood, is stable over time and leads to distress or impairment.

How it is manifested

At the present, eleven personality disorders are classified in the *DSM-IV-TR*:

- **ASPD (antisocial personality disorder):** Lack of regard for the moral or legal standards in the local culture, marked inability to get along with others or abide by societal rules. Sometimes called psychopaths or sociopaths.
- **AvPD (avoidant personality disorder):** Marked social inhibition, feelings of inadequacy, and extremely sensitive to criticism.
- **BPD (borderline personality disorder):** Lack of one's own identity, with rapid changes in mood, intense unstable interpersonal relationships, marked impulsivity, instability in affect and in self-image.
- **DPD (dependent personality disorder):** Extreme need of other people, to a point where the person is unable to make any decisions or take an independent stand on his or her own. Fear of separation and submissive behavior. Marked lack of decisiveness and self-confidence.
- **HPD (histrionic personality disorder):** Exaggerated and often inappropriate displays of emotional reactions, approaching theatricality, in everyday behavior. Sudden and rapidly shifting emotion expressions.

P

- **NPD (narcissistic personality disorder):** Behavior or a fantasy of grandiosity, a lack of empathy, a need to be admired by others, an inability to see the viewpoints of others, and hypersensitive to the opinions of others.
- **OCD (obsessive-compulsive personality disorder):** Characterized by perfectionism and inflexibility; preoccupation with uncontrollable patterns of thought and action.
- **PPD (paranoid personality disorder):** Marked distrust of others, including the belief, without reason, that others are exploiting, harming, or trying to deceive him or her; lack of trust; belief of others' betrayal; belief in hidden meanings; unforgiving and grudge holding.
- **SPD (schizoid personality disorder):** Primarily characterized by a very limited range of emotion, both in expression of and experiencing; indifferent to social relationships.
- **STPD (schizotypal personality disorder):** Peculiarities of thinking, odd beliefs, and eccentricities of appearance, behavior, interpersonal style, and thought (e.g., belief in psychic phenomena and having magical powers).

But the *DSM* sometimes brings up more questions than it answers, as, for example, with the following eleventh disorder:

- **PD–NOS (personality disorder—not otherwise specified):** diagnosed for disorders that do not fit into the other PD categories.

There are many who believe that some of the disorders relegated to this catch-all diagnosis are true stand-alones and point to the evolution of the *DSM* as a case in point. Those diagnosed with PD–NOS usually display the characteristics of multiple PDs, but not the full criteria of any specific one. Examples of PD–NOS include PAPD (passive-aggressive personality disorder) and DPD (depressive personality disorder).

Cause

The cause of these disorders is unknown, although many have a genetic link. Other factors such as biological aberrations, neurochemical abnormalities, or psychological trauma might be underlying causes as well.

Treatment

Treatment for most PDs is much more difficult than for most other psychological disorders because of the specific asocial symptoms associated with the PDs, such as chronic lying, paranoia, and inability to develop a trusting relationship, all qualities needed in a good therapeutic relationship. It is difficult to develop a workable patient–therapist relationship without trust or truthfulness.

Medication helps in many of the cases, and a multimodal approach of drug and psychological therapy usually works the best.

A large support system is helpful in getting a child with a PD to a point where he or she can function close to normal. That support should come from family, friends, teachers, psychiatric experts, medical doctors, and nutritionists. Single-, family-, and group therapy can help, depending on the specific disorder.

Sources and resources

Psychology Today, online dictionary
   (http://psychologytoday.com/conditions/histronic/html)

See the individual personality disorder chapters for information on the specific disorders, contacts, and sources used in this chapter.

PDD

Pervasive Developmental Disorder

Terms used in this chapter: ABA (applied behavioral analysis); ADHD (attention-deficit/hyperactivity disorder); AS (Asperger syndrome); ASD (autism spectrum disorder); DSM (*Diagnostic and Statistical Manual of Mental Disorders*); ICD (*International Classification of Diseases*); IEP (individualized education program); PDD (pervasive developmental disorder); PDD–NOS (pervasive developmental disorder–not otherwise specified)

Did you know?

PDD is a class of conditions that has the following characteristics in common: impairments with social interaction, imaginative activity, verbal and nonverbal communication skills, and a limited number of interests and activities that tend to be repetitive. PDD is, in itself, not a diagnostic label but rather refers to a broader group of neurobiological and developmental conditions known as ASDs. PDD manifests a wide range of delays of various depths of deficits in various areas. It is the specific PDDs that are diagnoses. The five disorders identified under the category of PDD listed in the *DSM* include autistic disorder, RS (Rett's syndrome), CDD (childhood disintegrative disorder), AS, and PDD–NOS. The *ICD* lists a few other disorders under the PDD umbrella, such as atypical autism (which usually involves the profoundly retarded) and elective mutism.

When parents deal with the PDD diagnosis, they have to be very clear about what the diagnostician is talking about. According to the National Dissemination Center for

Children with Disabilities (NICHCY), the general term PDD is often used to describe the specific disorders of PDD–NOS or ASD. Sometimes doctors will not want to be tied to a specific diagnosis like autism versus AS or PDD–NOS when the child is very young, so a blanket "diagnosis" of PDD is provided.

The *DSM* and *ICD* are supposed to be used as guides, so parents should keep in mind that the lines between disorders such as ASD, AS, PDD–NOS, and even high- and low-functioning autism can be very indistinct. Also the lines of what makes a PDD–NOS diagnosis can be unclear as well. Children diagnosed with autism can improve (or they might have been misdiagnosed in the first place) and then be rediagnosed with PDD–NOS, and vice versa with a PDD–NOS child's developing more clearly autistic symptoms and being rediagnosed with autism disorder. Parents must keep in mind that autism is a spectrum that ranges from mild to severe.

Although this might seem confusing, the bottom line is that early intervention is imperative and the basics of treatment are the same for all of the PDD disorders.

How it is manifested

PDD neurological disorders are often evident by age 3, although parents can notice PDD problems in infancy. Parents will notice their child's difficulty with general responsiveness, eye contact, relating to others, peer interaction, and speech. PDDs are characterized by severe and pervasive impairment in three major areas of childhood development: social interaction skills, communication skills, or the presence of stereotyped behavior, interests, and activities.

Symptoms may include problems with using and understanding language; difficulty relating to people, objects, and events; unusual play with toys and other objects; limited range of activities and interests; difficulty with changes in routine or familiar surroundings; and repetitive body movements or behavior patterns.

By the numbers

The rate of prevalence for PDDs is growing around the world. Some experts say the disorders are rising at alarming rates, while others say that more children are being diagnosed because of greater awareness.

It is a worldwide phenomenon. In Japan, for example, awareness is a factor in the numbers of rising diagnoses.

"The most prevalent developmental disorder [in Japan] may be ADHD followed by PDD. There is an increasing recognition of high-functioning PDD in Japan, and nowadays referral of children with PDD is increasing," states Yushiro Yamashita, M.D., professor of pediatrics at Japan's Kurume University.

As more and more children around the world are diagnosed with PDDs, the hope is that research will keep pace, and keys to these elusive disorders will be found quickly to open the locks that hold so many of these children within themselves.

But parents must watch out for wrong diagnoses. It is important to have a proper diagnosis and not have your child labeled with some other Alphabet Disorder when in fact the child has PDD—if for no other reason, the treatments and prognosis might be very different.

Cause

The cause of PDDs is one of the most volatile subjects in the medical field. While the disorder involves the biology and neurology of the brain, there might be numerous etiologies involved; ranging from genetic to environmental, from toxins to vaccines, from the age of the parent at conception of the child to hormonal factors, theories run rampant. What most researchers believe is that, despite the specific cause, the child must have a predisposition for this type of disorder. What might affect one child might not affect another. Parents should see the chapters for the individual disorders for more specific causes.

Treatment

There is no known cure for PDD, although there are many therapeutic treatments available that include behavioral (especially ABA), psychological, physical, therapeutic, occupational, social skills, pharmaceutical, and speech and language.

Early identification and intervention are most important in treating PDD. With early intervention and, often, extensive, wide-ranging therapy, there is promise for these children. Parents should be aware that, in the U.S., children with disabilities are entitled to free preschool services at 3 years of age under the Individuals with Disabilities Education Act (IDEA). A well-conceived IEP is essential for these children to succeed in the academic world.

There are numerous therapies that can be employed beside the traditional ones like speech-language and behavioral—music, art, and nutritional therapies are a few of the most effective ones. Again, parents are encouraged to see the chapter on an individual disorder for more specific treatments.

Sources and resources

National Dissemination Center for Children with Disabilities (www.nichcy.org)
National Organization for Rare Disorders (NORD) (for Rett's Syndrome and CDD) (203-744-0100; 800-999-NORD [6673]); (www.rarediseases.org)

See the individual chapters for PDD disorders mentioned in this chapter and "Autism" and in "General Resources" for more sources used in this chapter.

P

PDD–NOS

Pervasive Developmental Disorder–Not Otherwise Specified

Terms used in this chapter: ABA (applied behavior analysis); IEP (individualized education program); LD (learning disability); PDD (pervasive developmental disorder); PDD–NOS (pervasive developmental disorder–not otherwise specified)

Sound familiar?

Shirley has been falling through the cracks for fifteen years. Her parents have become great advocates for her, but they still feel there is something more they can do to make life easier for their daughter.

Shirley was born about three weeks early and appeared normal, except for a slight case of jaundice and a high bilirubin count, due to a hematoma on her head that was dissolving. At 6 weeks old, Shirley was rushed to the hospital because the pediatrician suspected sepsis. It turned out to be the flu, but she had already gone through a battery of tests, X-rays, and a spinal tap. For her first few years, the quiet, well-behaved girl was riddled with ear infections and allergies. She was often on antibiotics.

At 9 months, Shirley began talking—baby words, but still talking. At about 18 months, she completely stopped. Today, her mother, Tina, believes it was due to vaccines. Tina had brought Shirley for a speech evaluation in her school district's early-intervention program, and the speech therapist suggested speech therapy through the school district. The family opted against getting their daughter caught up "in the system," a decision they now regret. Little did they know what would be in store for them and how entwined in the system they would be.

Shirley did not start talking again until late in her third year. Her diagnosed disorders run the gamut of the Alphabet Disorders. "She's like A–Z," her father, Roy, jokes, rattling off deficits and diagnoses: expressive, receptive, and pragmatic speech; sensory integration problems; fine and gross motor deficits; anxiety; tics; auditory and visual-processing disorders; little imaginative play; social interaction problems; lack of emotion; aversion to being touched; repetitive routines; NLD (nonverbal learning disorder); several LDs ranging from writing to reading to math; attention and memory deficits; and OCD (obsessive-compulsive disorder).

"We kept thinking to ourselves, they all have to be connected," says Tina. "She can't really have all of these things and them not be connected." There must be one umbrella disorder, Tina believed, that could explain it all.

And she was correct. At age 13, Shirley was diagnosed as PDD–NOS by a pediatric neurologist, and although her parents were upset to hear the "autism" word in the description of the diagnosis, they were finally happy that their daughter would receive the right help, even if it was thirteen years late.

Today, Shirley is doing well, in general, although she is suddenly struggling in her academics. But with the help she is receiving from her school district and her IEP and her private therapies (occupational, psychological, speech-language), her family expects a good outcome.

"She has naturally almost grown out of so many of the scary things, especially a lot of the autistic behaviors," says Tina. "But they all still come and go. One day, she can appear totally normal, and the next symptoms will manifest themselves. But, for the most part, we see the light at the end of the tunnel and know we are on the right track."

Shirley has PDD–NOS—pervasive developmental disorder–not otherwise specified.

Did you know?

As described in the previous chapter, PDDs are a class of conditions that have the following characteristics in common: impairments in social interaction, imaginative activity, verbal and nonverbal communication skills, and a limited number of interests and activities that tend to be repetitive. PDD is not a diagnosis in itself; it refers to a broader group of neurobiological conditions, known as ASDs (autism spectrum disorders). PDD is a wide range of delays of various depths of deficits in various realms.

While PDD is not a diagnosis, PDD–NOS *is,* and it is more or less a catch-all for those children who have symptoms similar to PDD, but don't quite fit into the official diagnosis criteria for autism, mostly because of the degree or number of characteristics of autism observed. PDD–NOS is what's called a *subthreshold condition,* which really means that there are no specific diagnosis criteria. PDD–NOS is also sometimes referred to as "atypical personality development," "atypical PDD," or "atypical autism." It is also sometimes referred to as "autism lite." The Yale Developmental Disabilities Clinic reports that, in PDD–NOS, "while deficits in peer relations and unusual sensitivities are typically noted, social skills are less impaired than in classical autism."

This is obviously a very tricky disorder to diagnose, but when a parent comes to a doctor with a child who has numerous deficits in speech, language, and social interaction; behavior that's repetitive or displays unusual play; and exhibits sensory integration, auditory and visual-processing problems, lack of eye contact, attention deficits, and behavioral issues, then the doctor might conclude that the child has PDD.

PDD–NOS kids are often the ones who fall through the cracks with misdiagnoses or even no diagnosis. They are often the ones whose parents keep saying, "I know something is just not right with my child," but they keep getting a runaround from the medical community because any one of the symptoms (speech aptitude, for example) might not fall under the average score on its own. However, when compounded with other symptoms, the problem is greater than the parts. The same concerns are found with MSDD (multisystem developmental disorder).

When a parent is up all night desperately searching the Internet attempting to discover what is wrong with his or her child because the child doesn't seem to have *all* the symptoms of disorders that seem likely candidates or the parent scours through various autism organizations' Web sites, only to decide, "This seems so close, but it's not quite it," then PDD–NOS is usually a good place to restart the search. A large number of

P

PDD–NOS children might appear typical on the surface but suffer from numerous deficits and disabilities that, when brought together, form a unique, troublesome disorder.

PDD–NOS is one of the disorders that most exemplifies Alphabet Disorders—comorbid and interconnected and often exhibiting a wide spectrum of conditions.

But not all children with PDD–NOS have a history of being undiagnosed or misdiagnosed with other disorders. Since it is so difficult to fully assess a very young child with developmental disabilities, that child might easily receive a PDD–NOS diagnosis as a sort of "holding" diagnosis, prior to receiving an actual autism diagnosis, because, for example, communication development might not be assessable due to the child's young age.

One of the reasons that the autism numbers are rising dramatically is that PDD–NOS cases and diagnoses are rising dramatically. Many children who formerly would not have been regarded as "autistic" are now, through the diagnosis of PDD–NOS, being diagnosed as being on the autism spectrum, powerfully impacting autism prevalence statistics. One great concern raised by a growing number of parents of PDD–NOS children, (along with parents of children with HFA (high-functioning autism) and AS (Asperger syndrome), is that they feel that, while autism-awareness organizations are quick to use the PDD–NOS children in their statistics to raise awareness and money for research, they are not quick to provide information about or use that research money for PDD–NOS in any extensive way.

Signs and symptoms

Parents should keep in mind that PDD–NOS is a spectrum of disorders and severity of those disorders; for example, one PDD–NOS child might totally avoid eye contact, while another might avoid it only in certain situations, and a third might have very intense eye contact. One PDD–NOS child might be completely indifferent to affection, while another might be loving, affectionate, caring, and social. Below is the spectrum of symptoms and signs found in PDD–NOS children:

- appearance of talking "at" someone as opposed to talking "to" or "with"
- as an infant, demonstrates little interest in the human voice
- avoids eye contact
- avoids other children
- avoids physical contact
- babbling stops after first year
- behavioral inflexibility
- brief, telegraphic phrasing
- cognitive deficits
- collects odd objects
- craves certain foods or food textures or colors

- creates own words
- difficulty clapping hands
- difficulty following directions
- difficulty forming peer relationships
- difficulty with group games
- displays emotional extremes, not subtleties
- doesn't exhibit separation anxiety
- doesn't exhibit stranger anxiety
- doesn't follow parents around house
- doesn't imitate
- doesn't nod, shake head, or use gestures to express meaning or emotion
- doesn't raise arms to be picked up
- doesn't understand humor
- excessive talking about special interests
- failure to bond
- fearlessness
- hyperactivity
- inability to comprehend irony, sarcasm, or abstract thoughts
- inattentiveness
- indifferent to affection
- interrogative intonation when making statements
- lack of babbling in infancy
- lack of back-and-forth conversational skills
- lack of interest in peer socialization
- lack of response to other people's interests and emotions
- lack of social responsiveness
- lines up toys or objects
- little imagination in play or speech
- may passively accept physical contact
- mispronunciation problems
- mixing up words of similar sound or meaning
- monotonic, flat speech delivery
- motor skill impairments
- naïveté
- nonverbal communication impairment
- normal appearance
- objects are referred to by their use
- odd word pronunciations
- parts of speech such as pronouns or prepositions are dropped from phrases or used incorrectly

P

- passivity
- poor comprehension
- poor memory or good rote memory
- poor sequential logic
- preoccupations
- pulls adults by the hand to the object that is wanted
- quirkiness
- repetition of words or phrases (echolalia)
- repetitive play and actions
- resistance to change
- ritualistic or compulsive behavior
- seldom shows facial responsiveness
- self-stimulation (stimming), such as rocking, hand flapping, spinning, repeating words
- sensitive to noise, touch, or certain textures
- sing-song speech
- social immaturity
- sometimes appears blind
- sometimes appears deaf
- special skill abilities such as music, art, math, computers, mechanics
- speech-comprehension impairments
- staccato speech
- takes things literally
- toe walking
- unaware of potential dangers
- underresponsive or overresponsive to sensory stimuli
- unusual grammar

Cause

PDD–NOS is most likely caused by a neurological abnormality, but, as with its sister disorders, there has been no specific cause determined. But there are theories galore: vaccines; environmental toxins; genetics; age of parents at conception of the child (especially the father); hormonal factors, especially testosterone levels; jaundice at birth; strep and use of antibiotics as a child; physical trauma in either mother or child; diet; medications—the list goes on. All the theories could be correct, or none, but one thing on which many researchers and experts agree is that the child needs to be predisposed to this type of disorder. So, while a vaccine might not affect one child negatively, it might affect another completely differently.

There are many schools of thought in the autism community about cause, and there are debates on all sides of each theory. One—environmental toxins, or "environmental injury," as it is now being referred to—is one that is difficult to argue with. There is too much hard evidence showing the negative impact of toxins on the development of children. On their Web site, www.grassrootsinfo.org, the non-profit organization Grassroots Environmental Education provides a frightening list of environmental toxins impacting our children, as well as more hopeful alternatives.

And there is great interest in the genetic aspect with new promising research on chromosome 16.

Diagnosis

As with many of these Alphabet Disorders, the best medical specialist to see is one who specializes in developmental disorders, which would include a pediatric neurologist, neuropsychiatrist, pediatric psychiatrist or psychologist, or a developmental pediatrician. In many interviews conducted for this book, parents stated that it was an occupational therapist who first offered a suggestion of a PDD–NOS diagnosis for their child.

After a complete physical by the child's pediatrician, the initial assessment for PDD–NOS is conducted through a collection of information about the child's history: birth, developmental, and family history.

Sometimes a chromosome test is suggested to rule out genetic disorders. Diagnostic tests such as brain MRIs and EEGs are recommended to rule out other serious disorders or diseases. Often the child does not have to endure many of these tests because a trained doctor can observe the symptoms and determine a conclusive diagnosis, along with some psychological, cognitive, and developmental testing.

PDD–NOS is a phenomenon that is growing around the world.

"In the Netherlands, PDD–NOS has received very special interest," says Rutger Jan van der Gaag, M.D., Ph.D., of the Radboud University Nijmegen Medical Center, who specializes in child and adolescent psychiatry. "In many respects, children and adolescents in this country get a diagnosis of PDD–NOS, where in the U.K., they would be named Asperger." The catch-all nature of PDD–NOS is the same around the world.

Treatment

To help the child in the school setting, an IEP should be created around the child's abilities. In most cases, he or she should have structured classes and schedules; one-on-one opportunities with a teacher, inclusion teacher, or paraprofessional in a classroom to respond immediately to the child's particular needs; assignments provided and explained in a manner that the child can easily understand; class notes provided, especially before tests; information presented both visually and orally, or however the child best learns; an extra set of books at home; extra time between classes; reduced class size; quiet room for tests where general questions can be answered; extended time for tests; availability of communication devices such as FM amplifier; use of a calculator or tape recorder; seating in front of classroom with a clear view and close auditory proximity to the teacher; opportunities to interact with nondisabled peers; modified curriculum and assignments; speech, psychological, behavioral, auditory, social skills, sensory integration, and occupational therapies; and a team that includes the parents to monitor all aspects of the child's education.

ABA is a behavioral therapy that has also been proven effective for children on the autism spectrum. ABA breaks a skill down to its basic parts, and, as each part is worked on, positive reinforcement is employed when the child adapts his or her behavior. Other helpful therapies include occupational and physical therapy; psychological, especially group (peer), therapy; social skills therapy (SST); sensory integration therapy; music and art therapy; and even equine therapy.

Prognosis

PDD–NOS is a life-long disability, as are all disorders on the autism spectrum, but the disorder does not affect lifespan. There are no cures, although children can grow out of some of the symptoms as a normal course or because of intensive therapies. Still, the disorder stays with them, even if it is manifested in much more subtle and manageable ways. Early detection and intervention have changed the outcome for many of these children for the better. Depending on the severity of the disorder and the effectiveness of treatment, those with PDD–NOS can run the gamut of needing lifetime care to living completely independent, successful lives. The prognosis is decidedly better for the children who developed verbal language before the age of 5 years old.

Sources and resources

Grassroots Environmental Education (www.grassrootsinfo.org)
NYU Child Study Center (www.aboutourkids.org)
The Yale Developmental Disabilities Clinic (www.info.med.yale.edu/chldstdy)

See the "ASD: Autism Spectrum Disorder" and "AS: Asperger Syndrome" chapters, as well as "Autism" and in "General Resources," for more sources used in this chapter.

PHOBIAS

Terms used in this chapter: CBT (cognitive behavioral therapy); ERPT (exposure and response prevention therapy)

Did you know?

Just about everyone is afraid of something: the dark, storms, spiders, etc., but that fear becomes a phobia—specific or simple phobia—when the fear of an event, object, or situation is so intense and unrealistic that it interferes with the child's ability to conduct aspects of his or her everyday life. An immediate reaction is generated when exposed to the object or situation that will cause the child great anxiety, panic attacks, inability to function, and eventually avoidance of the situation at any cost. A child can have more than one specific phobia.

Phobic children, unlike adults, might not realize that their fear is irrational and might excessively avoid different situations; even worse, they will endure their fear in great silent, mental anguish.

These types of fears are often common in childhood and usually go away within six months. If that is not the case, parents should look into the situation with a professional.

It is believed that as many as 12 percent of the population have phobias and that the occurrence of specific phobias in children and adolescents is estimated as high as 9.2 percent.

Besides specific phobias, other phobias include PD (panic disorder), with or without agoraphobia (fear of open spaces or being in public); SP (social phobia), the fear of social or performance situations; and SM (selective mutism), the inability to speak in specific social situations when that child or adolescent can and does speak in other situations.

According to the Child Development Institute, in California, the most common phobias in children are darkness, being alone, angry people, rejection, disapproval, failure, making mistakes, dogs, public speaking, dentists, hospitals (blood), spiders, taking tests, police, school, and death. But remember, a child can develop a phobia about *anything*.

Signs and symptoms

- anticipatory anxiety
- avoiding the object or situation
- chest pain or discomfort
- chills
- clinging to parent
- crying

- diarrhea
- distress
- dizziness
- excessive or irrational fear of a specific object or situation
- fear of dying
- feeling like choking
- feeling of lose of control
- hot flashes
- hyperventilating
- lightheadedness
- nausea
- numbness
- pounding heart
- shaking
- shortness of breath
- sweating
- tantrums
- tingling
- trembling

Cause

Phobias have an inherited aspect to them, but it is not known if the specific fear is actually always inherited or it is learned behavior. Some phobias are caused by traumatic events like severe weather such as a tornado or hurricane or an animal attack.

Diagnosis

The first thing the child's pediatrician will do when presented with phobic symptoms is to conduct a physical examination to determine if there are any underlying medical conditions. The pediatrician will take a full history of the child and will refer the child to a mental-health professional if phobias are suspected.

There are no specific blood tests, but tests might be performed to rule out any other more serious disorders.

Treatment

There is good news regarding treatment for phobias because the therapies available are often very effective. They include CBT, which helps to change the child's negative thoughts and behaviors into more positive ones. This involves ERP therapy, which helps desensitize the child by gradually exposing them to the stressor that they are afraid of.

Although it is always the last resort for children, medication is sometimes necessary, if for no other reason than to provide some relief to the child when the phobias become disabling. Medication is useful in the short term (and sometimes in the long term) and is often used in conjunction with therapy. Anti-anxiety tranquilizers such as Xanax, Valium, Librium, and Ativan work well, as do SSRIs. (See the "SSRIs" section in "What You Need to Know" for more information.)

Other forms of therapy include relaxation, meditation, and yoga. Change of diet, taking vitamins and supplements, and exercising all add to the child's well-being.

Relaxation techniques, such as deep breathing, may also help to reduce anxiety symptoms.

Sources and resources

American Academy of Child and Adolescent Psychiatry (www.aacap.org)
American Psychiatric Association (www.psych.org)
American Psychological Association (www.apa.org)
Child Development Institute (www.childdevelopmentinfo.com)
DSM (Diagnostic and Statistical Manual for Mental Disorders)
National Institute of Mental Health (www.nimh.nih.gov)

See the mental-health contacts under "General Resources" for more sources used in this chapter.

PICA

Terms used in this chapter: ED (eating disorder); MR (mental retardation); NIH (National Institutes of Health); OCD (obsessive-compulsive disorder)

Did you know?

It is not unusual for a child to eat nonfood, nonnutritious items at some point in his or her childhood. But children with pica go beyond normal childhood curiosity when eating strange items. Indeed, they crave these items.

According to the NIH, the figures range as high as 32 percent of children aged 1–6 who suffer from this ED, which is the compulsive craving to eat nonfood items. This unusual craving must last longer than a month for the diagnosis of pica.

P

Pica is found mostly in children with developmental disabilities and usually between ages 2 and 3 (although the common age is 10–20 among those who are mentally retarded).

Children with pica frequently crave and consume nonfood items such as dirt, clay, soap, hair, glue, paint chips, soap, chalk, plaster, pebbles, needles, pencil erasers, paper, and many other items ranging from ice to feces. While some of these items are not necessarily a danger to the child's health, others are, and pica can be a very serious, life-threatening disorder. A child suffering from pica can be at risk for lead poisoning, bowel and intestinal obstruction or perforation, parasitic infections, and dental problems. Pica's definition has been broadened to include mouthing these items as well as ingesting them.

Cause

There really isn't a known cause for this disorder, but, in some cases, a nutritional deficiency can be the culprit. For example, the loss of minerals such as iron and zinc might trigger some cravings, so it is important to test the child's iron and zinc levels. If a child is suffering from malnutrition, then he or she might exhibit certain cravings. Brain abnormalities found in developmental disorders such as ASD (autism spectrum disorder) and MR also contribute to pica, as do psychological and personality disorders such as OCD and schizophrenia.

Treatment

Treatment for pica can be as simple as just hiding specific items from the child. But a doctor should be overseeing the child's progress, and a mental-health professional might also be needed to be brought on board. Mild aversion therapy is sometimes employed. There are some medications that might help the obsessive-compulsive aspects of the condition. See the "OCD: Obsessive-Compulsive Disorder" chapter.

Prognosis

The good news is that pica is treatable, and it is a condition that improves naturally as children grow older. If there is a developmental or mental-health proponent, then the child might have a more prolonged and complicated recovery.

Sources and resources

See the "ED: Eating Disorder" chapter and in "General Resources" for more sources used in this chapter.

PKU

Phenylketonuria

Terms used in this chapter: MR (mental retardation); PKU (phenylketonuria)

Sound familiar?

Zachary Sauder was born on June 24, 1996, a month earlier than expected. All went well except for a brief hospital readmission for dehydration from poor feeding related to his prematurity. When Zach was a week old, his pediatrician informed his father, Kurtis, that Zach's newborn screening revealed an elevated phenylalanine level. Phenylalanine is an essential amino acid. Kurtis, a pediatrician, panicked; he didn't quite know what that condition meant. He was also a little embarrassed because, as the chief resident in pediatrics at the University of Virginia at the time, he figured he should know more about the condition. It was arranged to have Zach's plasma amino acids checked the next day.

Kurtis and his wife, Cindy, spent most of that evening sitting on the couch, he recalls, "holding Zach, and staring into space." In an odd coincidence, it turned out that Cindy had written a report on this condition while in high school, but all she could remember from it were the words, "mental retardation." The next morning, Zach's test was conducted, and the Sauders received the official diagnosis.

A colleague of Kurtis, a metabolic specialist, visited them that evening to explain what they should expect.

"As he did the calculations to see how much phenylalanine-free formula and how much standard cow's milk formula Zach should eat, I realized that this was going to be more of a challenge than just avoiding hamburgers," Kurtis recalls.

Soon Kurtis and Cindy became experts in the diet: foods such as meat or eggs, which are high in protein, are forbidden. Dairy products, legumes, and flour, which are also relatively high in protein, can be eaten only in very small amounts.

Zach eats a lot of fruits and vegetables, as well as specially ordered low-protein foods such as bread and pasta. His blood is taken (finger sample) monthly (it started off as twice a week), and the sample is sent to a state lab to keep track of his phenylalanine level.

Keeping Zach healthy is constant work. Kurtis and Cindy "carefully calculate" Zach's daily intake of phenylalanine so that he does not exceed his limit. His food is weighed and the phenylalanine level is determined, all with the help of special cookbooks. To their dismay, they have found that foods that they didn't consider as suspect turned out to be on the "don't-eat" list. Many of the ones Zach could eat turned out to be very expensive.

While some states have legislation requiring insurers to pay for the formula and food products, in Zach's home state of Virginia, there is no such law, but there is a sliding scale. The blood monitoring is free.

"We wonder about the future," says Kurtis. "How and when do we explain this to him when he is older? For now, he knows that he eats special food because it is good for his brain. What about eating hot dogs at baseball games and frying our freshly caught fish over a fire? A lot of father–son bonding moments, which I had envisioned before his birth, involve ingesting protein. What if he eats something at school that he should not have? Will he rebel as a teenager by eating Big Macs? Will he have learning difficulties, hyperactivity, or psychological problems, all of which are reported to be more prevalent [with his disorder]?

"Others have many questions for us. 'Will he grow out of it?' Not really. The effects of hyperphenylalaninemia decrease with age, but he will never have the enzyme. 'How long does he need to stay on the diet?' Probably forever. Children who have come off the diet, even late in childhood, have been reported to have minor neurologic, cognitive, and psychological problems."

Kurtis and Cindy now have a one-month-old daughter, and she also has the same disorder. Kurtis: "A mild surprise to us since the chances of her having [this] were only one in four. This time around it is not a big deal. We know how to do the diet. We can look at her big brother and know everything is going to be fine. And Zach is proud to know that 'When Rachel gets big, she will eat special food like me.'

"Underlying our worries has always been a deep gratitude that Zach and Rachel were born in the era of routine newborn screening and effective dietary management and that they can be normal children on a weird diet instead of two of Dr. Asbjörn Fölling's [the Norwegian physician who first introduced the disorder] 'imbeciles' which he first described in 1934."

Kurtis has perspective on his children's disorder and advice to all parents who have a recently diagnosed child with any disorder—and for doctors as well: "I think of the parents of children to whom I have given very bad news—leukemia, severe brain damage, or the death of their child. I wonder how parents, many of whom do not have access to the same supports and resources that I do, deal with children with severe illnesses when a 'nuisance' diagnosis caused us so much worry. I understand why we need to repeat things over and over to parents who have just received an unexpected diagnosis. They need the diagnosis to sink in before they are ready to digest details and they need time to formulate all of their questions. I [now] understand why parents need reassurance for seemingly trivial things. If you think your child is at risk for developmental delay, any milestone not reached exactly on time is a potential life-long disability."

Zachary and Rachel have PKU—phenylketonuria.

Did you know?

PKU is a genetic disorder that occurs when the body is unable to utilize phenylalanine, an essential amino acid. In PKU, the enzyme that breaks down the phenylalanine is nearly deficient or completely missing. Essential amino acids are the body's protein building blocks that can only be obtained from the food we eat.

High levels of phenylalanine and some of its breakdown products can cause MR and neurological disorders if not treated within the first few weeks of life. If treated early, the

PKU child should lead a normal life. There is also a transient type of PKU that subsides over time.

Signs and symptoms

PKU children often have blue eyes, and hair and skin that is more fair than other family members.

Other than that, most of the symptoms associated with PKU are found in untreated children. But with current newborn-screening methods, children with PKU are often diagnosed at birth and do not go untreated. These are the *untreated* symptoms:

- active muscle tendon reflexes
- ADHD (attention-deficit/hyperactivity disorder) symptoms
- aggressiveness
- anemia
- anxiety
- behavioral problems
- decreased body growth
- depression
- eczema-like rash
- foul odor to the urine
- increased muscle tone (hypertonia)
- IQ decline
- irritability
- loss of appetite
- MR
- poor development of tooth enamel
- prominent cheek and upper jaw bones
- seizures
- sluggishness
- small head (microcephaly)
- twitching
- vomiting
- widely spaced teeth

Cause

PKU is an inherited, autosomal recessive metabolic disorder, which means the child inherited the traits from both parents. The incidence of carriers in the general population is approximately one in fifty people, and the chance of having a PKU child from two carriers is one in four. In order to know if you are a carrier, you must take a DNA test.

Treatment

In the U.S., all newborns have their blood phenylalanine level screened at about three days old. It is a simple test where the heel of the foot is pricked for a blood sample. If the initial screening test is abnormal, other tests will be performed.

While a PKU child still needs some phenylalanine for normal growth, the amount the child should be ingesting is restricted. The PKU diet minimizes or eliminates (depending on the severity) all of the very high-protein foods because protein contains phenylalanine. It is recommended that high-protein foods, such as meat, poultry, eggs, fish, cheese, milk, ice cream, dried beans, nuts, and legumes, and products containing regular flour, be avoided. Instead, the PKU child should eat well-measured amounts of cereals, starches, fruits, and vegetables. Most important to be avoided are Aspartame-based sweeteners, which contain 50 percent phenylalanine and are used in many foods. Phenylalanine-free formulas are also available.

Some states in the U.S. have laws mandating insurance coverage of special low-protein foods for PKU children's diets because of the food's high expense.

The PKU child might require a revised diet from his or her physician when the child has a fever or illness, since proteins break down in the body when this happens. The child's diet might need to be temporarily revised.

Maintaining phenylalanine blood levels is the key to a normal life for a PKU child, and he or she should have periodic developmental screenings to catch any unexpected problems that might occur.

If the PKU child has issues due to the restricted diet or any factor of having a chronic illness as he or she gets older, the child might benefit from mental-health counseling.

There are children who have been diagnosed with autism who, in fact, had untreated PKU and, when they were finally treated (put on the restricted diet), their autism symptoms improved.

There is now treatment, tetrahydrobiopterin supplementation, which may be helpful for some children with PKU.

Prognosis

If treated, the prognosis for the PKU child is excellent.

Sources and resources

Children's PKU Network (www.pkunetwork.org)
National PKU News Organization (www.pkunews.org)

PPD

Paranoid Personality Disorder

Terms used in this chapter: CBT (cognitive behavioral therapy); PPD (paranoid personality disorder)

Did you know?

PPD is characterized by a pervasive distrust of others; the PPD child believes that those around him or her have ill will. The PPD child appears cold and distant and lives in a world that continuously throws hostility his way.

Signs and symptoms

- detachment
- distrust of others
- dwells on trivial things
- feeling of being exploited, without reason
- feeling that others are trying to deceive, without reason
- feeling that others want to do harm or betray, without reason
- holds grudges
- hypersensitive
- jealous
- lack of trust
- misperceives attacks on character
- poor sense of humor
- quick to react angrily
- reads hidden meanings into innocent comments or actions
- scheming
- secretive, reluctant to confide in others
- suspicious of others' intentions
- unforgiving

Similar disorders include delusional disorder (persecutory type), schizophrenia (paranoid type), mood disorder with psychotic features, STPD (schizotypal personality disorder), SPD (schizoid personality disorder), BPD (borderline personality disorder), HPD (histrionic personality disorder), AvPD (avoidant personality disorder), ASPD (antisocial personality disorder), NPD (narcissistic personality disorder), and personality change due to a general medical condition.

Cause

There is no known specific cause of PPD, but studies have shown that it might be genetic since it seems to increase in prevalence in families with a family member who is schizophrenic. It can also occur due to environmental reasons such as a violent home life or other domestic causes for childhood insecurity.

Treatment

There are effective treatments for PPD children, but getting them to accept the treatment is problematic—due to the nature of the disorder, they won't trust the doctors. PPD is treated both with pharmaceuticals and through psychotherapy.

Talk therapy and CBT work well. CBT helps the child change his or her negative behaviors into positive ones, while the talk therapy will help alleviate the child's paranoia and dig to the deep roots for the cause of the disorder. Individual, family, and group therapies all work for the PPD child. It is good to get the child into therapy early while the parent still has control because, once a PPD child grows up, he will most likely not initiate therapy on his own as an adult due to the nature of the mistrust issues of the disorder.

The drug of choice is usually diazepam (Valium), which helps ease the anxiety aspect of the disorder. If there are concerns about severe anxiety and delusional thinking, then antipsychotic medications such as thioridazine (Melleril) or haloperidol (Haldol) may be prescribed. Drugs should never be given to a child without consulting with a doctor first.

Prognosis

The long-term prognosis for PPD is not very promising. Although PPD is treatable, the symptoms remain throughout life, and the patient will often require ongoing therapy.

Sources and resources

American Academy of Child and Adolescent Psychiatry (www.aacap.org)
American Psychiatric Association (www.psych.org)
American Psychological Association (www.apa.org)
DSM (*Diagnostic and Statistical Manual of Mental Disorders*)
Mayo Clinic (www.mayoclinic.com)
National Institute of Mental Health (www.nimh.nih.gov)
psychologytoday.com

See the mental-health contacts under "General Resources" for more sources used in this chapter.

PWS

Prader-Willi Syndrome

Terms used in this chapter: AAFP (American Academy of Family Physicians); FISH (fluorescent in situ hybridization); IEP (individualized education program); LD (learning disability); MR (mental retardation); OCD (obsessive-compulsive disorder); PWS (Prader-Willi syndrome)

Sound familiar?

This letter was written by John Hudson Symons of Ontario, Canada. It was provided by the Prader-Willi Syndrome Association.

"We have feelings, dreams and personal thoughts. We have a heart, a soul, mind and spirit and we need you to understand us. Understanding and caring are two of the most important things you can do for us. In high school the students did not understand me either. I loved to learn. I went through so much pain and harassment at school because I wanted to learn so much. The hunger urges at school were difficult to control. It was hard to watch other students eat snacks. I tried to ignore the snacks the best I could but then I became agitated and started constantly trying to sneak food at school and at home. I didn't mean to be a sneak, but I could not help myself. The food desire was in control! My father was a doctor and my mother was a nurse. If I was left alone I would eat every thing I could. I would think about food all the time, food is everywhere—on TV, at school, at home and in the junk mail. I would even hide food and sneak food that belonged to my brothers and sisters. I had no control. I could feel sharp teeth tearing at my stomach like piranhas—and still do. I know that I need someone to keep the cupboards locked and I need someone to keep me active to control my weight. I want to have some fun in my life. I have the right to have the same choices in life that you do. If the government has money to fund crisis situations why can they not prevent situations from becoming a crisis? I need full support NOW before I get into a crisis situation. I want to live and I am sure that you want the same for your child."

John Hudson Symons died of obesity related causes shortly after he wrote this. John Hudson Symons had PWS—Prader-Willi syndrome.

Did you know?

PWS is a genetic disorder that was first described by a group of Swiss doctors in 1956, including pediatrician/endocrinologist Andrea Prader, M.D.; pediatrician/neonatologist Heinrich Willi, M.D.; as well as Alexis Labhardt, M.D., and Gido Fanconi, M.D. (The disorder is sometimes referred to by any combination of the above surnames, but most popularly by PWS.)

The genetic defect of PWS is based on chromosome 15, inherited from the father, and the syndrome displays characteristics of low muscle tone (hypotonia), sex glands producing little or no hormones (hypogonadism), the compulsive need to eat and obsession with food (hyperphagia), cognitive impairment, difficult behaviors, and obesity. It affects both sexes. Most cases of PWS are the result of new spontaneous genetic errors that occur some time around the point of conception.

PWS is identified in about one in 25,000 births, but the AAFP believes that this is an underestimate because of the many children undiagnosed at an early age. The AAFP believes the statistic is more like one in 10,000 to one in 15,000.

One of the more curious aspects of PWS is the hyperphagia, which usually occurs before age 6. Since these PWS children have hypotonia and remain fairly inactive, it compounds the overeating problem and morbid amounts of weight are gained.

When PWS children are young, they are like other children when it comes to temperament; but, as they grow older, their behavior starts to take a turn for the worse. Certain factors, such as change in routine, trigger their behavioral outbursts; and since the behavioral problems often manifest at the same time as the hyperphagia, it becomes a double whammy—trying to keep the child away from food and disciplining the child's difficult outbursts. Strong and consistent rules are highly suggested.

Working with a mental-health professional along with a nutritionist, physical therapist, and occupational therapist is important to the child's success, and the mental-health specialist might very well suggest putting the child on medication. SSRIs have proven very successful in aiding the PWS child with behaviors such as OCD, repetitive questioning or actions (perseveration), anxiety, and mood swings. (See the "SSRIs" in the section "What You Need to Know" for more information.)

Signs and symptoms

- almond-shaped eyes
- antisocial behavior such as lying and stealing
- argumentative
- cross-eyed (esotropia)
- curvature of the spine (scoliosis)
- decreased fetal movement
- delayed or incomplete gonadal maturation
- delayed pubertal signs after age 16
- diabetes type II
- distinctive facial characteristics
- excessive or rapid weight gain between ages 1 and 6
- fair skin and hair compared with family (hypopigmentation)
- feeding problems in infancy

P

- food foraging/obsession with food (hyperphagia)
- global developmental delay before age 6
- good long-term memory
- high blood pressure (hypertension)
- hypothalamic dysfunction
- incomplete or cessation of development of genitals (hypoplasia)
- LDs
- lethargy in infancy
- long, narrow head (dolichocephaly) in infants
- low sex-hormone levels
- manipulative
- mild to moderate MR
- motor milestones are typically delayed one to two years
- mouth that appears small, with down-turned corners
- narrow face
- narrow hands
- nearsightedness (myopia)
- neonatal and infantile central low muscle tone (hypotonia), improving with age
- obesity
- OCD
- oppositional behavior
- osteoporosis
- poor coordination and balance
- poor short-term auditory memory abilities
- poor weight gain in infancy
- possessiveness
- repeated behaviors (perseveration)
- rigid behavior
- round back (kyphosis)
- short stature
- short-term memory problems
- skin picking (dermatillomania)
- sleep apnea
- slight or no menses in adolescent girls
- small feet
- small hands
- speech articulation problems when younger
- strong reading skills
- strong receptive language skills
- strong verbal ability, even after speech delays

- strong visual-perceptual skills (e.g., jigsaw puzzles)
- stubbornness
- teeth grinding (bruxism)
- temper tantrums
- thick saliva with crusting at corners of the mouth
- thin upper lip
- underdeveloped sex organs (hypogonadism)
- undescended testes
- violent outbursts
- weak abstract thinking
- weak cry in infancy

Diagnosis

Genetic testing is the most fool-proof, specific way to diagnose PWS. Methylation analysis confirms diagnosis of PWS as does the FISH test, which utilizes fluorescently labeled DNA probes to detect or confirm gene or chromosome abnormalities. FISH and DNA techniques can identify the specific genetic cause and associated recurrence risk.

Treatment

Diet and exercise are key components of keeping a PWS child healthy. Speech therapy is indicated for poor oral-motor skills and speech delays. Products to help increase saliva production will also help speech problems. Physical and occupational therapy can help a PWS child strengthen his or her coordination and motor skills. Social-skills training can also be useful. Sex-hormone treatment has good results, but it is sometimes accompanied by side effects.

Academically, the children need a very structured special-education program, and they should fare well. The Prader-Willi Syndrome Association reports that an IEP is "the most important tool created in helping the student with PWS in the school setting."

Prognosis

There are numerous complications involved with PWS, such as diabetes and heart problems, but the most common concern is avoiding the complications that come with morbid obesity. The PWS child who is under a strict diet and exercise program will have a chance at a much better quality of life, with a normal life expectancy. Few PWS children and adults can live independently without supervision, and depending on IQ, the child might end up in a residential facility or might be able to live at home.

Sources and resources

American Academy of Family Physicians (www.aafp.org)

Prader-Willi Alliance of New York (716-276-2211; 800-442-1655);
  (www.prader-willi.org)

Prader-Willi Syndrome Association (800-926-4797); (www.pwsausa.org)

R

RAD (Reactive Attachment Disorder)

RS (Rett's Syndrome)

RAD

Reactive Attachment Disorder

Terms used in this chapter: ADHD (attention-deficit/hyperactivity disorder); RAD (reactive attachment disorder)

Sound familiar?

Kevin was 4½ years old when he was adopted from a Romanian orphanage. His parents expected he'd be a handful, but they never expected the aggressive, defiant, and hyperactive behavior he had demonstrated from the day he moved in.

From the start, he didn't eat and showed intense oppositional behavior toward his new mother and father, Jam and Scott. Kevin would show absolutely no affection, at least toward his parents. He would often seem fine with absolute strangers or other members of his family.

Scott noted odd behaviors aside from the hyperactivity. Kevin would rock back and forth, eyes shut tight. When he did open his eyes, he would not make eye contact.

He was argumentative and bossy, becoming what Jam calls "just plain unlikable."

Talk therapy didn't help—Kevin could just not bond with his therapist, and behavioral therapy didn't seem to make a dent. When he started school, he was a discipline problem and was moved to three different preschools before starting kindergarten where his behavioral problems continued.

Then Scott was told by a coworker of a support group of parents of international adoptees. It didn't take long before Scott and Jam found themselves in the company of many parents in the same situation with their once-long-term-institutionalized children.

At this group Jam and Scott learned what was wrong with Kevin, and with that information they went to a recommended psychiatrist and left with a diagnosis that has helped them since make some therapeutic progress with their son.

Kevin has RAD—reactive attachment disorder.

Did you know?

RAD is a condition that is a disturbance of social interaction, characterized by the inability of a child to form healthy social relationships, particularly with a primary caregiver. RAD is often found in children who have had little human affection and contact or abusive care in early childhood. Many children adopted from orphanages or hospitals are RAD children. These children are reacting to formative years of abuse, neglect, or untreated illness.

It is very simple how a child becomes so disordered. Attachment is the intimate bond between the child and his or her primary caregiver. It is normal for children who cry to have their needs met by their caregiver—being soothed, in most cases, by the mother. When those needs are met, the child is able to learn affection and trust. When no attachment is formed, the child's basic emotional needs are not met and the child becomes detached, with rage and mistrust developing instead of the trust and love. The normal child also learns limits from proper caregiving because, once an attachment is formed, a parent can say "no" to certain demands without being neglectful or abusive. Children learn those limits in a reciprocal relationship, enabling them to function properly in the give-and-take social world. Through these positive interactions with his or her caregiver, the normal child will learn about love, responsibility, self-esteem, and empathy and will develop a full set of emotions, self-control, sense of safety, and a conscience.

Children with RAD do not form any of the positive behavior or emotions. To them, the world is cold, uncaring, and sometimes violent. So, to cope, they take on those attributes.

There are two main subtypes of RAD—inhibited (emotionally withdrawn) and disinhibited (overly sociable)—as well as several other "styles" of RAD—ambivalent (angry, oppositional, and violent), anxious (clings and does not like to separate); avoidant (puts on a front, no depth to emotions); and disorganized (inappropriate and unusual symptoms).

Signs and symptoms

- ADHD
- anger
- antisocial behaviors such as lying and stealing
- argumentative
- avoids caregiver
- avoids physical contact
- bossy
- defiant
- demanding
- destructive
- difficult to comfort
- disinterest in peer friendships
- distrustful
- eating disorders
- has control issues
- hides and hoards food

- inability to give and receive affection
- indifference to others
- indiscriminate sociability with strangers
- isolated
- lack of conscience
- lack of eye contact
- lack of impulse control
- learning delays and disorders
- manipulative
- no reciprocal smile response
- poor sucking response in infants
- rage
- self-injurious
- sensitivity to touch, cuddling, and hugging
- separation anxiety
- shows no remorse
- speech and language problems
- superficial friendliness and charm
- unresponsive
- unusual speech patterns and modality
- violent
- weak crying response in children
- whining

Cause

There are a variety of suspected causes for RAD, most having to do with early-childhood situations. In particular, the mother–child (or primary caregiver) relationship is at the heart of this disorder. The mother may have had a drug addiction or suffered from depression, including postpartum depression, resulting in her being unable to care adequately for her newborn. The newborn may not have received the proper care for his or her physical needs and comfort from either parent and may not have received the proper loving interaction necessary for bonding—touching, cuddling, stimulation, and play. There may also have been physical abuse in the home.

As the opening story shows, many RAD children have experienced their early months or years in an orphanage or state-sponsored facility, where the one-to-one interaction is limited. In this situation, the child becomes anxious, may suffer from PTSD (post-traumatic stress disorder), or may have an undiagnosed physical ailment. Other causes may include changes in or separation from primary caregiver, frequent institutional or foster home placements, frequent moves, lack of food, no childhood play, or young and inexperienced parents with poor parenting skills.

Diagnosis

The child's complete history will be taken by his or her pediatrician, and a physical exam will be performed to rule out any other underlying medical concerns. A mental-health specialist will then evaluate the child. Once the diagnosis of RAD is given, the child should be seen by a pediatric psychiatrist or psychologist who specializes in attachment issues. Since there are so many potential comorbid disorders that might accompany a RAD child, especially one who is adopted or has been in foster care, other specialists such as a pediatric neurologist and speech-language pathologist should be seen.

Other Alphabet Disorders can be mistaken for RAD, including ADHD, ASPD (antisocial personality disorder), CD (conduct disorder), ODD (oppositional defiant disorder), FAS (fetal alcohol syndrome), receptive language disorders, MR (mental retardation), schizoid syndrome of disorders, RS (Rett's syndrome), ASD (autism spectrum disorder), and other PDDs (pervasive developmental disorders).

Treatment

It might be natural to think that the best treatment for a RAD child is love and a safe environment, but, while these are paramount, psychological help is also necessary. Therapy will help your child eventually accept your love, but your affectionate, safe home and good intentions will not erase your child's problems.

For both biological and adoptive parents, counseling and parenting-skills classes should be considered.

Therapy is problematic and challenging for the RAD child because these children are unable to form a bond, and they will be resistant to a therapist. If that bond is formed with a therapist—and it can happen—then the child is lucky to have that avenue of treatment. The therapist, along with the parents, will help remodel behavior and will use cognitive behavioral therapy (CBT), a type of therapy that is extremely effective with numerous psychological disorders, to help reshape the child's behaviors, turning negative behaviors and thoughts into positive ones.

This will be an ongoing collaboration between the parents and the therapist.

Prognosis

Depending on the severity of the disorder, with the proper treatment, interventions, and a safe, loving home, the RAD child can show great improvement. Other seriously ill RAD children do not show improvement.

Sources and resources

Adopting.org (www.adopting.org)
Attachment Disorder Site (www.attachmentdisorder.net)
RadKid.org (www.radkid.org)

See the mental-health contacts under "General Resources" in the appendix for more sources used in this chapter.

RS

Rett's Syndrome

Terms used in this chapter: MR (mental retardation); PDD (pervasive developmental disorder); RS (Rett's syndrome)

Sound familiar?

Eleven-year-old Kaitlyn Tovey, with her short, dark brown hair and 4-foot, 4-inch frame, at first appears like a typical teenager—she has teen moodiness down pat; if her mom, Jana, says something Kaitlyn doesn't like, Jana says Kaitlyn will give her "the typical teenager stare."

But Kaitlyn is not a typical teenager.

She walks with the aid of someone shadowing her, she cannot speak, she eats through a tube, she drools (although her mom emphatically jokes, "not around good-looking boys"), she suffers from anxiety, and she wears diapers.

Life has not been easy for Kaitlyn. She has endured a bit more than a decade of surgeries and other medical procedures—three ear tubes; a fundoplication (a surgery that strengthens the valve between the esophagus and stomach, which prevents the backing up of acid into the esophagus); a "G" or gastronomy button that allows access to the stomach for medications and/or feedings; removal of her tonsils and adenoids; vagus nerve stimulator implanted for seizures; hysterectomy; and three Botox procedures, twice with serial casting (a well-padded cast that immobilizes a joint that helps improve range of motion).

Jana says Kaitlyn is "tired of being poked and prodded. She is tired of it being so physically hard."

Kaitlyn weighed only 4 lbs., 13 oz. when she was born. Jana had intrauterine growth restriction (IUGR), where the fetus is smaller than expected, and she says that the doctors blamed Kaitlyn's initial difficulties on that.

Kaitlyn began occupational therapy at 10 months because she was not crawling or sitting up independently. The family was told by the doctor and therapists that she would soon catch up, but, at each six-month review, she would be given another therapy.

By 12 months, Kaitlyn was sitting up, and two months later, she began crawling and rolling around. The following year she was holding onto objects to help her stand, moving things around, using assistive communication devices, and saying five words.

The last word she said on a regular basis was "Amen."

Her parents were beginning to relax when Kaitlyn reached 2 years old, thinking that all would be well because Kaitlyn was making "amazing strides."

At 26 months, however, Kaitlyn began to put her hands in her mouth continuously and suffered increased anxiety. She also started to have screaming and biting spells and began to lose some of her skills; she was beginning to appear autistic—losing eye contact and retreating into her own world.

When Kaitlyn was 3, her family was watching some home movies of her childhood activities. The family friends who were also watching the video commented on how they never knew Kaitlyn was once able to perform some of the actions she did in the video. Jana and Dave, Kaitlyn's father, had forgotten how much she had changed. While watching the video, they began to notice habits exhibited by the young girl such as "increasingly prevalent hand movements," which now they realized were autistic-like behaviors. They silently wept to themselves, thinking about how they hadn't even noticed the skills lost.

The following day, Kaitlyn's mother had what she calls "a special talk" with her daughter, telling her how she realized that it must be so difficult and frightening with everything that was happening to her. Kaitlyn stopped rocking, was still for a moment, and gave her mother a look Jana has never forgotten to this day.

It was then when Jana told Kaitlyn about her disorder in detail. She explained to her why it had sidetracked the family so badly. Jana made Kaitlyn a promise: "I told her I would make sure I remembered everything for her."

Jana then began to explain to the young girl everything that was happening with her body.

"It sounds like a big conversation for a 3-year-old," Jana now says, "but I knew she got it."

Today, Kaitlyn makes her likes and dislikes clearly known through her expressive eyes that change between brown, hazel, and green. Communication is something Dave and Jana are very excited about. In one month, Kaitlyn will start working with a DynaVox, a piece of equipment that will eventually allow her to communicate with her parents. And they are sure she will have a lot to say.

Meanwhile, Kaitlyn attends public school, where she is in a "life-skills" class. Dave and Jana say they "wish she was learning more literature and math and cultural things," but, as surprising as it may sound, their school district is resistant. Jana and Dave know those are skills that will greatly benefit their daughter, especially after she begins the DynaVox.

One of the most evident things about Kaitlyn, who is completely nonverbal, Dave says, is "her wicked sense of humor"—her parents can tell from her reactions and facial movements.

The Toveys feel blessed because there are many other girls with the disorder who are in much more serious shape, completely immobile and shut off from the world, let alone being able to display the type of sense of humor they see in their daughter.

And although Kaitlyn usually travels in her wheelchair, when she does take a walk with her parents, as with any other preteen, she will push their hand away from her when they walk together.

But taking care of Kaitlyn is a twenty-four-hour a day job, and it is hard for an outsider to imagine how they cope.

Not only do they cope, they have an even more amazing revelation: "We're hoping to bring other girls with this disorder into our home as foster children," says Dave.

Kaitlyn has RS—Rett's syndrome.

Did you know?

RS is a genetic-based disorder that is one of the most physically disabling of all the five PDDs that are part of the autism spectrum. This childhood neurodevelopmental condition that mostly occurs in females affects one in 10,000–15,000 girls by the age of 12, although many advocates and RS organizations believe the statistics are higher and that many girls are not diagnosed properly.

RS, first introduced in 1965 in Vienna, Austria, by Andreas Rett, M.D., is characterized by normal early development with an onset of the disorder between six and eighteen months. At the start, RS girls (a very slight percentage of boys are diagnosed with RS, and most die in utero) will exhibit appropriate speech (using words or phrases) and motor development as well as age-appropriate sitting and walking. But, eventually, the child will lose use of her hands and exhibit distinctive repetitive hand movements, slowed brain and head growth, abnormalities when she walks, seizures, and MR. The girl enters a period of regression, losing speech and motor skills. This period of regression between 1 and 4 years old can be sudden, but it can also be slow and indistinguishable from normal behavior and be missed in diagnosis if the symptoms come on singularly and slowly. The regression can last for a few days or it can go on for months. Whatever the case is, as soon as parents suspect that anything is wrong, they should seek help and be persistent until they get the right answers. These early years are a critical time period for the child to have the RS detected and to begin intervention.

Signs and symptoms

- autistic behaviors
- bone fractures
- cessation of social interaction
- cold, sometimes bluish-red or purple extremities
- constipation
- decreased body fat and muscle mass
- diminished eye contact
- EEG abnormalities and changes
- extreme motor control problems
- gait abnormalities (unsteady, wide-based, and stiff-legged)

- hand tapping and handwringing
- irregular breathing patterns such as hyperventilation
- irritability
- loss of motor skills
- loss of speech
- MR
- muscle rigidity
- normal development before symptoms arrive
- obsessive-compulsive behaviors
- persistent clapping
- persistent hand washing
- reflux
- scoliosis
- seizures
- sleep apnea
- slowed growth (after 1 year old)
- slowed head growth (after 3 months old)
- slowed weight gain (after 1 year old)
- small feet
- small head (microcephaly)
- spasticity
- swallowing problems
- teeth grinding (bruxism)
- toe walking
- torso shaking
- weak muscle tone (hypotonia); dangling arms, legs, and head are usually the first symptoms
- well behaved

Cause

Professor Alan K. Percy, M.D., scientific director of the International Rett Syndrome Association, says the cause of RS is genetic.

"In more than 95 percent, RS is due to mutations in the gene, MECP2, otherwise known as methyl-CpG-binding protein 2," he explains. "About two hundred different mutations are known, but eight common-point mutations and a group with large-scale deletions of the gene account for 75–80 percent of those with mutations."

The remaining 20 to 25 percent, it is believed, may be caused by partial gene deletions, by mutations in different parts of the gene, or by unidentified genes.

The MECP2 gene, which is found on the X chromosome, is thought to control the functions of other genes and the switching on and off of various proteins.

Diagnosis

Besides clinical observations of the stereotypical hand movements, loss of developmental skills and speech, small head size, and decrease in growth, genetic tests can be conducted to obtain a diagnosis. The discovery of the MECP2 gene has made possible the development of a blood test for RS. The diagnosis of the disorder, however, is still based on observation of those distinctive symptoms and the child's clinical history.

At this time, approximately 85 percent of those diagnosed with RS also test positive for an MECP2 mutation.

"Rett syndrome remains a clinical diagnosis," says Dr. Percy. "Finding a mutation confirms the diagnosis but is not required. Indeed, some females have mutations in this gene but do not have RS, yet may have a variety of neurodevelopmental problems.

"It is diagnosed typically now in early childhood, but after age 12–18 months. Because it is not recognized by many physicians and other health-care providers, diagnosis may be delayed even into adulthood."

Treatment

"There is no effective treatment or cure known for RS," says Dr. Percy. "Treatment generally involves management of accompanying problems such as epilepsy, gastroesophageal reflux, constipation, scoliosis, other orthopedic issues, sleep problems, and intervention therapies include physical, occupational, speech, music, and hippo [use of a horse as a therapeutic tool] and aqua therapies. Speech therapy should include augmentative communication to take advantage of the intense eye-gaze that is present. Nutritional supplementation may be required, including the use of gastrotomy feeding."

The treatment is all about managing the symptoms. Many aspects of it have to be constantly monitored to make sure existing symptoms don't degenerate—such as heart abnormalities, scoliosis, breathing problems, and epilepsy.

Since scoliosis is such a serious aspect of RS and since it is progressive, a bendable support is often used adjacent to the spine to relieve pressure on the lungs.

Medications are sometimes used for breathing irregularities and motor difficulties, and anti-epileptic drugs may be used to control seizures, which are progressive with onset in teen years. Occupational therapy will teach the child life skills such as dressing, eating, toilet training, etc.

Physical therapy and hydrotherapy (therapeutic use of water) can help with the child's mobility, while some children might need devices ranging from braces to wheelchairs. Splints are used to control the RS child's many hand movements.

The multitherapeutic approach also involves nutritional assistance, to maintain the general health of these children who have many potential eating problems.

Of course, special-education services should be employed, which might also include vocational training.

Prognosis

RS children become profoundly disabled and require full assistance with every aspect of their daily lives. There is no cure for RS.

"We are currently near the end of an update on life expectancy," says Dr. Percy. "Based on somewhat old information, longevity may be well into adulthood and even into the sixth decade of life or beyond. However, sudden, unexpected deaths do occur, even in childhood and generally without evident cause. This older information suggested 70 percent survival to age 35 compared with 98 percent of all females."

Some very promising news was announced by the Rett Syndrome Research Foundation in February 2007, when RS was reversed in a study done on mice. This study has a profound effect on many Alphabet Disorders, especially those on the autism and schizophrenia spectrums.

Sources and resources

International Rett Syndrome Foundation (1-800-818-RETT); (www.rettsyndrome.org)
Rett Syndrome Research Foundation (513-874-3020);
    (www.rsrf.org/parent_resources/9.5.html)
We Move (www.wemove.org)

See "Autism" and "General Resources" for more sources used in this chapter.

S

SAD (Seasonal Affective Disorder)

SAD (Separation Anxiety Disorder)

SID (Sensory Integration Disorder)

SLD (Speech-Language Disorder)

SLOS (Smith-Lemli-Opitz Syndrome)

SM (Selective Mutism)

SMS (Smith-Magenis Syndrome)

SPD (Schizoid Personality Disorder)

SPLD (Semantic Pragmatic Language Disorder)

STPD (Schizotypal Personality Disorder)

SAD

Seasonal Affective Disorder

Terms used in this chapter: SAD (seasonal affective disorder)

Sound familiar?

Maggie started off her freshman year of high school with great energy. The New Jersey high schooler had no trouble keeping up with her classwork and was involved in several after-school activities. But after the Thanksgiving break of her freshman year, she began to have trouble getting through her assigned reading and had to work harder to apply herself. She couldn't concentrate in class, and, after school, all she wanted to do was sleep. Her grades began to drop, and she rarely felt like socializing anymore. Even though Maggie was always punctual before, she began to have trouble getting up on time for school and was absent or late many days during the winter.

At first Maggie's parents thought she was slacking off. They were upset with her, but they figured it was just a phase—especially because her energy finally seemed to return in the spring. But when the same thing happened the following November and Maggie's mood and her grades plummeted again, they took her to a psychiatrist.

The doctor learned that Maggie was so depressed at times that she was unable to leave her house. She was often sick to her stomach and suffered headaches. She started drifting away from her friends and began to let her appearance slide, which was a red flag to her parents because she was an actress in local theater and was always conscious of keeping up a good appearance. Her depression would have been obvious, her mother now says, but her mental state changed for the better during the course of the year—her parents were perplexed.

It didn't take long in therapy for the doctor to determine what was wrong. Now, with the awareness of her disorder and the use of full-spectrum (daylight) lamps during the winter and occasional medication, Maggie is doing very well.

Maggie has SAD—seasonal affective disorder.

Did you know?

The aptly named acronym SAD is depression that follows a seasonal pattern. It manifests itself and disappears at the same times each year. In the U.S., it usually starts in October and November and lasts about six months. In the U.K., it starts in September and lasts through April.

The typical manifestation is the depressive symptoms occurring when winter arrives and there are fewer hours of daylight. SAD children get reinvigorated with the arrival of spring when the daylight hours become longer. The children are more energetic and display normal mood behaviors. What distinguishes SAD from other mood disorders is that it annually occurs in a specific season—a few months each winter—and not during any other time of the year.

It is estimated that 6 percent of people suffer from SAD, and, in children, it mostly affects older teens. It is believed to affect between 2 and 10 percent of northern Europeans, and it has been reported that as many as one in fifty people in the U.K. suffer from the disorder. Ten percent of Americans suffer from the disorder, while it is estimated that, in the U.K., Canada, and Australia, the rate is 5 percent. Many feel the discrepancy is due more to awareness and mis- or undiagnosed cases in those latter countries.

As with other forms of depression, this disorder is often inherited.

Signs and symptoms

- agoraphobia
- bowel irregularities
- changes in eating patterns and tastes
- changes in sleep patterns
- craving comfort- and sugary foods
- crying
- difficulty with schoolwork
- disinterest in socializing
- dissatisfaction
- fatigue
- feeling of hopelessness and worthlessness
- feelings of enjoyment diminish
- guilt
- headaches
- heart palpitations
- hypersensitivity
- irritability
- lack of confidence
- lethargy
- loss of energy and interest
- lowered self-esteem
- mood changes
- muscle and joint pains
- no motivation
- overeating
- oversleeping
- phobias

S

- procrastination
- restless sleep
- sadness
- self-criticism
- suicidal feelings
- tension
- weight gain

Cause

SAD is believed to be the result of how the brain responds to the decrease in sunlight in the winter months. Theories are wide-ranging, including its being an interruption in the brain's ability to regulate hormones, therefore disrupting the energy, mood, and sleep–wake cycles those hormones regulate. Melatonin and serotonin, two brain chemicals associated with sleep and mood, are involved in SAD responses.

Sleep-linked melatonin is produced in greater quantities when the daylight hours shorten; with the darkness, the body believes it should be asleep. Serotonin—which, when decreased, causes depression—increases with sunlight exposure, enabling the child to sleep, and helps fight depression. So shorter, darker days will decrease serotonin and increase melatonin, causing depression.

There are many other potential causes for SAD besides individual biology and brain chemistry. As with other depressive and anxiety disorders, SAD runs in the family—it could be inherited or a learned behavior. Obviously, not everyone develops SAD from changes in daylight, so it is believed that those who do have a certain sensitivity to variations in sunlight.

There is also a regional aspect to SAD. According to the Nemours Foundation, a nonprofit dedicated to children's health,

> the prevalence of SAD varies from region to region, and it's far more abundant among people who live in higher latitudes. For instance, one study found the rates of SAD [in the U.S.] were seven times higher among people in New Hampshire than in Florida, suggesting that the farther someone lives from the equator, the more likely they are to develop SAD. Interestingly, when people who get SAD travel to lower latitude areas during winter where there is more daylight, they don't experience their seasonal symptoms.

Diagnosis

The child's pediatrician or a pediatric psychiatrist or psychologist can diagnose SAD from clinical observations and a history of the child's symptoms.

Treatment

There are several ways to treat SAD.

One major form of therapy is simply increasing light exposure. Depending on the severity of the disorder, a SAD child might need only to go out into the sunlight for a few extra hours or be exposed to full-spectrum (daylight) light bulbs. These bulbs can be found in most supply stores and can be used in most lamps.

Light- or phototherapy can be effective with more severe symptoms of SAD. The child sits in front of a lightbox device that simulates daylight for a brief period during the day; since light is absorbed through the retina, it is suggested that the child glance at the light every once in a while. These are specialized lights—they are not tanning lights—and they should, without exception, always be utilized under a doctor's supervision.

As with other depressive disorders, there is also a pharmacological avenue of therapy. SSRIs are the new drug of choice. (See the "SSRIs" section in "What You Need to Know" for more information.)

St. John's Wort is a herbal remedy that has also been used to help SAD and other mild depressive disorders. Parents should discuss any herbal supplements, as well as any medications your doctor suggests, very carefully with him or her because these drugs and supplements usually have side effects.

And, of course, psychological therapy will help the SAD child.

Prognosis

The prognosis is usually good for those with SAD if they are receiving ongoing treatment. The proper therapy (or therapies) will help ease the symptoms and enable the SAD child to lead a normal life. For many children, SAD is a lifelong disorder.

Sources and resources

American Academy of Child and Adolescent Psychiatry (www.aacap.org)

American Psychiatric Association (www.psych.org)

American Psychological Association (www.apa.org)

Mayo Clinic (www.mayoclinic.com)

National Institute of Mental Health (www.nimh.nih.gov)

The Nemours Foundation (www.nemours.org)

See the mental-health contacts under "General Resources" for more sources used in this chapter.

SAD

Separation Anxiety Disorder

Terms used in this chapter: CBT (cognitive behavioral therapy); CHB (Children's Hospital Boston); *DSM* (*Diagnostic and Statistical Manual of Mental Disorders*); SAD (separation anxiety disorder)

Sound familiar?

When Tony, a charming, smart boy with wild, curly, reddish-blond hair, had to be anywhere without his parents, well … he just wouldn't do it. He wouldn't stay at his grandparents' condo; he fought about going to school; he wouldn't participate in play dates. From as early as his parents can recall through fifth grade, when Tony was 11, separating was "an ordeal."

"He never liked being away from us," says his father, Ritter, who operates a business from the family's Cincinnati, Ohio, home, with Tess, Tony's mother, who once suffered from agoraphobia.

Tony never had a babysitter outside of his grandparents. And trouble started early.

"My wife had to sit outside his nursery-school classroom for the duration of the day," Ritter says of the preschool years. "As long as she was there, outside the door, Tony was OK, and it never really got better."

In fact, according to Tess, it got worse.

"We had to peel him out of the car every morning [for] school. The principal had to help. The school psychiatrist had to help. The teachers had to help. The custodian had to help. He would not leave the car. He was often dragged in screaming and crying."

The reason Tony was in the car? He wouldn't get on his school bus, of course.

"I gave him a family photo to take with him, and that helped for a while," Tess says. "We brought him for all sorts of help, and most of it didn't help. In fact, some of the testing results were downright scary. They told us he was almost psychotic in his separation fears." Tony's parents thought their child had a severe lifelong problem on his hands.

"We were truly terrified that we had this child who would not be able to function in the real world," Ritter says.

But with the right therapist and therapy (Tony spent a year in CBT and game therapy) and with what his parents felt were normal changes when puberty hit, Tony got better. He also became a vegetarian at this time, but his parents don't know, to this day, if that had any effect.

"He became a totally normal, obnoxious teenager," Tess says, with a laugh, "but along with that came a sociability that we never saw before. He started hanging around with friends, got involved in sports, and suddenly was like a 'normal' teenager."

"And it's been uphill ever since," Ritter adds.

Tony became extremely active and popular throughout junior high and high school, he has a longtime girlfriend, and he currently attends college—a local one.

But this is a new Tony.

"Ever since he was, like, 14, he has been out more than he's home," says Ritter. "We thought we'd never get past those early days, but we have, and Tony is amazing now—he is so self-confident and social.

"I don't think he will be completely rid of that fear. Even now, we still see a strong connection between him and us. He likes being around things that are familiar—his home base, so to speak. Even though he still hates to separate, he has learned to control his fear, and even though he still has that residue, he's a million times better than when he was suffering so badly when he was younger."

Tony has SAD—separation anxiety disorder.

Did you know?

It is not unusual for young children to exhibit anxiety when a loved one or caregiver like a parent, grandparent, aunt, uncle, or sibling leaves them. It is unusual, however, when the anxiety starts becoming age-inappropriate and begins to interfere negatively with the child's daily life. The older the child or adolescent is, the more concern the parent should have.

SAD is diagnosed when children are excessively anxious about separating from their caregivers and other authority figures or from a safe place like home. The children become afraid that harm might befall them as well as those they love.

According to the *DSM*, separation anxieties become a disorder when the child's anxiety or fear causes anguish and starts to affect social, academic, or, for adolescents, work-related situations, and this anxiety lasts at least one month.

Children with SAD fear the loss of their parent; for example, they worry that the parent might become ill or die in an accident. This should not be confused with the anxiety of children who live in dangerous areas because of crime, natural disasters, war, etc., where there is a real fear of leaving the house or losing loved ones.

About 4 percent of children and young adolescents suffer from SAD according to the *DSM*, which also reports that, in survey samples, the disorder is more prevalent in girls.

Signs and symptoms

- apathy
- aversion to school
- bedtime fears
- clinging to parents
- crying
- depression and sadness
- desire to sleep in parents' bed

S

- difficulty concentrating
- difficulty falling asleep
- dizziness
- excessive worry
- fear of carpooling
- fear of getting sick on school bus or in school
- fear of meeting new people
- feeling unsafe being alone
- headaches
- hiding, especially behind parent
- nausea
- shadowing parents
- shortness of breath
- sleep disorders such as inability to sleep and nightmares
- stomachaches
- sweating
- tantrums at school
- trembling
- unreasonable fear of harm or death
- unwillingness to interact with anyone other than parents
- wanting to be held
- whining
- withdrawal

Cause

There isn't a known cause for SAD, although there are several common triggers. SAD can be engendered by an event that the child has experienced, such as an illness or death of a loved one; moving to a new neighborhood and starting new school; having a new nanny or babysitter; hearing frightening news such as a kidnapping; the loss of a pet; divorce or military deployment of a parent or guardian; or the birth of a new sibling. But there's a physiological aspect to this as well—a norepinephrine and serotonin chemical imbalance, which is common to many other anxiety disorders. Genetic connections have shown up in twin studies and familial connections are very strong in anxiety disorders. A child of parents who suffer from such disorders is more likely to suffer from them as well. It can also be a learned behavior.

The CHB, part of the Harvard Medical School, reports that, in cases where separation anxiety interferes with an older child's normal activities, it can be the sign of a deeper anxiety disorder, or, if it appears "out of the blue," it can be an indication of another type of problem such as bullying or abuse.

The "Helpguide" by the Rotary Club of Santa Monica and Center for Healthy Aging offers this developmental guide in terms of separation anxiety:

First few months: Babies don't differentiate much among caregivers and usually can be calmed by any loving person, regardless of relationship.

7-14 months: By about 7 months, babies realize that there's only one Mommy and/or Daddy, but they don't have a sense of time, so even if parents step into the next room for a minute, all the baby knows is that they're gone—maybe forever!—and they're going to cry or cling or do whatever it takes to keep that from happening. This phase is often called "stranger anxiety," because even the happiest child becomes shy or fearful around everyone but the primary caregiver, and generally peaks before 18 months.

Toddler/preschool years: Children can be anxious and become emotional when a parent or primary caregiver leaves, but can be distracted by activities with the caregiver or other children.

By age 5: Most children are secure enough to be left with a babysitter or dropped off at school without distress.

Treatment

As with most other anxiety disorders, CBT is the best form of treatment. Children learn how to recognize their specific feelings of anxiety and how to separate their physical symptoms from those feelings. They think about and act out their particular anxiety-provoking situations, and they learn coping skills in how to adapt to those anxious situations, with alternative behaviors. They take their negative thoughts and create positive new thoughts to replace them.

Other behavior-modification strategies include play therapy, which uses puppets, toys, and games (which was so successful for Tony); biofeedback; behavior-modeling therapy, which reinforces positive behavior, along with role-playing; and relaxation techniques like deep breathing and self-calming techniques. Reading books on the subject (bibliotherapy) proves to be helpful, and family therapy is also very highly recommended.

The good news is there are lots of things a parent can do to make the child's difficult journey with SAD an easier one.

The CHB offers the following tips:

Timing is everything. Try not to start day care or child care with an unfamiliar person between the ages of 8 months and 1 year, when separation anxiety is first likely to present itself. Also, try not to leave your child when he or she is likely to be tired, hungry, or restless. If at all possible, schedule your departures for after naps and mealtimes.

Practice. Practice being apart from each other, and introduce new people and places gradually. If you're planning to leave your child with a relative or a new babysitter, then invite that person over in advance so they can spend time together while you're in the room. If your child is starting at a new day care center or preschool, make a few visits there together before a full-time schedule begins. Practice leaving your child with a caregiver for short periods of time so that he or she can get used to being away from you.

Be calm and consistent. *Create a goodbye ritual during which you say a pleasant, loving and firm goodbye. Stay calm and show confidence in your child. Reassure him or her that you'll be back and explain how long it will be until you return using concepts your child will understand; for example, don't say, "I'll be back after lunch," because your child can't yet understand time. Give him or her your full attention when you say goodbye, and when you say you're leaving, mean it; coming back will only make things worse.*

This is good. *Try to keep in mind that your child's unwillingness to leave you is a good sign that healthy attachments have developed between the two of you. Eventually your child will be able to remember that you always return after you leave, and these memories will be enough to comfort him or her while you are gone. This also gives your child a chance to develop his or her own coping skills and a little independence. Leaving your photo with your child, or letting them take it to school, can work wonders.*

Follow through on promises. *It's important to make sure that you return when you have promised to return. This is critical, and there can be no exceptions. This is the only way your child will develop the confidence that he or she can make it through this time.*

Praise and reward *the child for overcoming his fears.*

If you are caring for another person's child, and that child is experiencing separation anxiety, it's a good idea to try to distract the child with another activity or toy, by being outside, or with songs, games, or anything else that works. You may have to keep trying to distract the child over and over until something just clicks with the child.

Prognosis

As with other anxiety disorders, with the right therapy and treatment, there is a hopeful prognosis for children with SAD, but the remission rate for this disorder is high. The illness can fluctuate in severity, and it can come and go, lasting for long periods of years or a short amount of time. It can also be a lead-up to more severe anxiety disorders such as PD (panic disorder), phobias such as agoraphobia, and OCD (obsessive-compulsive disorder).

Adults who had the disorder as children, who have been illness-free in terms of symptoms for years, can have it return when they must separate from their own children or spouse. The disorder, as with other anxiety disorders, also has a tendency to run in families.

Sources and resources

American Academy of Child and Adolescent Psychiatry (www.aacap.org)

American Psychiatric Association (www.psych.org)

American Psychological Association (www.apa.org)

Children's Hospital Boston (617-355-6000); (www.childrenshospital.org)

DSM (*Diagnostic and Statistical Manual of Mental Disorders*)

National Institute of Mental Health (www.nimh.nih.gov)

Rotary Club of Santa Monica (www.rotaryclubofsantamonica.org/index.htm)

See the mental-health contacts under "General Resources" for more sources used in this chapter.

SID

Sensory Integration Disorder

Terms used in this chapter: ADHD (attention-deficit/hyperactivity disorder); *DSM* (*Diagnostic and Statistical Manual of Mental Disorders*); LD (learning disability); OT (occupational therapist); SID (sensory integration disorder); SPD (sensory processing disorder)

Sound familiar?

The best way to tell Tamara's story is through the points her mother, Michele, an occupational therapist, provided.

From the moment she was born, she wouldn't stop crying.

In the months following, she hardly slept … well, unless I held her through the entire nap until even my arms fell asleep.

She was allergic to every formula except the one that cost $16 a can.

The pacifier became her best friend until 3 years old, and she never found any replacement afterwards to help her soothe herself.

There were nights she spent the entire night in a vibrating baby seat so she would stay asleep.

I would literally spend hours gently shaking her in my arms until she fell asleep.

She startled with every noise she heard.

She gave up (or I gave up?) naps at 1 year old.

As she grew, she became a shy observer, always on the outside watching with pure anxiety as to what might happen (a noise, a touch, a loud voice etc.) next within her environment.

She decided whether she liked people based on the sound of their voice.

She feared family activities because of the unpredictable noises and laughter that were inevitably a part of it (she cried every time a sudden burst of laughter happened).

She hated public bathrooms, covering her ears and crying with the sound of a flushing toilet.

She only ate about five different foods (refuses sight, smell, and taste of meat to this day) and bases decisions purely on smell, texture, and appearance of food before she will even try something new.

She likes certain brands of food prepared a specific way.

Falling asleep required all lights on, rubbing her back and head literally sometimes for one-to-two hours, playing an ocean-wave tape the entire night or she would wake up as soon as it stopped, room-darkening shades or the sun would wake her up in the morning, sleeping in our bed or my being in her room with her, or at least visible to her.

She would only wear soft clothes, no jeans or "itchy shirts" … stretch pants and cotton shirts were the staples.

It took five-to-six years before she started not fearing and becoming adventurous on playground equipment.

She fears being tipped upside down/sideways, any unexpected movement.

She has daily anxiety about the unknown/unpredictable.

She will become nauseous/disgusted by certain smells … our dinners sometimes needed to be accompanied by air-freshener sprays.

She dislikes firm hugs and will avoid people who want to hug her or turn backwards for them to hug her.

She is excessively ticklish.

She wouldn't tolerate the feeling of water spraying on her in the shower until about 8 years old … and still prefers baths.

Even gentle brushing of her hair, crying—"Ow, Ow … you're hurting me, stop it!!!!!"

She doesn't go to the hairdresser because of the feeling of the hair falling on her body and the pain of someone else brushing her hair.

For the first seven years of her life, we had to sing "Happy Birthday" and clap for her extremely quietly.

She couldn't stand the beach due to the feeling of the sand blowing on or sticking to her legs or feet.

Dental work requires hospital sedation due to oral and tactile hypersensitivities and anxiety.

Tamara has SID—sensory integration disorder.

Did you know?

SID or SPD is the inability of the brain to properly process information brought in by the senses—and it can manifest itself in many different ways. SID is a neurological disorder originally called sensory integration dysfunction by A. Jean Ayres, Ph.D., OTR, the doctor who first researched the disorder forty years ago.

A child's brain organizes and interprets movement, smells, sounds, tastes, touch, space, sight, and body awareness. When this breaks down, all hell can break loose.

Each sense works in conjunction with the others to form an amalgamated picture that gives the child a sense of who he or she is, where he or she is, and how that all fits together. Sensory information is organized in order for the child to function properly. While SID is often noticed in autistic children, it is also found to be comorbid with other Alphabet Disorders such as ADHD, APD (auditory processing disorder), VPD (visual processing disorder), and other LDs, especially motor disabilities. Indeed, studies have shown that SID can be found in 70 percent of children who are labeled LD by their school.

In children with typical sensory function, the integration of the senses is a normal, involuntary activity; for those with SID, it can be devastating. The child doesn't look sick and often goes undiagnosed or misdiagnosed. The longer this disorder goes unattended, the worse it is for the child. Early intervention is the key to success because, when the integration does not occur, it can result in learning, behavioral, mood, eating, and psychological and developmental disorders.

How it is manifested

SID manifests itself in several ways: auditory (sounds), olfactory (smell), proprioception (sense of where the body is and what it is doing), tactile (touch), vestibular (balance, coordination), and visual (sight).

SID kids can be either undersensitive or oversensitive. They might be bombarded by stimuli or not get enough. The underreactive child will avoid stimulation by becoming a picky eater or by not wearing certain uncomfortable (to them) clothes, while the oversensitive child will crave stimulating activities like spinning, eating only crunchy food, craving hot baths, listening to loud music, or eating spicy food. Some children are both under- and overreactive.

SID children are often the sloppy ones at the table with food all over their faces, hands, arms, and hair. They don't feel the food, and they spread it from one body part to another without realizing what they are doing.

Besides the more obvious sensory issues like aversion to touch, tastes, smells, and sound, SID children might have difficulty telling where they fit in the world around them. They might not be able to tell what arm is being touched or how many times they were touched (if they let you touch them at all) or what direction a sound is coming from. They are unsure of their own body space—"Did I move my leg to the right or the left?"

They have difficulty manipulating themselves in the space around them—"I want to climb into that box like my friends did, but I'm not sure how to do it." Or "My friend just drew a smiley face, but I don't know how to copy it."

Most children with SID are just as intelligent as their peers. Many are intellectually gifted—their brains are simply wired differently.

Signs and symptoms

- aversion to being touched
- aversion to new situations
- aversion to touching anything messy
- clumsy, bumps into things
- covers ears to shut out noise at inappropriate times
- covers eyes
- craves heat or cold
- craves spicy foods
- difficulty dressing him- or herself
- difficulty imitating movements
- difficulty in transitioning
- difficulty playing with toys
- difficulty tying shoes
- difficulty using writing implements
- does not react, or reacts strongly, to odors
- drops things
- easily distracted
- emotional problems
- enjoys spinning, swinging
- falls often
- fearful reaction to ordinary movement activities like playground activity
- high tolerance for pain
- impulsive
- inability to calm down
- inability to wear clothes that are tight or that have tags, tight waist bands
- inability to wear shoes or socks with seams
- insensitive to heat or cold
- intolerant of certain textures of clothing
- intolerant of certain textures of food
- jumps often
- lack of balance
- lacking in self-control
- language and speech delays
- LDs
- learning delays
- low activity level
- low tolerance for pain
- motor-skill delays

- overactive
- overly sensitive to movement, sights, and sounds
- overreacts to touch (tactile defensiveness)
- picky eater
- poor motor skills
- poor self-esteem
- reacts to the suggestion of sensory input
- seemingly careless
- single food preference
- sniffs people, objects, and food
- social problems
- tires easily
- uncoordinated
- underactive
- underreacts to movement, sights, sounds
- walks on tiptoes

Cause

As with other neurological disorders, there is no known cause or cure for SID. It is believed that there is a miswiring in the brain, and, as with so many related Alphabet Disorders, SID can be the result of genetic, biological, or environmental causes. Some experts think that uncovering the secret behind SID will someday provide the secret to many other Alphabet Disorders such as ADHD and autism.

Diagnosis

If a child is suspected of having SID after an examination by his or her pediatrician, an evaluation can be conducted by a qualified occupational or physical therapist or pediatric psychiatrist. There is no one standardized medical test for SID, but evaluation usually consists of both standardized testing and structured clinical observations of responses to sensory stimulation, posture, balance, coordination, and eye movements. After carefully analyzing test results and other assessment data along with information from other professionals and parents, the therapist will make recommendations regarding appropriate treatment.

Sensory integration and sensory-processing problems are not regarded officially as diagnoses, but this is one of those disorders that many parents and experts feel will be fully accepted in time. The American Psychiatric Association is being heavily lobbied by a growing number of SID advocacy groups to include SID as an official disorder in the next edition of the *DSM*, the *DSM-V*, which will be published in 2012.

Treatment

The SID child needs a specific type of therapy—sensory integrative therapy—in a sensory rich environment. While activities such as gymnastics are good for any child, the SID child should not be taking specific-skills classes in lieu of proper sensory-oriented therapy.

An OT has been proven to provide the best therapy for SID. Besides working with all the senses, the OT might focus on balance training and therapeutic body brushing for SID children (not infants). A nonscratching surgical-type brush is used over the child's body (arms, legs, back, feet, hands—but not the stomach) in very specific prescribed movements. Deep-joint compression—mostly of the shoulder, elbow, and wrist but also of the legs and feet—should follow. The OT will teach the parents how to do this. It helps organize the sensory system, providing the child with focus, balance, and a sense of well-being.

Touch and movement are keys for successfully treating an SID child. Here are a few examples: back rubs; balancing on a therapy ball; barefoot play; bicycle riding; brushing skin; carrying heavy items; climbing; crawling through tunnels; dancing; drumming; eating snacks with different textures; finger painting; going through an obstacle course; hammering; hopping; hugging; jumping; karaoke; kneading dough; manipulating small objects such as jigsaw puzzles and pegs; oral activities (flutes, bubble blowing); playing dress-up in different textured clothes; playing catch; playing with and petting animals; playing with different tasting foods; playing with different textured foods; playing with Play Doh; playing with water, sand, bean bags, and pillows; pushing against walls; pushing and pulling items; ripping and tearing different textures; rocking; rolling; roughhousing with peers; running; sliding; somersaulting; spinning; swaddling; swimming; swinging; tickling; walking and balancing on uneven surfaces; walking up and down stairs; washing and drying hands in game play—all activities that stimulate the senses.

Prognosis

Depending on the severity and cause of the disorder, with early intervention and the correct type of therapy, the prognosis for children with SID is hopeful. Some children have dramatic improvement, while others might improve in only some areas. For some parents of SID children, the diagnosis is a godsend, after having the child misdiagnosed with autism or another disorder that is not as easily responsive to treatment.

Sources and resources

Sensory Processing Disorder Foundation (303-794-1182); (www.spdnetwork.org)
Sensory Processing Disorder Resource Center (www.sensory-processing-disorder.com)
Vestibular Disorders Association (800-837-8428); (www.vestibular.org)

See the mental-health contacts under "General Resources" for more sources used in this chapter.

SLD

Speech-Language Disorder

Terms used in this chapter: ASHA (American Speech-Language-Hearing Association); DAS (developmental apraxia of speech); LD (learning disability); NIDOCD (National Institute on Deafness and Other Communication Disorders); RELD (receptive-expressive language disorder); SLD (speech-language disorder); SLP (speech-language pathologist)

Sound familiar?

Fifteen-year-old Elizabeth has never been able to get one full, clear sentence out, says her mother, Jeanette, who self-admittedly also "flubs" her own speech.

In her South Florida neighborhood, where E, as her family calls her, was born and raised, there are many children who are first-generation Americans, from non-English-speaking homes representing several nationalities. Jeanette says E, who is native born, has the worst speech pattern of the lot.

"Ever since she started speaking at about 2½ years old," Jeanette says, "E never sounded right. We never made a big deal about it because her cousin had a terrible stutter [when he was 3, before E was born], and his therapist told [the cousin's] parents, 'Just let it slide. Encourage him positively, but don't bring attention to it.' So that's what we did with E."

When E was just starting to talk, she began transposing some of her sounds and soon "began to sound like a character from a Bugs Bunny or Tweety Bird cartoon," her mother says, with a laugh.

But it wasn't all laughs. E's speech errors began to affect her in her academic life and with social interaction. It started off with kids not quite understanding her to kids making fun of her, which caused anxiety and stress.

"It's, like, cleared up a lot," E says, sounding like a typical tenth-grade teen. "But I still trip over my words, and I pause a lot to think of the correct ones."

Jeanette, who is a social worker, and her husband, who is a history professor at a local college, continuously butted heads with the school speech-language pathologist.

"The school speech therapist was awful," Jeanette recalls. "It was a constant battle."

So they brought their daughter to a private speech therapist, who immediately yielded positive results. In addition, getting an official diagnosis was very helpful in terms of getting appropriate help and accommodations from the school.

"I hated speaking ... taking speech in school," says E, tripping over her tongue. And she proceeds to tell a story about how difficult it has always been for her to understand what was being said to her and also to articulate what she needed to say. In a rambling monologue, dotted with many speech errors and disfluencies, E talks about the frustrations of having impaired speech; she talks about her "frat fend," who has an eating disorder, and mentions a "term praper" she has due.

S

Many of her words had transposed sounds, and she stopped herself numerous times, stammering and attempting to correct her words.

"This is a million times better," Jeanette says. "Sho youda … you shoulda heard her two years ago. And I know how lucky, he … we are because my nephew has a child who cannot speak at all."

Elizabeth has an SLD—specifically, RELD. Her mother probably does as well.

Did you know?

With a typical child, receptive abilities (understanding language) and expressive skills (vocabulary, the production of complex sentences, and recall of words) usually develop at the same pace. However, when there is broad disparity between the two and when a child's communication is noticeably lagging behind his or her peers in the attainment of these skills, a serious disorder is indicated and red flags go up.

When a child's ability to understand language is in the normal range but his or her expressive ability, speech, is critically inadequate—it might be completely absent, somewhat impaired, or just difficult to understand—then they have a speech or language disorder.

According to the National Dissemination Center for Children with Disabilities (NICHCY), it is estimated that communication disorders (including speech, language, and hearing disorders) affect one of every ten people in the United States.

The rise in prevalence has become a major concern.

"We have observed over the past decade that the proportion of children (all under 3 years of age) referred to that agency primarily for speech/language concerns has risen from about 20 to well over 50 percent," says the report, "The Early Intervention Strategies in Communication Disorders," by Sheila Daly Russo, M.Ed./CCC-SLP, and David W. Bailey, M.D., both affiliated with the Early Intervention Program at the University of Florida Health Science Center/Jacksonville.

Speech problems are prevalent around the world, despite language differences.

In Finland, according to Pirjo Korpilahti, professor in logopedics at the University of Turku, "It is estimated that about 10–15 percent of children have developmental language problems. Some of them are, of course, 'late learners' and do not need intensive speech therapy. So many of them just meet the speech-language therapist only few times and perhaps the day care gets some consultation on how to support the development."

The Alphabet Disorder aspect is clearly seen in Finland. "In early years of life, specific language impairment is reported in 2–3 percent of children. So this group includes children with developmental verbal/motor dyspraxia, central auditory processing disorder, and severe receptive/expressive language problems. CAPD [central auditory processing disorder] can be the primary diagnosis, but many of these children also have other learning disabilities, ADHD [attention-deficit/hyperactivity disorder], Asperger-type of behavior, for example. The diagnosis 'developmental dysphasia' is commonly used in clinical practice."

Having access to early intervention seems to be a key to success around the world. According to Veronika Raudsalu, president of the Estonian Logopedists Union, the estimated statistics for Estonia regarding speech and language disorders is "similar to that of other nations. Central speech problems [is at a] 5–7 percent rate and all speech problems [are at a] 12–17 percent [rate]."

"Environment and genetics" is what she regards as the cause for the rise in rates.

How it is manifested

Agrammatism—telegraphic speech. ("Me, you, uh, watch television.")

Anomia—difficulty in retrieving or recalling a specific word.

Aphasia—problem with language caused by brain damage. The National Aphasia Society is quick to remind us that this is a disability that affects communication, not intellect. Depending on where on the brain the damage is and the severity of the damage itself, language can be affected in many ways, from the lack of ability to produce language to the lack of ability to understand language. Relatively few cases of aphasia strike children and adolescents, but it can. The concern is that not enough is known about it when it does. When speaking with a person who has aphasia, it is suggested that it helps to minimize distractions and speak slowly and clearly. If they have comprehension difficulties, use short simple sentences and pause between sentences. Pair gestures with your speech to aid comprehension. Allow them more time to respond. If you need to find out information, ask questions that can be answered easily with a yes or no or other single word. Remember that a person with aphasia has not lost his or her intellectual abilities, just the speech- and language-making skills.

Apraxia—a neurological disorder that occurs when a child is unable to execute speech movements—the specific sequence of movements that result in proper speech—because of problems with coordination and motor planning. Apraxia does not involve muscle weakness. The child's brain is unable to plan and order motor activities so that the mouth can form the correct shapes to form words. The apraxic child knows what he wants to say, but his mouth isn't getting the correct messages to be physically able to say the desired words or sentences. **Oral apraxia** affects the child's ability to move his or her mouth muscles for intent other than speech, e.g., coughing or blowing out birthday candles. **Verbal apraxia** is identified when the child's ability to sequence speech sounds is impaired, again, not resulting from muscle weakness. Children who have apraxic speech search with several attempts for the correct word to say before it is said correctly.

Apraxia develops in two ways: AAS (acquired apraxia of speech) occurs from an injury that causes brain damage. DAS (developmental apraxia of speech) or CAS (childhood apraxia of speech) is present from birth, and its etiology is not quite understood. Many other types of developmental delays, such as impairment with expressive speech or auditory processing, might affect and confuse the apraxia diagnosis. With DAS kids, the muscle incoordination might be more systemic than with just the mouth. Young children with verbal apraxia will point and use vowel sounds when their typically developing peers are speaking in short phrases.

APhD (articulation-phonology disorder)—a child with an articulation problem can be hard to understand. A child with a phonology disorder lacks the ability to use speech sounds that are expected for the appropriate developmental age and language expectations. Articulation-phonology is the production of speech sounds; how intelligible those sounds are determines the extent of the child's disorder. Some children distort the sound, but it is still understandable, such as in a lisp. Some transpose letters; others substitute one letter sound for another. Some will just not say the sound at all. Some children just make up their own phonological rules, creating their own sounds and sound patterns. When they do create their own rules that are different from the traditional rules of their own language, it is considered a phonological disorder. These are not single sounds involved; these are groups or classes of sounds. The child, for example, may have created a whole set of rules for sounds influenced by tongue movement or produced in a certain area of the mouth.

Circumlocation—describing or defining a word instead of saying the word.

Cluttering—language disorder that is unintelligible speech due to the child's using poor syntax or grammar; speaking too fast, or speaking in an inconsistent rhythm—or both. Children who demonstrate cluttering will use irrelevant words or word groups that are completely unrelated to the sentence they are trying to get across. Sometimes they don't finish their words, or they use spoonerisms, interjections, and phrase repetitions and revisions. There are many reasons for this type of speech including attention deficits, inability to concentrate or organize, or auditory-processing problems. The child will often be clueless as to his or her erratic speech problem. Screening is difficult for cluttering, because it depends on the subjective judgment of the listener/tester, and cluttering children do not always exhibit their symptoms in the typically short evaluation period. Tape record the cluttering child at home, and bring that tape to the diagnostician.

DLD (developmental language disorder)—when a child's language skills do not appropriately relate to his or her age, the child is regarded as being language disordered or delayed. This can be caused by numerous factors including environmental ones, being hearing impaired, cognitive disabilities caused by physical injuries or malfunctions, and suffering from syndromes such as PDD (pervasive developmental disorder). Because of the nature of language and what is expected at different stages of childhood, a child can lose one type of delay or disorder and in a few years develop a new one. Children with delayed language can even, and often, end up meeting the milestones of their peers, but others with more serious disorders often continue to fall behind. Early intervention is the key.

Dysarthria—a speech disorder that is the result of some sort of neurological injury that can affect the throat, tongue, lips, or organs such as lungs that play a part in the speech process; the injury, in turn, can affect many aspects of speech from articulation to intonation. Speech dysarthria is an oral motor weakness that causes sluggish and often nasal-sounding speech. The dysarthriac child's speech becomes slow, frail, inexact, or clumsy. Childhood dysarthria can be either congenital or acquired and is usually associated with a disease or head injury. There are several parts of the body (respiratory system, larynx, soft palate, lips, tongue, teeth, and jaw) that must work in concert to produce clear and proper speech; and when any one of the parts fails, the result is dysarthria. The respiratory system supplies the power (the air) to generate speech. The larynx, or voice box, vibrates the air and the voice is formed. The soft palate is the portal between the nasal and oral cavities, and it enables the different sound qualities in the voice. The articulatory system (tongue, teeth, etc.) helps to form the different consonants and vowels.

Echolalia—the immediate repetition or echoing of words or phrases verbalized by another person.

Expressive-language delays and disorders—simply put, problems in how a child speaks. There are many types of expressive-language problems, and these problems go well beyond just misusing a word. It is the basis of how children relate to each other, and a child with impaired speech will almost always have impaired social relationships. While they might have limited vocabulary, tell rambling stories filled with confusing pronouns, use short sentences, leave off part of a word, transpose phonemes (the smallest units of sound in language), or grope for a specific word to get across their thought, Li Kan, M.D., a pediatric neurologist at Schneider Children's Hospital in New Hyde Park, New York, says the problem can be easily missed by a professional. She suggests that often other children's reactions to the speech-impaired child can be a good warning sign for parents "because the child's peers might be more sensitive to the problem" than even the child's speech therapist.

Grammatism—the excessive and stringent use of using proper grammatical rules.

Jargon disorder—similar to grammatism with lengthy and fluently articulated speech, but unlike grammatism it makes no sense to the listener.

Lisp—speech impediment, when a child is unable to pronounce sibilant sounds, like the letter "s," and instead replaces those sounds with "th" (interdental) sounds. Lisping can occur in several ways: the tongue protrudes past the front teeth; the tip of the tongue just touches the front teeth; the tongue is in contact with the palate; and the "wet" lisp when "s" and "z" sounds are produced because air is passing across the sides of the tongue.

Malapropism—word expressed is either different from the word meant or it sounds similar to the word meant, as in Boston Mayor Thomas Menino's famous statement about a predecessor: "He was a man of great statue," of course, meaning "stature." For a more familiar example, President George W. Bush uses so many malapropisms that they have begun to be known as "Bushisms."

Metathesis—linguistic process whereby a sound alteration changes the order of phonemes within a word. Some popularly mispronounced examples of metathesis include the words *asterisk, integral, nuclear, often, realtor, vegetable,* and *Wednesday.*

S

Morpheme errors—transpositions of morphemes (the smallest meaningful unit in the grammar of the language) between words. An example of a morpheme error, offered by language expert Gary Dell, Ph.D., is when the phrase "self-destruct instructions" becomes "self-instruct destructions."

Paraphasia—according to the 1983 BDAE: Boston Diagnostic Aphasia Examination by Harold Goodglass, Ph.D., and Edith Kaplan, Ph.D., a paraphasia is the "production of unintended syllables, words, or phrases during the effort to speak." There are three types of paraphasias: **Phonemic**: replacing words with sound-alike words, where more than half of the word is said correctly (*bike* for *bite*, *pisghetti* for *spaghetti*); **Verbal**: replacing a word with another that has a semantic or thematic connection; it can range from a direct connection (*girl* substituted by *boy*) to a more remote connection (such as *milk* for *juice*); **Neologism**: a word that the child has invented and is not identified as coming from their language, where less than half to no part of the word is said correctly.

Perseveration—in speech, the unnecessary repeating of a word or phrase. This disorder is often found in children on the autism spectrum.

Phoneme anticipations—a word influenced by a phoneme that comes later: *a big doll* becomes *a dig doll*.

Phoneme deletions—an aspect of a word is lost: *a pretty plate* becomes *a pretty pate*.

Phoneme perseverations—a later word is affected by an aspect of a previous one: *a big doll* becomes *a big boll*.

RLD (receptive language disorder)—when a child has an RLD it means, simply, that he or she has difficulty understanding spoken language. This results in many potential problems from not comprehending subtleties in speech—such as a parent saying, "It's noisy," and the child's not realizing it means "turn your extremely loud radio down"—to having an impaired vocabulary. These children might have difficulty with grammatical rules, such as possession and tenses, and have difficulty understanding sarcasm or nonverbal signals.

RELD—when a child is impaired in both receptive (understanding) and expressive (speaking) abilities.

Rhotacism—occurs with the overusage of the letter "r," an inability to pronounce the letter "r," or converting other consonants into the letter "r." Think of Elmer Fudd chasing that "wabbit."

SM (selective mutism)—characterized by a consistent failure to speak in social situations in which a child would be expected to speak. These children have the ability to speak and understand but do not use their abilities because of social anxiety. SM is regarded as more of an anxiety disorder and not a communications or developmental disorder. These children can be normal in all other aspects of their lives.

SPLD (semantic pragmatic language disorder)—the social aspect of language. It refers to how language is used appropriately within the context in a social setting. Children with SPLD demonstrate the inability to communicate efficiently with others.

The problem is believed to be in the processing ability of the child. SPLD children have difficulty pulling out the meaning of the relevant part of a story, conversation, or event. They are detail oriented and will focus on those details as opposed to the full conversation. A child with SPLD has difficulty with two-way conversation. They are sometimes unemotional, and often do not understand body language, nor do they know how to read facial expressions. They will often use unintentionally aggressive language, ask an excessive amount of questions, and talk about specific things in an incredibly detailed manner. Their talk can be self-centered, the only perspective being their own, and they might show no interest in relating to other children. They can view things in a very literal way and do not comprehend abstractions, innuendos, subtleties, jokes, double meanings, sarcasm, etc. SPLD kids have difficulty with open-ended questions; they need strict boundaries. They question directly—"Why is that?" "How do you know that?"

Sound error—those transpositions of sounds between words (*claw hammer* will become *haw clammer*).

Spasmodic dysphonia—a disorder characterized by involuntary movements of one or more muscles of the larynx or voice box, which can result in a hoarse, jumpy, quivering voice or no sound at all, along with periods of normal vocalization. This is usually found in adults.

Spoonerism—words or phrases in which letters or syllables are swapped. While funny sounding, when it publicly disrupts a child's speech, a tendency toward spoonerism can be very embarrassing. The affliction was named after British academic Reverend W.A. Spooner, who produced one of the most famous spoonerisms when he toasted Queen Victoria: "Three cheers for our queer old dean!"

Stammering—flow of speech is interrupted by abnormal repetitions: *st-st-st-stammering.*

Stuttering—unlike the erratic rhythms of the communicative problem of cluttering, stuttering is a disorder that is a disruption of fluent speech. It is the involuntary repetitions, disruption of forward-moving speech, and drawing out of sounds, syllables, words, and phrases: *sssstuttering*. It might be accompanied by various physical disruptions that appear tic-like, such as blinking or head jerking. There is no single known cause of stuttering; and although it is affected by psychological issues, it is not a nervous disorder. It has, however, been regarded as a neurological concern.

Fluent speech is smooth, forward-moving, unhesitant, and effortless. A disfluency is any break in fluent speech. Everyone has disfluencies from time to time, and they are not uncommon in normal speech. Children often go through a disfluent stage between ages 3 and 5. Stuttering is speech that has more disfluencies than is considered average. The average person will have between 7 and 10 percent disfluency in his or her speech. These disfluencies are usually word or phrase repetitions, fillers such as *like, uhm, you know, ah*, the well-known Canadian *eh*, and other interjections. When a speaker experiences disfluencies at a rate greater than 10 percent, chances are he is stuttering.

Stuttering is often accompanied by tension and anxiety. There are three theories about the cause of stuttering, and it is believed that all three could be factors: genetic (it runs in families), environmental, and biological—malfunctions in the timing and coordination of muscles involved with speech, auditory processing, and language function. A stutter can last from one-half of a second to thirty seconds and is accompanied by physical and emotional rigidity and tension.

Vocal disorder—What is a normal voice? It's hard to say because everyone's voice is unique. A normal voice is pleasant sounding and has age- and sex-appropriate pitch and loudness. When a voice is not pleasant sounding or is too loud, soft, high, or low for the child's age and gender, a voice problem may be present. Voice disorders fall into two categories: functional disorders, which are caused by misuse of the voice and can be helped with voice therapy; and organic disorders, which are pathological and require medical attention.

Word errors—transpositions of words as in "I'm taking my dog to the vet" becoming "I'm taking my vet to the dog."

What are the most common speech errors? Expert in the field, Gary S. Dell, Ph.D., professor of psychology at the University of Illinois at Urbana-Champaign, says, "Phonological speech errors (movement, addition, deletion, substitution of phonological material) are somewhat more common than lexical speech errors (same categories for whole morphemes or words). Within phonological speech errors, anticipations of consonants are probably the most common."

Examples of how these speech problems exhibit themselves are best demonstrated in Dell's example from his 1986 paper, "A Spreading-activation System of Retrieval in Sentence Production," which gives different examples of the different ways the sentence "Some swimmers sink" might fall into speech errors:

Error	Type
Sim swimmers sink	phoneme anticipation
Swum simmers sink	phoneme shift
Some simmers sink	phoneme deletion
Sim swummers sink	phoneme exchange
Some swummers sink	phoneme perseveration
Some swinkers sink	cluster anticipation
Some sinkers swim	stem exchange
Some swimmers swim	stem perseveration or word substitution
Some swimmers drown	word substitution

Signs and symptoms

- articulation impairments
- awkward and clumsy physicality
- delayed first words with many sounds omitted or replaced by easy-to-pronounce consonant sounds
- difficulty imitating sounds and words
- difficulty understanding spoken language
- difficulty with nursing or feeding during infancy
- distractibility
- fine motor problems
- groping for words while speaking
- grunting instead of using first words
- handwriting problems
- high frequency of vowels and voicing errors
- history of ear infections
- improper use of words
- inability to express ideas
- inability to follow verbal directions from ages 2 to 3
- inappropriate grammatical patterns
- inappropriate responses to simple questions from ages 2 to 3
- inattention to spoken language
- late onset of first words
- LDs
- little or no cooing or babbling in infancy
- not using two-word phrases by 24 months
- pointing instead of using first words
- poor organizational skills
- reduced vocabulary
- repeating words and phrases but not comprehending them
- saying easy sounds (b, m, p, t, d, and h) from ages 2 to 3 but unable to use them in words
- seeing a word but not understanding its meaning
- sensory problems, such as being sensitive to touch
- slow, halting speech that is full of effort
- slow or no progress with traditional speech therapy
- trouble getting across what they are trying to say
- unable to use consonants ·
- unintelligible speech
- unpredictable speech errors
- voice fluency not present

Children with any combination of these red flags should be immediately referred to a speech-language pathologist for testing.

Speech and language milestones

While it is certainly helpful to know the signs and symptoms of SLDs, it is equally helpful for parents to be aware of normal speech-language development. The following milestones are provided by the NIDOCD:

Birth to 5 months

- reacts to loud sounds
- turns head toward a sound source
- watches person's face when he or she speaks
- vocalizes pleasure and displeasure sounds (laughs, giggles, cries, or fusses)
- makes noise when talked to

6 to 11 months

- understands "no-no"
- babbles (says "ba-ba-ba" or "ma-ma-ma")
- tries to communicate by actions or gestures
- tries to repeat sounds

12–17 months

- attends to a book or toy for about two minutes
- follows simple directions accompanied by gestures
- answers simple questions nonverbally
- points to objects, pictures, and family members
- says two to three words to label a person or object (pronunciation may not be clear)
- tries to imitate simple words

18–23 months

- enjoys being read to
- follows simple commands without gestures
- points to simple body parts such as nose
- understands simple verbs such as *eat* and *sleep*
- correctly pronounces most vowels and the letters "n," "m," "p," and "h," especially in the beginning of syllables and short words. Also begins to use other speech sounds.
- says eight to ten words (pronunciation may still be unclear)
- asks for common foods by name

- makes animal sounds such as *moo*
- starting to combine words such as *more milk*
- begins to use pronouns such as *mine*

2–3 years

- knows about fifty words at 24 months
- knows some spatial concepts such as *in* and *on*
- knows pronouns such as *you, me,* and *her* and begins to use more pronouns such as *you* and *I*
- knows descriptive words such as *big* and *happy*
- says around forty words at 24 months
- speech is becoming more accurate but may still leave off ending sounds. Strangers may not be able to understand much of what is said.
- answers simple questions
- speaks in two-to-three word phrases
- uses question inflection to ask for something (e.g., "My ball?")
- begins to use plurals such as *shoes* or *socks* and regular past tense verbs such as *jumped*

3–4 years

- groups objects such as foods, clothes, etc.
- identifies colors
- uses most speech sounds but may distort some of the more difficult sounds such as "l," "r," "s," "sh," "ch," "y," "v," "z," and "th." These sounds may not be fully mastered until ages 7 or 8.
- uses consonants in the beginning, middle, and ends of words. Some of the more difficult consonants may be distorted, but attempts to say them.
- strangers are able to understand much of what is said
- able to describe the use of objects such as *fork, car,* etc.
- has fun with language. Enjoys poems and recognizes language absurdities such as "Is that an elephant on your head?"
- expresses ideas and feelings rather than just talking about the world around him or her
- uses verbs that end in "ing," such as *walking* and *talking*
- answers simple questions such as "What do you do when you are hungry?"

4–5 years

- understands spatial concepts such as *behind* and *next to*
- understands complex questions
- speech is understandable but makes mistakes pronouncing long, difficult, or complex words such as *hippopotamus*

- says about two hundred to three hundred different words
- uses some irregular past tense verbs such as *ran* and *fell*
- describes how to do things such as painting a picture
- defines words
- lists items that belong in a category such as animals, vehicles, etc.
- answers "why" questions

5 years

- understands more than two thousand words
- understands time sequences (what happened first, second, third, etc.)
- carries out a series of three directions
- understands rhyming
- engages in conversation
- sentences can be eight or more words in length
- uses compound and complex sentences
- describes objects
- uses imagination to create stories

Cause

Some speech-language disorders are caused by brain injury, a traumatic physical event, or motor impairment. In many other cases, the disorder is neurologically based, without a specific cause. As with most other Alphabet Disorders, there are many suspected factors including genetics, environment, and neurobiological reasons, such as anxiety disorders.

Diagnosis

Most often it is the parent or caregiver who will first notice potential speech-language problems, and the child will be initially examined by a pediatrician to rule out any other medical conditions. The child will then be referred to an SLP who will assess the child and help determine the extent of the disorder and further course of action, which should include a pediatric neurologist and an audiologist—to test for the often comorbid APD (auditory processing disorder).

As with most Alphabet Disorders, early intervention is the most important thing a parent can do for a child. Some speech and language problems, such as DAS, can be diagnosed in children as young as 18 months of age.

Treatment

Early intervention is the key to treating SLD in any of its manifestations.

According to ASHA, "All communication disorders carry the potential to isolate individuals from their social and educational surroundings," and because of this, the association suggests early intervention. What might appear as just an early delay can very well turn out to be a severe and pervasive disorder, affecting a wide variety of aspects of your child's life, from his or her academic success to social interaction.

ASHA reminds us that "because of the way the brain develops, it is easier to learn language and communication skills before the age of 5. When children have muscular disorders, hearing problems or developmental delays, their acquisition of speech, language and related skills is often affected."

There are several keys to early intervention success at both home and school.

School intervention

The school's SLP is there to evaluate and help your child, and they often perform miracles, but sometimes he or she can also get in the way. They might be tied down to very limiting district regulations, or rely solely on abbreviated testing that does not show the child's full range of problems. There are those professionals, such as Larry B. Silver, M.D., an expert on LDs and the author of *The Misunderstood Child*, who complain that school officials involved in special education and connected services are too tied to budgetary concerns and are often caught up in an evaluation that averages out a child's testing, wholly disregarding the high highs and especially the low lows. Many advocates in the field recommend that parents bring their child to a private speech-language pathologist and then have the school SLP follow up on the outside expert's assessment and recommendations.

Once there is a proper diagnosis, the SLP will develop a program that will include speech therapy. The therapist will provide assessments and consult with the parents and the child's teachers and help to create the proper classroom environment for the SLD child. This team might also suggest or provide certain communication devices to assist the child. Make no mistake: the child needs a team. His or her teacher, along with the therapist, should be concentrating on enhancing the child's vocabulary and concept abilities. They will work on reading and writing skills, while a psychologist and occupational therapist might be brought in to help work on psychological issues like anxiety and self-esteem as well as social and life skills.

The child's pediatrician or school district will recommend an SLP who will provide recommendations to use at home and for school, which should be added to the child's IEP.

In school, aside from speech-language therapy, the best generally accepted tips for a child with a speech and language disorder include the following:

- avoid correcting the child's speech difficulties outside of the therapeutic environment
- be at eye level with the child, face to face
- build vocabulary
- constantly focus and refocus the student
- create proper speech models

- display patience when the child is speaking and do not hurry the child when he or she is struggling
- do not call on a student who has a speech problem unless he or she has been given ample time to prepare
- expand on what the child says. If the child says, "Flower," say, "Yes, pretty flower." If the child says, "Dog," say, "It is a brown dog."
- follow the child's lead
- group speech might lessen pressure on an individual child, while individual speech therapy concentrates on the child without any distractions
- let the child pick the topic to discuss
- maintain a positive learning environment
- overarticulate
- pause before key words
- practice speech and oral-motor activities
- provide a quiet area in which child can work
- provide detailed step-by-step directions
- provide positive reinforcement
- provide visuals to help enhance the lesson
- reduce extraneous classroom noise so that the child can focus without having to sort through irrelevant distractions
- reinforce the student's strengths
- repeat instructions, make sure child understands what's going on in the lesson
- repeat the same sentence but changing the inflection, thereby changing the sentence's meaning (contrastive stress drill).
- seat the child close to the teacher so the child can have direct visual and auditory contact with the teacher
- tap or clap out the rhythm of speech
- take focus off child by using pictures or puppets that can "speak" for the child
- take frequent pauses for breath
- take turns when communicating
- teach routines, like songs or memorizing books
- teacher should be in touch with the SLP and parents
- teacher should speak slowly and clearly to child
- use alphabet board, pointing to letters or black-and-white picture symbols (pic-syms)
- use computers with predictive text
- use language on a level that is equal to or slightly higher than the child's
- use physical gestures to enhance lesson
- use tactile, visual, or auditory cues
- use voice output devices

The SLP's work goes beyond actual speech and language therapy. The pathologist will also evaluate the child's executive functioning, in which he or she assesses the child's ability to plan, organize, and attend to details. The types of activities the therapist might conduct include problem solving and reasoning: "Your cat ran away. What do you do?" The SLP will also read a story fragment and ask the child to complete the story, adding a beginning, middle, and end that make sense. The therapist will also attempt to build up the child's vocabulary and teach him or her social speech cues.

Other programs or therapies the SLP might incorporate include the following:

Fast ForWord is an Internet and CD-ROM-based training program that has been successful with some children with speech, language, and reading problems. It uses acoustically processed speech and speech sounds.

Lindamood-bell Learning Process has helped children with language and literacy by stimulating basic sensory functions.

Motokinesthetic therapy directly manipulates the child's articulators like tongue, lips, etc.

Oral-motor therapy has proved helpful.

Oro-facial exercises may be employed, if the problem is due to muscle weakness.

PROMPT (Prompts for Restructuring Oral-Muscular Phonetic Targets) is a multidimensional, multisensory therapeutic system that can be used.

The teacher might employ touch cues (e.g., by stating, "Let's put your glove on" and then touching the child's hand).

Home intervention

Many of the above-mentioned school tips should also be used at home. In addition, however, parents should also pursue the following:

- ask the child questions that involve problem solving and reasoning
- elaborate on the child's simple statements
- maintain eye-to-eye contact
- play music for and sing to your child
- play simple directional games like "Peek-a-Boo" and "Pat-a-Cake"
- point out sounds and explain what they are—dog barking, doorbell ringing
- point out logos and signs
- read, read, read:
    - read to your child as often as you can
    - have the child act out a story they are reading
    - let the child see *you* read
    - have the child retell the story you are reading
    - have the child name items in the book
    - have the child describe what is taking place in the illustrations
    - ask your child predictive questions regarding the book
    - leave books and writing implements around the house

- remain positive with your child; never say, "wrong"—instead, correct incorrect speech through modeling your own speech
- repeat what your child says, using correct grammar or pronunciation
- respond to all of your child's noises and sounds
- speak in brief sentences using simple and concrete words so the child can model his or her speech after yours
- stimulate all of the child's senses
- talk to your child constantly, in the car, in the stroller, in the playpen and crib
- teach your child the names of everyday items throughout the day
- write notes to your child

Prognosis

Depending on the severity of the disorder, for the most part with the proper intervention—especially early detection and intervention—a child can overcome many speech and language disorders and symptoms. Some symptoms linger and might cause slight problems in adulthood, but there are often ways to compensate, or the child may simply learn to live with the disorder. For the most part, however, the prognosis is excellent.

Sources and resources

Alliance for Technology Access (707-778-3011); (www.ataccess.org)
American Speech-Language-Hearing Association (ASHA) (800-638-8255); (www.asha.org)
BDEA-3 (Boston Diagnostic Aphasia Examination, 3rd edition) (Baltimore: Lippincott, Williams & Wilkins, 2001)
Childhood Apraxia of Speech Association (412-767-6589)
Gary S. Dell, "A Spreading-activation System of Retrieval in Sentence Production," *Psychological Review* 93 (1986): 283–321.
The National Aphasia Association (800-922-4622); (www.aphasia.org)
The National Center for Stuttering (800-221-2483); (www.stuttering.com)
National Dissemination Center for Children with Disabilities (NICHCY) (800-695-0285); (www.nichcy.org)
National Institute on Deafness and Other Communication Disorders (NIDOCD) (www.nidcd.nih.gov)
Sheila Daly Russo and David W. Bailey, "The Early Intervention Strategies in Communication Disorders" (www.dcmsonline.org/jax-medicine/2000journals/march2000/commdis.pdf)
Scottish Rite/RiteCare Childhood Language Program (202-232-3579) (www.scottishrite.org)

SpeechPathology.com (800-242-5183); (www.speechpathology.com)
The Stuttering Foundation (800-992-9392; 901-452-7343); (www.stutteringhelp.org)
Trace Research and Development Center (www.trace.wisc.edu)

SLOS

Smith-Lemli-Opitz Syndrome

Terms used in this chapter: LD (learning disability); MR (mental retardation); NIH (National Institutes of Health); SLO/RSHF (Smith-Lemli-Opitz/RSH Foundation); SLOS (Smith-Lemli-Opitz syndrome)

Did you know?

Named after pediatrician and dysmorphologist David Weyhe Smith, M.D., pediatrician Luc Lemli, M.D., and geneticist John Marius Opitz, M.D., SLOS is a metabolic genetic disorder (formerly called RSH syndrome, after the initials of the first three patients) that causes the body to produce or synthesize cholesterol incorrectly. Studies have shown that children with SLOS usually have cholesterol levels less than 50 mg/dL (normal is greater than 100 mg/dL) and abnormally high levels of a potentially toxic enzyme called 7DHC-reductase.

"Currently, the reason defects in cholesterol synthesis cause congenital malformations is not known," says Robert D. Steiner, M.D., and professor of pediatrics and molecular and medical genetics at the Oregon Clinical and Translational Research Institute. But research is now focusing on the role of cholesterol in early human development.

Cholesterol is essential to the body's cells; it affects all aspects of the body's health and growth, with a deficiency of cholesterol causing developmental problems.

There are wide-ranging symptoms in this syndrome, and the condition can itself range from normal development to severe impairment and death. There is a high fetal loss, but experts such as Dr. Steiner say that the majority of SLOS children live to adulthood with the proper cholesterol monitoring and treatment.

By the numbers

According to NIH studies, the prevalence of SLOS is approximately one in 20,000 to 40,000 live births. In the U.K., it is believed to have a prevalence of one in 60,000 and a carrier frequency of one in 122. For Canada, the prevalence rate is estimated at one in 26,000.

Dr. Steiner reports that one in thirty persons of northern European extraction are carriers and that the frequency is one per 5,000–18,000. The Genetic Science Learning Center at the University of Utah supports Steiner's statistic regarding northern European ancestry as well as a lower frequency in people of Asian or African background.

Since the syndrome is wide-ranging with some children developing normally with only a few minor abnormalities, SLOS sometimes goes undiagnosed or misdiagnosed, so many experts and advocates believe the prevalence numbers are even higher than reported. Also affecting the rate is the fact that many SLOS babies are stillborn or are miscarried.

SLOS carriers are asymptomatic, and a sibling of an SLOS child has a 25 percent chance of having SLOS, while 50 percent become asymptomatic carriers and the remaining 25 percent are neither affected nor a carrier.

Signs and symptoms

- aberrant behavior
- abnormally placed urethral opening in males (hypospadias)
- absence of nerves in the colon (Hirschsprung disease)
- absent testes
- adrenal underdevelopment and insufficiency
- allergies
- ambiguous genitalia
- androgen deficiency
- antisocial behavior
- autism
- behavioral problems: violent, self-destructive
- bluish coloration of skin (cyanosis), nailbeds, and lips
- brain malfunctions
- brittle bones
- broad nasal tip with slanted nostrils
- cataracts
- cleft palate
- club foot
- congenital heart disease, congestive heart failure, heart murmur
- coma
- complete sex reversal
- constipation
- cystic kidneys
- distinctive, shrill cry
- drooping eyelids (ptosis)

- dysmorphic facial features
- edema of the fetus (hydrops fetalis)
- estrogen deficiency
- excema
- extra digits (postaxial polydactyly)
- eyes improperly aligned (strabismus)
- failure to thrive
- feeding difficulties
- gastroesophageal reflux
- good receptive language abilities, but unable to communicate well
- hammer toes
- hearing loss
- high palate
- inability to absorb fat and fat soluble minerals (abetalipoproteinemia)
- inability to sleep
- jaundice
- language disorders
- LDs
- lethargy
- liver failure
- low muscle tone (hypotonia)
- low-set ears
- malformation of the airway (bifid epiglottis)
- mouth anomalies
- MR
- neonatal sepsis
- obstruction of the anal opening (imperforate anus)
- ophthalmologic problems: poor visual tracking, loss of vision, optic nerve abnormalities
- osteoporosis
- photosensitivity
- pneumonia
- prematurity and breech presentation
- projectile or forceful vomiting
- pulmonary anomalies
- reduced alertness or consciousness (obtundation)
- respiratory failure
- second and third toes are joined (syndactyly)
- self-stimulation (spinning, rocking, hand flapping, etc.)
- short stature

S

S

- short sternum
- short thumbs
- slanted ears
- small head circumference (microcephaly)
- small jaw (micrognathia)
- small penis (microphallus)
- small veins, making it difficult to draw blood
- sporadic red cheeks
- toxic dilation of the colon
- upper eyelid fold covering inner corner of eye (epicanthic folds)
- weaker immune systems
- withdrawal

Diagnosis

Dr. John L. Opitz, one of the doctors for whom the disorder is named, explains the diagnostic procedure and the difficulty in ascribing proper prevalence statistics: "In the U.S., we do not have newborn screening for RSH; hence, we lack total ascertainment, and these percentages [are unavailable]. It should be the pediatrician to first suspect the condition in an infant and to order tests."

The tests get a bit technical. According to the Smith-Lemli-Opitz/RSH Foundation (SLO/RSHF), there are two ways to test for SLOS. The first a specialized blood test to measure the level of 7-DHC is the most common test with tandem mass spectrometry (MS/MS) breaking down the cholesterol into sterol cholesterol, 7-DHC and 8-DHC.

SLO/RSHF reports that there are approximately a dozen labs in the United States that can perform this test, including the Kennedy Krieger Institute in Baltimore, Maryland; Baylor University, College of Medicine in Houston, Texas; Mayo Clinic in Rochester, Minnesota; and Oregon Health & Science University in Portland, Oregon.

The second way to test is through molecular or DNA testing to search for the SLOS mutations. SLO/RSHF states that most families get the diagnosis of SLOS by way of the 7-DHC test and then have the DNA testing done, so that they can properly warn other family members who are thinking of starting a family.

Dr. Steiner provided the following suggestions for diagnosis: "A diagnosis of SLOS is usually made postnatally after a clinician has become suspicious of the disorder based on clinical findings that match some of those described in SLOS. Diagnosis is best confirmed biochemically by analysis of sterols in blood, typically by gas-chromatography-mass spectrometry (GC-MS). Specifically, elevated levels of 7- and 8-dehydrocholesterol in blood along with low or low-normal levels of cholesterol are diagnostic. DNA mutation analysis is also available and can be used to confirm the diagnosis, but this is complicated by the fact that many different mutations have been shown to cause SLOS.

"Prenatal diagnosis is also possible and routinely performed for SLOS [which] may be suspected prenatally based on abnormal ultrasound findings with clinical features that match SLOS or when maternal serum screen for trisomies [trisomy is the presence of three copies of a chromosome instead of the normal two] is abnormal but trisomy is ruled out, or when a previous sibling was affected with SLOS. Prenatal diagnosis may be confirmed by analysis of sterols in amniotic fluid by GC-MS as above or analysis of sterols in chorionic villi. In addition, Shackleton pioneered a method that is being more widely applied of measuring unique sterols in maternal urine found in appreciable amounts only when SLOS is present in the fetus."

Despite the technical difficulties of the tests, as with so many of the other Alphabet Disorders, parents need to become lay scientists in order to help their children. However, parents should not worry: your doctor will explain this all to you.

Other diagnostic tools include abdominal ultrasound and X-ray, adrenocorticotropic hormone (ACTH) testing, audiogram, barium enema and swallow test, brain MRI or CT scanning, brainstem evoked response, chest X-ray, cortisol testing, ECG, echocardiography, electrolytes testing, enzyme analysis, genitourinary ultrasound, IQ test, low-density lipoprotein (LDL) cholesterol levels, rectal biopsy, renal ultrasound, skin biopsy (for culturing fibroblasts that can be used in enzymatic testing to provide diagnostic confirmation in atypical cases)., and slit lamp opthalmagic test SLO/RSHF suggests that since testing centers for some of these tests are hard to come by, parents should check out the Web site www.genetests.org for more information on SLOS testing.

Treatment

There isn't a specific recognized treatment for SLOS children, although one obvious direction would be to supplement the child's cholesterol levels that need to be raised in their plasma and tissues and reduce the toxic 7-DHC levels through synthetic or high-cholesterol foods like egg yolks, cream, and meat.

Dr. Opitz says, "Cholesterol has been used for treatment in RSH (or egg yolks); however, its effect in severe cases is doubtful."

Fetal therapy is another area that is being aggressively researched.

Other treatments and accommodations include antibiotics for ear infections, behavioral therapy, cleft-palate repair, comfortable clothing, communication systems, constipation medication, correcting pyloric stenosis (pyloromyotomy), early repair of polydactyly, gastrostomy feeding, hearing aids, hormone supplementation, hydrotherapy, immune system supplements, incontinence medication, limited exposure to the sun, motor therapy, pasteurized egg supplements, reflux medications, repair congenital heart defects, seizure medication, sensory therapy, sign language, sleep medications, and sun screen. Specialists who can help include an audiologist, developmental pediatrician, dietician or nutritionist, facial and plastic reconstructive surgeon, medical geneticist, metabolic-disease specialist, occupational therapist, ophthalmologist, pediatric cardiologist, pediatric gastroenterologists, pediatric neurologist, pediatric otorhinolaryngologist, pediatric psychologist or psychiatrist, pediatric surgeon, pediatric urologist, and physical therapist.

Prognosis

Depending on specific health issues of this wide-ranging disorder, it is difficult to suggest one prognosis. Depending on the severity of their symptoms, SLOS children often grow into adulthood and succeed in academic and work settings, as long as they have a strong support team. However, in many cases, an SLOS child will not make it past the fetal stage. Dr. Opitz says, "Many affected embryos must die prenatally."

Dr. Steiner explains how different aspects of the SLOS spectrum affect the prognosis: "At the mildest end of the spectrum, affected individuals may have only subtle LD and dysmorphic features. Severe SLOS, therefore, is associated with markedly shortened lifespan. Survival is less likely when the plasma cholesterol level is less than approximately 20 mg/dL as measured by gas chromatography.

"Those with mild SLOS can probably enjoy a normal lifespan. Moderately affected individuals often have growth and mental retardation, and the expected lifespan of such moderately affected individuals is unknown, but may be normal or nearly normal."

Sources and resources

Children's Hospital Boston (www.childrenshospital.org)
GeneTests (www.genetests.org) (site sponsored by NIH)
Kennedy Krieger Institute (443-923-9200; 88-554-2080); (www.kennedykrieger.org).
National Institutes of Health (www.nih.gov)
John M. Opitz, M.D., Division of Medical Genetics, University of Utah,
     Salt Lake City, UT 84132 (801-581-8943); e-mail: john.opitz@hsc.utah.edu.
Oregon Health & Science University (OHSU) (www.ohsu.edu)
Dr. Robert Steiner (503-494-7859)
The Smith-Lemli-Opitz/RSH Foundation (www.smithlemliopitz.org).
     For family support, general information, or to join the group, contact the Smith-Lemli-Opitz/RSH Foundation, c/o Cynthia Gold, P.O. Box 212, Georgetown, MA 01833 (978-352-5885); e-mail: cgold@smithlemliopitz.org

SM

Selective Mutism

Terms used in this chapter: ASD (autism spectrum disorder); CBT (cognitive behavioral therapy); *DSM* (*Diagnostic and Statistical Manual of Mental Disorders*); ERPT (exposure and response prevention therapy); *ICD* (*International Classification of Diseases*); SM (selective mutism); SMF (Selective Mutism Foundation)

Did you know?

SM, as classified by the *DSM*, or EM (elective mutism), as classified by the *ICD*, is a psychiatric disorder that is selective (or elective) silence—an anxiety disorder that is characterized by a child's failing to speak in social situations when fully able to speak. Anxiety disorder is the most common form of psychiatric disorder. SM children are very comfortable speaking to close family members; but outside of that circle, they go mute and do not make eye contact. They often do not use gestures or change their facial expression while in this mute mode. Sometimes they will depend solely on gestures.

Children with SM are socially phobic, anxious, and afraid of being judged negatively or that they will embarrass themselves in public. School and social situations are the most common settings in which this disorder is exhibited, but it can happen at home as well, with the child's selecting a particular family member to whom he or she doesn't speak.

These children usually are normal functioning aside from the speech, but they also often have other comorbid Alphabet Disorders such as OCD (obsessive-compulsive disorder), phobias, and depression. The SMF reports that, as related in anecdotes collected from parents, SM is also often comorbid with TS (Tourette syndrome), SID (sensory integration disorder), schizoid spectrum disorders, speech-language disorders, ASD, and phobias.

SM is often mistaken for ASD, but the difference between the two disorders is that the ASD child has limited verbal abilities and the SM child has the ability to speak. It is important to note that the SM symptoms are not a result of willfulness, as was believed for many years, but a reaction to growing anxiety. The nonverbal behavior is not intentional, but rather reactive. The SMF has gotten the official diagnostic wording changed from "refusal to speak" to "failure to speak."

Some children will stop speaking for a wide variety of reasons, but, until this behavior affects their daily functioning, it is not considered a disorder. But the trouble with waiting is, the earlier the intervention, the better the prognosis.

Signs and symptoms

- aversion to touch
- cries easily
- fear of people
- freezes up in social situations
- heightened sensory reactions
- immobility
- introspection
- lack of smiling
- moodiness
- nervous fidgeting
- no eye contact
- no facial expression
- not speaking in some settings
- often sociable and talkative at home
- plays with hair
- sensitive
- separation anxiety
- shyness
- sleeping problems
- speech-language problems
- stiff posture
- turns head away when spoken to

Cause

The cause of SM is not yet known, but most research indicates that SM is a social phobia that grows out of anxious and shy behavior in early childhood and that it has a genetic link. The majority of SM children are said to have an inherited link and that the child's parents might suffer from a social phobia or anxiety disorder. Some children develop it out of trauma—which had been the widely held belief in the past—but most SM children have not suffered a traumatic event.

Children with social inhibitions have exhibited an impaired excitability activity in the amygdale section of the brain, which is the part of the brain that processes indicators of danger that set off reactions to allow the body to protect itself. With anxiety-predisposed children, there is an overreaction in the amygdale, with the danger reaction's being set off when there isn't danger.

Some studies have shown that anxious children are born with their social inhibitions.

S

Diagnosis

The major factor for diagnosis is that the child being evaluated has the ability to speak and to understand speech and just chooses selected situations in which he or she does not use that ability. A visit to the pediatrician should be set up and the child evaluated, with a full physical exam to see if there are any underlying medical problems. If SM is suspected, the child should be sent to a speech-language therapist and a mental-health professional such as a pediatric psychiatrist or psychologist for a complete assessment.

Treatment

The SM child should be helped by CBT, which will help convert negative behaviors and thoughts into positive, productive ones. The therapist will work on reducing anxiety through another therapy, ERPT, which helps to desensitize the child to various fears by subjecting the child to those fears in a graduated manner. The therapist will also encourage the child to model his or her behavior on positive role models.

Relaxation and meditation techniques are also very helpful and effective in helping a child with SM.

Medications are usually not the first course of therapy, but they can be important in treating an SM child. The most successful medications for SM are the SSRIs, which increase the serotonin in the brain. The brain chemical serotonin has been shown to help decrease anxiety. (See the "SSRIs" section in "What You Need to Know" for more information.)

Other drugs such as Effexor XR, Serzone, Buspar, and Remeron work on the brain's chemical transmitters other than serotonin. Nardil, a monoamine oxidase inhibitor (MAOI), has also proven effective. Parents should get several doctors' opinions when they begin to consider a pharmaceutical route for their child. A drug treatment plan usually lasts between nine and twelve months, with the hope that the child will have become comfortable enough to speak on his or her own. Beginning drug therapy, revising drug therapy, and ending drug therapy should always be conducted under a physician's care.

Encouraging the child to speak as opposed to forcing the child to speak is the direction that SM treatment is heading. Much of the therapy is geared toward encouraging speech, whether through play, whisper therapy, or positive reinforcement. This is a group effort that involves the family, medical professionals, teachers, and various therapists.

A combination of therapies is usually the best way to approach this disorder.

Prognosis

SM *can* be treated, and there is a good prognosis, especially if there is early intervention.

Sources and resources

American Speech-Language-Hearing Association (ASHA) (800-638-8255); (www.asha.org)

Selective Mutism Foundation (www.selectivemutismfoundation.org)

Selective Mutism Group (www.selectivemutism.org)

See the mental-health contacts under "General Resources" for more sources used in this chapter.

SMS

Smith-Magenis Syndrome

Terms used in this chapter: ADHD (attention-deficit/hyperactivity disorder); FISH (fluorescence in situ hybridization); MR (mental retardation); NIH (National Institutes of Health); OCD (obsessive-compulsive disorder); ODD (oppositional defiant disorder); PRISMS (Parents and Researchers Interested in Smith-Magenis Syndrome); SMS (Smith-Magenis syndrome)

Sound familiar?

Tony and Barclay Daranyi of southwest Colorado never thought they'd conquer the trials and tribulations that their daughter Ali's mysterious syndrome had presented them with.

"Conquering implies control," says Tony, "something we don't feel we've gained."

Ali, who is now a teenager, has demonstrated extreme self-abusive behaviors since she was about 2 years old. Her episodes have dramatically decreased in frequency, but not necessarily in intensity, over time. Along her parents' journey, they learned about and eventually employed the Skinner Behavior Model and have found it to be the most effective way of coping with Ali's behaviors.

"We completely, 100 percent disengage and ignore the harmful self-abusive behavior once it has escalated, and redirecting [the initial strategy] has failed," explains her father.

What does that mean in real terms? No eye contact, no changes in body language or facial expressions, and no verbal communication. At the same time, the parents also have a reward strategy in place to get Ali to do what they want of her. "We continually reward the positive behaviors," says Tony.

Tony and his wife are the primary advocates for Ali, but they know they cannot do it alone— they receive help from a strong support network, including friends, the state of Colorado, a live-in helper, Big Brother/Big Sister programs, a full-time aide at school, family, and counseling. "We strive to remain positive by looking at the glass as half-full, not half-empty," Tony says. Ali has a sister, Tasha, who is two years younger, and who Tony describes as "abnormally normal."

No matter how dire matters may seem at any one time, Tony believes, "There is/will be light at the end of the tunnel." They always have a contingency plan in place in the event the worst-case scenario—a full-blown, self-abusive episode (they refer to them as "fits")—is experienced.

Tony's advice to other parents with a similar problem is to "always create a safe place, or have one available (e.g., at home, while traveling, at school, shopping, etc.)." Tony has "Ali-proofed" his daughter's room (turned locks inside out, taken out all lights, boarded up windows, put in wainscot along the walls, anchored bookshelves and dressers to the wall). When she was little, they created a 4x4x4 padded box to place Ali in a safe place for her fits. They also use the automobile "as a sacrificial safe haven when traveling."

"For safety's sake, we have to be able to separate ourselves and others from Ali when she is tantruming," explains Tony.

But Tony and Barclay realize that taking care of Ali also means thinking of their own wellbeing.

"We strive to take care of ourselves. If we're not healthy, we cannot expect to have a healthy household. We schedule a night out one day a week; we try to take one day off a week, usually on the weekends; we exercise or pursue a vocation to try to achieve balance in our lives and diffuse the stresses that raising a child with this syndrome presents." This is good advice for all parents of Alphabet Kids.

Ali isn't all about fits and tantrums. Ali has what her father calls "a unique, if not amazing, sense of humor. [She] want[s] nothing more than for us to laugh, out loud, with [her]."

Besides their tough-love policy of ignoring Ali's bad behaviors, a strict routine is in place. "Ali functions best when we adhere to a strict schedule on a day-to-day basis," Tony explains.

Since Ali is not wholly proficient at expressing her needs, her parents have had to anticipate her hunger and sleep needs, as a means of heading off her self-abusive behaviors.

Tony says he and his wife "try to celebrate our child, although we definitely don't do this often enough. The successful small steps in her life—learning how to dress herself, bathe, etc.—are actually large stepping stones to what we hope will be a life of self-actualization and completeness. For this, we must be celebratory.

"Most importantly, we have tried to tap into the incredible love that Ali pours out. She personifies unconditional love in the purest sense. That is her blessing. That can become our blessing, too, if we're ready to surrender."

Ali has SMS—Smith-Magenis Syndrome.

Did you know?

SMS is a chromosomal, developmental syndrome that affects many areas of a child's physical, behavioral, and developmental being. It is characterized by mild-to-moderate MR, delayed speech and language skills, distinctive facial features, numerous sleep disturbances, distinctive behaviors like self-hugging, and intense behavioral problems.

The distinctive facial appearance includes a broad, square-shaped face with deep-set eyes, full cheeks, and a prominent lower jaw. The middle of the face and the bridge of the nose often appear flattened. The mouth tends to turn downward with a full, outward-curving upper lip. SMS children have dental abnormalities, dark eyebrows that meet midline, and prominent, rosy cheeks. These facial differences can be subtle in early childhood, but they usually become more distinctive in later childhood and adulthood.

It was Ann C.M. Smith, M.A., D.Sc., a genetic counselor, and Dr. R. Ellen Magenis, a physician and chromosome expert, who described the first group of children with this disorder in the 1980s. Most people with the diagnosis have been identified since 1995 as a result of improved genetic-testing techniques. It is estimated that SMS occurs in one out of 25,000 births, but it is widely believed that SMS is underdiagnosed and that, as awareness increases, the prevalence rates will rise. The NIH reports that researchers believe the rate might actually be closer to one out of 15,000.

As with other Alphabet Disorders, early intervention is important, from providing physical, psychological, and occupational therapies to teaching sign language. Progress is being made in another aspect of SMS—sleep problems. One of the unusual and distinctive aspects of SMS is the disturbed sleep pattern. It has been discovered that SMS children have an inverted circadian rhythm (the normal twenty-four-hour cycle) of melatonin. Although the cause is not known, therapeutic melatonin has helped with reversing the abnormal sleep patterns.

Signs and symptoms

According to the NIH and the SMS advocacy group PRISMS, the following symptoms and signs are prevalent in those affected with SMS:

- abnormal EEG
- affectionate, endearing personality
- aggressive behavior
- articulation problems
- attention seeking (especially from adults)
- awaking in early morning
- broad-based gait
- cherubic, rosy-cheeked faces in infants
- chronic ear infections
- chronic sleep disturbances
- cleft lip
- cleft palate
- complacency in infancy
- congenital heart defects
- constipation

- curvature of the spine (scoliosis)
- damaged body communications system (peripheral neuropathy)
- daytime sleepiness
- decreased sensitivity to pain
- delayed fine motor skills
- delayed gross motor skills
- delayed toileting skills
- destructive behavior
- developmental delays
- diminished vocalizations in infancy
- distractibility
- early speech/language delay
- excellent long-term memory for names, places, events
- excitability
- explosive outbursts
- eye that turns in or out (strabismus)
- feeding problems as infant
- flat feet
- forearm abnormalities
- frequent drooling
- frequent nap taking
- frequent nighttime awakenings
- good sense of humor
- hand biting
- head banging
- hearing impairments
- heart murmurs
- high blood cholesterol
- high level of triglycerides in blood
- hoarse voice
- hugging their own arms
- hyperactivity
- hypernasal speech
- impulsivity
- infrequent crying as infant
- inserting foreign object into ears, nose, or other body orifices
- inverted circadian rhythm of melatonin
- iris anomalies
- laryngeal anomalies
- lethargy in infancy

- "lick and flip" (licking fingers and rapidly flipping pages of a book or magazine)
- low muscle tone (hypotonia)
- lowered immune function
- middle-ear problems
- MR (mild to moderate)
- nearsightedness (myopia)
- nighttime bedwetting
- open mouthed
- picking at skin, sores, and nails
- prolonged tantrums
- pulling off finger- and toenails (older ages)
- putting objects and hands in mouth, beyond childhood years
- reduced sensitivity to pain and temperature
- reflex response decreased (hyporeflexia)
- renal/urinary track defects
- repetitive behaviors
- retinal detachment
- seizures
- self-injurious behaviors
- sensory aversions and integration problems
- short fingers and toes
- short stature (especially in early childhood)
- skeletal anomalies
- small cornea
- speech delay
- squeezing own hands
- suck/swallow ability impaired
- sudden mood changes
- teeth grinding
- thyroid function abnormalities
- tongue strength and movement decreased

As with many Alphabet Disorders, there are several psychiatric disorders that are associated with SMS—ADHD, OCD, and ODD.

Cause

SMS is caused by a missing piece of genetic material from chromosome 17, referred to as deletion 17p11.2. Although SMS is caused by a deletion of genetic material, it usually does not run in families. In most cases, the deletion occurs accidentally in a child around the time he or she is conceived without being inherited from either parent. For this reason, SMS appears clearly genetic, but not usually familial. Families are advised to consult a genetic counselor or specialist for further advice regarding their own particular family situation.

Diagnosis

PRISMS describes how SMS should be diagnosed:

A diagnosis of SMS is usually confirmed by a clinical laboratory test that is performed in a cytogenetics laboratory. Cytogenetics labs perform blood tests called chromosome (cytogenetic) analysis and utilize a technique called FISH to diagnose SMS. FISH is a technique or process which vividly paints chromosomes or portions of chromosomes with fluorescent molecules. People with SMS are born with a small deletion (missing section) of one member of their 17th pair of chromosomes. It is the lack of this specific section, known as 17p11.2, which causes a child to develop the features of SMS. The genes commonly deleted in persons with SMS have been narrowed down to a "critical region" and encompass approximately 25 genes.

Until the mid-1990s, SMS was not well known, even among genetics professionals. The tiny 17p11.2 deletion was often overlooked in the laboratory and chromosome results were reported as "normal." The recent development of FISH for 17p11.2 deletion has allowed more accurate detection of SMS. Thus, a repeat cytogenetic study including FISH is indicated for individuals with prior "normal" routine cytogenetic analysis in whom a diagnosis of SMS is strongly suspected.

If you need help finding a genetic counselor in your area, please see the National Society of Genetic Counselors. A genetics counselor may refer you to a geneticist, a medical doctor or medical researcher. While a genetic counselor may help you with testing decisions and support issues, a medical geneticist will make the actual diagnosis of a disease or condition such as SMS.

Treatment

SMS cannot be cured, but its symptoms can be managed. SMS children require much support, including physical and speech/language and occupational therapy. Psychological and/or psychiatric therapy is also required to help control bad behaviors and comorbid disorders such as ODD and OCD. Support for those with SMS is a lifetime concern.

Medications are also often required to manage some SMS symptoms. Melatonin supplements and trazodone, a psychoactive sedative and antidepressant, are used to help regulate sleep problems. Risperdal is becoming the most common way to help control the violent behaviors associated with SMS.

Prognosis

Life expectancy for a child with SMS is normal. The prognosis is a promising one for many with SMS—they can attend school, find employment, and enjoy a productive life with the support of their family, school, and residential programs, as long as they have the proper intervention and treatment.

Sources and resources

Chromosome Disorder Outreach, Inc. (561-395-4252); (www.chromodisorder.org)
National Institutes of Health (www.nih.gov)
National Society of Genetic Counselors (312-321-6834); (www.nsgc.org)
PRISMS (Parents and Researchers Interested in Smith-Magenis Syndrome)
        (972-231-0035); (www.prisms.org)
Smith-Magenis Syndrome Foundation/UK (www.smith-magenis.co.uk)

SPD

Schizoid Personality Disorder

Terms used in this chapter: CBT (cognitive behavioral therapy); *DSM* (*Diagnostic and Statistical Manual of Mental Disorders*); SPD (schizoid personality disorder)

Did you know?

SPD is characterized by the avoidance of social activities and the profound inability to form relationships; it is often misdiagnosed. Even the current *DSM-IV-TR* suggests that there is a "great difficulty differentiating" between SPD, mild autism, and children with AS (Asperger syndrome).

SPD children have flat demeanors, appearing aloof, disinterested, unemotional, and humorless, and since forming a personal relationship is a two-way street, SPD children are at a disadvantage. They seem as if they are acting detached, so the child's peers are turned off by the behavior. But it is important to know that, although they seem so "empty" to an outsider, these children are filled with rich fantasy and very strong emotional needs.

SPD is on the mildest end of a biologically related spectrum of disorders; STPD is in the middle, while schizophrenia is found on the more severe end. All of these disorders result in an incapacity for social relations and emotional expressiveness. The main difference is that SPD kids don't usually experience the perceptual distortions, paranoia, or delusions characteristic of STPD (schizotypal personality disorder) or the psychosis experienced in schizophrenia.

Signs and symptoms

- appears dull and indifferent
- confused
- craves independence
- detached
- fear of dependency
- follower rather than leader
- general feeling of discomfort or restlessness (dysphoria)
- hypersensitivity in adolescence, despite actions that would appear otherwise
- inability to experience pleasure (anhedonia)
- inability to read social cues
- indifferent to praise or criticism
- lack of expressiveness
- lack of interest in other people's feelings
- lack of motivation
- lives in fantasy world, has imaginary friends
- loner
- longs for intimacy, despite actions
- poor academic performance
- seeks solitude
- social anxiety
- unsociable

Cause

The cause of SPD is not known, but, as with similar disorders, it is believed that it is a combination of genetics, neurodevelopmental aberrations, and environmental factors such as having emotionally detached parents, being neglected or abused, or being scorned or teased for behaviors exhibited as a child.

Diagnosis

If your child is experiencing symptoms such as those listed above, his or her pediatrician will conduct a full physical examination to rule out any underlying medical condition and then refer you to a mental-health professional—a pediatric psychiatrist or psychologist. This specialist should be expert in the schizoid spectrum of disorders.

Treatment

Psychotherapy would be the best course of action for an SPD child, but the very nature of this disorder makes therapy difficult because these children have a difficult time forming relationships, so they are apt to reject speaking with a therapist or forging a meaningful and helpful relationship with one. But when that relationship is successful, it can be a very positive step for the SPD child.

A universally well-accepted type of psychological therapy, CBT helps the child readjust his or her thinking so that negative behaviors are replaced by positive behaviors.

Antidepressants and/or anti-anxiety drugs are often used successfully for any comorbid anxiety or depressive conditions that the child has. For those mood and anxiety disorders, SSRIs are recommended. (See the "SSRIs" section in "What You Need to Know" for more information.)

Distorted thinking, flattened emotions, and some social problems can be controlled by clinical low doses of antipsychotic medications like Risperdal and Zyprexa. The SPD child's inability to experience pleasure can be treated with Wellbutrin.

More serious behaviors such as violent outbursts or severe detachment should be treated with antipsychotic drugs and sometimes hospitalization. It is suggested that those children be reevaluated, because those more extreme symptoms could indicate a different diagnosis than SPD.

Since SPD children manifest odd behavior and don't pick up on social cues, teaching social skills should be another important focus of therapy.

Early intervention is an important aspect to the SPD child's future success.

Prognosis

Of all the disorders on the schizophrenic spectrum, SPD is the most treatable. With early intervention, the proper therapies or medication, the eventual willingness of the child to accept help, and constant vigilance, there is hope for improvement in the SPD child.

Sources and resources

American Academy of Child and Adolescent Psychiatry (www.aacap.org)
American Psychiatric Association (www.psych.org)
American Psychological Association (www.apa.org)
DSM (*Diagnostic and Statistical Manual of Mental Disorders*)
Mayo Clinic (www.mayoclinic.com)
National Institute of Mental Health (www.nimh.nih.gov)
psychologytoday.com

See the mental-health contacts under "General Resources" for more sources used in this chapter.

SPLD

Semantic Pragmatic Language Disorder

Terms used in this chapter: ADHD (attention-deficit/hyperactivity disorder); ASD (autism spectrum disorder); HFA (high-functioning autism); IEP (individualized education program); LD (learning disability); PDD (pervasive developmental disorder); SPLD (semantic pragmatic language disorder)

Sound familiar?

When Jeffrey was a toddler, his parents knew something was wrong but just couldn't put their finger on what it was exactly. At first, they were concerned that he might have visual problems and that he might be deaf.

They noticed that, when Jeffrey played with his toys—during which time he appeared as if he were totally absorbed—he didn't seem to be doing much more than surface play. He would line his videos up and line up his plastic cowboy-and-horse toys, but there was no imaginative or interactive play. One pediatrician told Jeffrey's parents that he believed Jeffrey was autistic because of the child's obsessiveness, constant focus on the same interests, repetitive movements, and continuous jumping, spinning, and hand flapping.

"I was devastated," says his mother, Jillian. "But then I did my homework and not only did I realize that autism was not a death sentence, I also began to realize that what he had was not quite autism."

Meanwhile, Jeffrey was a happy, contented boy. If he could watch his cartoons all day long and not eat, sleep, or interact with humans, he'd be thrilled, his parents would say.

When Jeffrey started speaking, he was well past 3 years old. He hadn't babbled much as an infant. His first words were echoed from TV or his parents. Sometimes he would repeat the last few words of someone else's statement, not really meaning or understanding what he was repeating. His speech had very little meaning, and he would become frustrated when someone didn't get his intent. He would cry and throw a tantrum.

Jeffrey began speech-language and occupational therapy at age 3, and he progressed in that he expanded his vocabulary over the next couple of years, but there was still a flat affect to his speech.

He attended a special-education preschool in San Francisco where he received extensive therapy, but he was still far behind his peers in many developmental ways. By the time kindergarten began, he was just becoming toilet trained. But soon, Jeffrey began progressing and even surpassing his peers. Although he was clumsy and was not very good at riding his bike or playing soccer with the neighborhood kids, he was becoming very verbal, adept on the computer, and a whiz at math—as long as it wasn't word problems.

English lessons were difficult, and he had problems with creative writing.

S

At home, Jeffrey was very sweet and sociable, Jillian says, but, in public, he was shy and withdrawn. His mother, an office worker, says she thinks his attitude was due to his constant rejection by other children, who often made fun of his in-your-face lectures on dinosaurs and other subjects unrelated to anything his peers were interested in.

"Jeffrey loves talking to adults," his mother says. "Well, actually it is talking at adults. He will tell them in excruciating detail everything that interests him on a subject."

His speech is also muddled. He mixes up or drops his pronouns, starts in the middle of a story, and transposes sounds. But his vocabulary is "genius-level," Jillian says.

Jeffrey is in a public-school inclusion class and seems to be progressing very well, thanks to speech and occupational therapy. He especially likes the fact that he has the modification of being allowed to use a computer in class, because his handwriting is, as Jillian says, "totally illegible."

"I am very filled with promise," says Jillian. "Through his social-skills classes and in school in general, I see so many children who came around the other end of this. He even has a physical therapist who had some of the same problems when he was a child."

Jeffrey's parents are thrilled with his progress.

"If you didn't know what he went through to get here," says his mom, "and you just met him, you would think that he is just a quirky kid."

Jeffrey has SPLD—semantic pragmatic language disorder.

Did you know?

SPLD is a language/communication disorder characterized by a child's having difficulty in communication skills and social language. SPLD is diagnosed when a child has his or her language intact and an average-to-high IQ, but the communications aspect does not correlate to verbal ability. SPLD is often found in children with PDD and is usually considered interconnected with ASD (children with SPLD have the same types of difficulties as those on the autism spectrum: deficits in communication, social interaction, and imagination), but it is actually a separate disorder. SPLD is a spectrum disorder that appears to be a blend of autistic-like and normal behaviors. It is sometimes confused with HFA, ADHD, AS (Asperger syndrome), hyperlexia, PDD–NOS (not otherwise specified), and LDs. As the autism spectrum broadens, there are some experts who believe that SPLD might one day be blended with HFA.

How it is manifested

Let's break down SPLD: *semantics* is the meaning of words, and *pragmatics* is the social use of language. It is believed that the problem SPLD kids encounter is a processing one.

The SPLD child does start developing language, but it is often impaired, especially in conversational speech—the child has difficulty understanding and using language rules. The child's speech patterns will appear peculiar, and the language is stiff, inappropriate, rote, off topic, and one-sided. The child will not understand subtleties, sarcasm, and humor, often taking statements literally. You can ask an SPLD child, "What's up?" and they will respond, "The ceiling, the sky, the sun."

These children will tell a story without proper names or specific details, initiating a sentence without any context: "So she told them that they can't do that." Who told them, and who is them?

SPLD children will give away secrets: "My mother drinks beer all day long," or will make comments about someone's physicality out loud, "That man has really funny-looking big ears."

They might go on and on about baseball stats or dinosaurs without any regard for the interest or boredom level of the listener.

They cannot assess the emotional impact of a statement. For example, a child without SPLD might say, "My house burnt down last night." The SPLD child might respond, "Well, my house has the prettiest rooms, and I have so much fun living there."

Salient points of conversation are missed on SPLD children, and they will not be able to move beyond one linguistic rule to another.

SPLD also affects nonverbal abilities. These children use inappropriate body language, usually talking straight into someone's face or avoiding eye contact. They might even walk away from someone in mid-conversation. These children have good grammar and vocabulary, but they have no context in which to use those skills.

Pragmatics in language involves following a set of social expectations, following the listener's needs and expectations, and providing enough coherent information to get a point across. SPLD children have a difficult time with the subtleties of language—abstractions, irony, sarcasm, idioms—and they are unable to get beneath the obvious or understand what is implied.

SPLD children will sometimes assume prior knowledge and begin to lecture a listener. They will also talk over others, which often appears rude, but is not. Remember, these children do not know the social rules of conversation.

It is obvious that these children will be singled out by their peers and have great social difficulties including being bullied, teased, and shunned.

Signs and symptoms

- anxiety
- appears deaf
- assumes listener's knowledge, without providing details or background information
- attention problems
- confuses pronouns
- delays in gross motor skills such as riding a bike

- detailed memory
- difficulty answering open-ended questions
- difficulty following instructions
- difficulty with change
- doesn't stay on point when speaking
- doesn't take turns when speaking
- fine motor difficulties
- flat voice
- groping for words
- inability to maintain focus in conversation
- incessant chattering
- lack of insight into others' emotions or intent
- little babbling in infancy
- makes up words (neologisms)
- needs routine
- no imaginative play
- obsessive interests
- odd gait
- parroting (echolalia)
- poor handwriting
- poor language processing
- poor social skills
- prefers cartoons to live action
- repetitive behaviors
- repetitive speech
- scripted language
- self-stimulation (stimming—rocking, spinning, hand flapping, etc.)
- sing-song speech
- speaks in jargon
- takes expressions literally
- talks in details
- tantrums
- uses wrong words (paraphasias)
- will reveal secrets

Cause

There is no one concrete theory on what causes SPLD, but, as with autism and other speech, language, and processing disorders, it is suspected that genetic, biological, and environmental factors might affect a predisposed child.

Diagnosis

Delayed language development raises the first red flag with an SPLD child. It's often a gut feeling that parents have, thinking that something is "off" about their child. When this occurs, the child should be brought to a pediatrician for a full physical evaluation to rule out any medical condition, and then be referred to a speech-language pathologist, developmental specialist, pediatric neurologist, or neuropsychiatrist. These professionals will rely on standardized testing, developmental history, and clinical observations.

Treatment

The team of specialists who will work with the child might include a pediatrician, speech-language pathologist, pediatric psychiatrist or psychologist, social-skills specialist, and occupational therapist, among others.

Developing social and conversational skills will be the key to success for SPLD children. They will learn simple things such as knowing that they have to respond to someone when asked a question, taking turns in conversation, sticking to a topic, responding to nonverbal language such as body language, making eye contact, and understanding language subtleties.

Play and imagination therapy help the SPLD child loosen up and learn to be less rigid, while also teaching the child how to give and take.

There are modifications in school that will prove very helpful and obtaining an IEP is a must. Besides providing specific therapies, there are things that can be done in the classroom, especially an inclusion classroom, where a teacher can help explain things to the SPLD child that he or she just might not "get" or even "hear" because of processing problems. Having the child sit in front of the classroom near the teacher will make a profound difference. Sometimes the teacher will have to make eye contact with the student or even tap the student to refocus his or her attention. Tests should be taken in a designated "quiet room," where a teacher can help redirect the student's attention and makes sure the child properly comprehends the subject matter.

Directions have to be very specific, and simple: "Please take the red crayon that is in the yellow box and put it on top of your desk next to the green book."

There is a growing belief that children with SPLD should be in social groups together, group therapy and the same classroom, so they can feel a part of a group without the social pressures and social problems brought in by children without the disorder.

Therapists, especially speech-language therapists, will help SPLD children with skills such as greetings, initiating a conversation, observing situations, commenting on things, rejecting and accepting others' ideas, joining in on other people's conversations, zeroing in on and sticking to one topic, changing a topic and following when someone else changes a topic, understanding the other person's intent, manipulating conversation, mending misinterpretations or misunderstandings, making a point, and knowing when someone wants something from you and what they want.

Prognosis

Depending on the severity of the disorder, the prognosis can be quite positive. Early intervention is very important, and obtaining the correct diagnosis is crucial. Some SPLD children can resolve their issues with a prognosis of normal ability, while others might improve upon their symptoms but still remain odd and stiff in terms of their speech and affect.

Sources and resources

American Speech-Language-Hearing Association (www.asha.org)
SPD Support Organisation (www.spdsupport.org.uk)

See the "SLD: Speech-Language Disorder" chapter and the "Autism" contacts in "General Resources" for more sources used in this chapter.

STPD

Schizotypal Personality Disorder

Terms used in this chapter: CBT (cognitive behavioral therapy); COS (childhood-onset schizophrenia); PD (personality disorder); PD (personality disorder); SPD (schizoid personality disorder); STPD (schizotypal personality disorder)

Did you know?

STPD is characterized by deficits in social and interpersonal relationships as well as the manifestation of eccentric behaviors. STPD children have great difficulty forming and maintaining close relationships and tend also to have a distorted reality. Sometimes it is regarded as a milder form of the much more serious COS, which is a debilitating brain disorder that severely distorts a child's reality and the way he or she acts and thinks. STPD can turn into schizophrenia in rare cases.

Much of the disorder is manifested by odd behaviors such as being lost in fantasy worlds or believing in extra-sensory perception (ESP), which, it should be noted, can be signs of normal behavior as well—but when it begins to interfere with a child's daily functioning and negatively impacts the child's mental well-being, it is time to consider it a disorder and not normal behavior.

STPD is in the middle of a biologically related spectrum of disorders with SPD on the mild end and COS on the more severe end. Although all three of these PDs share genetic commonalities, it is not known why one child will develop a specific one that is more or less severe than another.

Most children with STPD will have problems with attention, memory, and learning, and distorted perception. They do not manifest the psychotic symptoms of schizophrenia such as hallucinations. STPD symptoms are often described as subtle.

STPD children range in severity of the disorder and some might be able to lead relatively normal lives while others will not be able to work or live independently.

Signs and symptoms

- anxiety
- attaching personal meaning to outside events
- attention problems
- avoids social situations
- awkward and eccentric social behaviors
- bizarre fantasies
- daydreaming
- disrupted sensory/reality communication (mistaking sounds for voices)
- distrust
- dresses oddly
- emotionally aloof
- inability to form intimate relationships
- inability to function
- inability to make and sustain friendships
- magical thinking (if I do action "A," it will prevent action "B")
- memory problems
- odd preoccupations
- odd speech (overly elaborate, metaphorical, nonessential details, etc.)
- paranoia
- stiff, rigid affect
- strange speech patterns
- superstitious

Cause

This is a disorder that can be found in family members of schizophrenics, so there is a strong sense that it is genetic, as well as neurodevelopmental and environmental.

Diagnosis

If a child is presenting symptoms of this disorder, he or she should have a full physical evaluation by a pediatrician to rule out any other medical problems. That doctor will then refer the child to a pediatric psychiatrist, who will evaluate the child. Since these schizophrenic spectrum disorders are often overlooked in children, it would make sense to find a doctor who is familiar with them.

To help differentiate STPD from SPD and COS, the diagnostician will examine signs in the child for the presence of symptoms such as mood and anxiety disorders as opposed to psychosis and delusions.

Treatment

It is common for a child to be sent initially for treatment for one of the comorbid disorders that often accompany STPD, such as depression or anxiety. Although it is daunting, the first course of treatment is psychotherapy. Through CBT, the doctor will work with the child to help change his or her bad habits and replace them with better, more beneficial, ones. Psychotherapy is problematic for these children because STPD kids don't form good relationships and might not be able to bond with the therapist. But the good news is that a child with STPD can be shown that his or her reality has been distorted. Family therapy has also been found helpful.

Antidepressants and/or anti-anxiety drugs are often used successfully for STPD and certainly for any additional anxiety or depressive conditions that the child has. For those mood and anxiety disorders, SSRIs are recommended. (See the "SSRIs" section in "What You Need to Know" for more information.)

Distorted thinking can be controlled by antipsychotic medications like Risperdal and Zyprexa; in the case of STPD, even clinical (low) doses can be effective. More serious behaviors such as violent outbursts or severe detachment should be treated with antipsychotic medication and sometimes hospitalization. It is suggested that children with serious behavior problems be reevaluated because those more extreme symptoms could indicate a different diagnosis than STPD.

Since STPD children manifest odd behavior and don't pick up on social cues, teaching social skills should be another important focus of therapy.

Prognosis

STPD is a chronic condition. Children with STPD cannot be cured, but they can be treated. The results of the treatment can range from being very successful to not having much of an impact. The earlier the disorder is caught, the better. In rare cases, the STPD can turn into full-fledged schizophrenia.

Sources and resources

American Academy of Child and Adolescent Psychiatry (www.aacap.org)

American Psychiatric Association (www.psych.org)

American Psychological Association (www.apa.org)

DSM (Diagnostic and Statistical Manual of Mental Disorders)

Mayo Clinic (www.mayoclinic.com)

National Institute of Mental Health (www.nimh.nih.gov)

psychologytoday.com

See the mental-health contacts under "General Resources" for more sources used in this chapter.

T

TS (Tourette Syndrome)

TS

Tourette Syndrome

Terms used in this chapter: ADHD (attention-deficit/hyperactivity disorder); *DSM* (*Diagnostic and Statistical Manual of Mental Disorders*); ERPT (exposure and response prevention therapy); *ICD* (*International Classification of Diseases*); LD (learning disability); OCD (obsessive-compulsive disorder); PANDAS (pediatric autoimmune neuropsychiatric disorders associated with strep); TS (Tourette syndrome); TSA (Tourette Syndrome Association)

Sound familiar?

Jennifer Zwilling is the middle of three children.

Her development was normal. Her mother, Jane, says that Jen reached many milestones early, including walking before ten months.

"She was always a very cuddly child," recalls Jane. "The only significant issue early on was that Jen was a very irritable baby and cried for fourteen weeks straight. But after that, she was a delight."

There was nothing out of the ordinary in regard to Jen's development until one day during her kindergarten year when she was 5½ years old after she had been sick with a bad cold and had been absent from school for several days. The day Jen returned to school, Jane received a phone call from the school nurse saying Jen had a rash and needed to go home.

Jen went to the pediatrician who said the rash was nothing to be concerned about. It was only later that Jane began to suspect that Jen's illness was a case of untreated strep. Sure enough, when Jen's blood work was eventually analyzed by NIMH revealing extremely elevated strep titers, Jane's suspicions were confirmed.

The next morning, Jen woke up with a very noticeable eye tic. The tic persisted, and Jane decided that Jen must have been anxious about an upcoming move, so she brought her to a psychologist. After several sessions, the psychologist terminated the treatment saying that Jen was not anxious at all about the move and that she seemed perfectly well adjusted.

The tic soon began to include Jen's nose—she wiggled it—and then it moved to her mouth. A pediatrician suggested the cause was allergies and gave Jen eye drops and antihistamines. Jen began to "cough," clear her throat, and seemed to be bothered by her eyes. An ophthalmologist found nothing wrong.

The symptoms got better and then turned worse. Sometimes the movements included Jen's head nodding, and soon her arms were affected. Jane began reading up on symptoms and disorders. She took Jen to a neurologist who confirmed that the girl had tics, but no diagnosis was made because she had

T

exhibited them for less than a year, the time allotted before a diagnosis can be made.

First grade was better for Jen—just some throat clearing persisted. In second grade, she developed eye-rolling. As with so many parents of Alphabet Kids, Jane kept reading as much as she could to determine what was wrong with her daughter. One strange thing she noticed was that, whenever Jen was ill, her tics got better.

Jane came upon some research that was being done with sudden onset of tics and its relation to untreated strep infections. She convinced Jen's pediatrician to look into this research. Jen's blood sample was sent to researchers at the National Institute of Mental Health who felt that she fit the diagnosis of PANDAS, which is associated with streptococcal infections. This diagnosis is used to describe a set of children who are thought to have developed OCD and/or tic disorders such as TS following group A beta-hemolytic streptococcal (GABHS) infections such as strep throat and scarlet fever. The treatment for PANDAS includes high doses of antibiotics (Jane remembered that Jen always seemed to be symptom-free when she was ill and on antibiotics).

At age 7, Jen was officially diagnosed with PANDAS. She now takes a prophylactic dose of antibiotics every day. Jane says that "to this day, when [Jen] is exposed to strep, she does seem to tic more."

It had taken two years to get that diagnosis of TS, which her mom knew instinctively was the case, and during that time, Jen was being treated for allergies instead of TS.

Jen never had any tics while she slept. "It was almost like her body had to wake up before the tics would begin again," according to Jane.

Each morning Jane would stare at her blonde-haired, blue-eyed daughter at the breakfast table, and now recalls: "[I was] hoping that this was the morning that the tics went away. So many times I have told Jen and other parents that, if I could do anything to take her tics, I would."

"We have been very lucky," Jane says. "Jen is a beautiful child with a winning smile who has always had great friends. She has always been included." Jen, an athlete, was on a competitive gymnastics team, played travel softball and basketball when she was younger, and played tennis and lacrosse for her high school. She is an honor student and does not have the comorbid disorders that so many kids with TS have. As a teenager, Jen's tics are mostly internal, so not really obvious to others. This, of course, makes a huge difference in her life, compared to others with her disorder. Jane says, "[Jen] has never let her disorder interfere in anything that she has set out to do."

Jen has graduated high school, where she was a National Merit scholar, and member of the National Honor Society. She will now be attending Duke University.

Jen is the founder of the TSA's National Youth Ambassador Peer Training Program, and she is the only student member of the executive board of the Long Island chapter of the TSA. As a teen ambassador, Jen has spoken at more than 50 schools, spoken four times at congressional receptions, and visited individual members of congress. She was also the recipient of the 2008 Prudential Spirit of Community Award for demonstrating outstanding volunteerism.

Jen has TS—Tourette syndrome.

Did you know?

TS is named for the French doctor Georges Gilles de la Tourette, who first described the condition in 1885. The exact cause of this neurological disorder is not known, but it is believed that TS is an inherited genetic condition. It is found throughout the world. The *ICD* classifies it as combined vocal and multiple motor tic disorder.

In the simplest terms, TS is a dysfunction in which the brain's neurotransmitters (chemicals in the brain that carry nerve signals from cell to cell) suffer some sort of disturbance. TS is a common childhood-onset disorder distinguished by its unrelenting vocal and motor tics as well as obsessions, compulsions, and attention problems. It is now regarded as a spectrum disorder with a wide range of manifestations.

Between one in 1,000 and one in 2,000 people have TS, and their symptoms usually become apparent in childhood or in the teenage years. Many children with mild and simple TS are never diagnosed, so the statistics are skewed, indicating many more people have the disorder than statistics show.

TS appears more often in boys than girls, and its course is erratic, whether worsening or subsiding. And it is prevalent around the world.

Dr. Roger D. Freeman, M.D., clinical head, Neuropsychiatry Clinic, British Columbia Children's Hospital, Vancouver, British Columbia, and chair of the Tourette Syndrome Foundation of Canada, explains the difficulty in diagnosing TS: "Tourette syndrome is not a disease; it is a syndrome, a cluster of recognizable patterns. There are no tests for it. The diagnosis is by history and observation only, and the boundary is fuzzy. No one has decided how many tics a day are necessary to call it a tic disorder. [Spitting three times in school, for example, will probably result in a phone call, whereas 10,000 eye-blinks won't!] Although tics are often described as 'rapid' or 'sudden,' not all are; some tics are 'held' or 'tonic' movements involving freezing in a position for a few seconds. 'Purposeless' is another descriptor, but because many tics are preceded by an uncomfortable feeling to which the tic is a response, this word also isn't very satisfactory. The definition is simply a multiple, changing pattern of tics [not necessarily at the same time] for at least twelve months, including at least one noise-making tic. [There is no requirement for severity or impairment.] You can have Tourette syndrome and function normally."

Huei-Shyong Wang, M.D., is the president of the Taiwan Tourette Family Association: "Most TS is mild. Only 10 to 25 percent of TS patients are severe and even morbid. Even in the same family or identical twins, they may have very different presentations."

Signs and symptoms

The main symptoms of TS are motor tics and vocal tics.

At certain times, such as when a child is overly anxious or under a lot of stress, the tics can change in frequency and severity. Some children are able to suppress their tics

T

for short periods of time; but, as anxiety and stress build, the child needs to release the tension—it is released as a tic. This is where the social component comes in: as a child is concentrating on his tic, he is shutting out everything else, like a teacher's lecture or a friend's conversation.

What is a tic?

The Tourette's Information Center defines tics as sudden, repeated, involuntary movements or vocal sounds. There are two classifications of tics: simple and complex.

Simple motor tics involve only a few muscles, occur suddenly, are often inconsequential, and are separate from other tics the child might have. An example of a simple tic is sniffing, shrugging, or blinking. Complex motor tics are obviously more complicated, usually involving several muscle groups. Facial and motor tics may include eye blinking, head movements, stomping, or sudden arm movements. For example, a child with a complex motor tic might repeatedly hit another person or twirl around while walking. Simple vocal tics may include coughing, barking, or humming. The complex vocal tic can involve echolalia (the repetition of words or sentences), palilalia (the constant repetition of syllables), or coprolalia, the "cursing disorder."

One of the biggest misconceptions about TS is coprolalia, which involves the screaming out of curse words or phrases or other inappropriate utterances. It is what the vast public thinks of when they hear the term *Tourette*. However, it is estimated that only between 5 and 15 percent of those diagnosed with TS have tics that involve coprolalia.

TS's age of onset, according to the *DSM*, "may be as early as 2 years, is usually during childhood or early adolescence, and is by definition before age 18 years. The median age at onset for motor tics is 7 years. The duration of the disorder is usually lifelong, though periods of remission lasting from weeks to years may occur. In most cases, the severity, frequency, and variability of the symptoms diminish during adolescence and adulthood. In other cases, the symptoms disappear entirely, usually by early adulthood."

For many TS children, the first symptoms to appear are bouts of a single tic, most frequently eye blinking, as was the case with Jen; less frequently, tics involve another part of the face or the body.

It is important to know that many tics involved in TS are very subtle or go largely unnoticed. And children's tics often change. Sometimes the tic is short-lasting, staying with the child for a few days or weeks, while other tics may be chronic. They are sometimes stress related and can often disappear for a while.

Tics are involuntary, and while the child might feel a "build-up," almost a premonition they are coming, he or she often can't control them. Some children learn how to compensate or suppress the tic. After the tic occurs, there is a feeling of relief.

This is a list of tics compiled from various TS organizations. Parents should keep in mind that some of the below-listed "tics" on their own are perfectly normal behaviors.

Physical motor tics

- abdominal jerking, tension
- arm—extending, flailing, flapping, flexing, jerking, rotating, squeezing, touching
- banging items, body parts, and self against other objects
- bending at waist
- biting—self, mouth, lip, nails, arm, others
- bladder tic
- blowing in air, on fingers, on objects
- blurring or doubling objects by staring
- body jerking
- bowel tics
- breath holding
- buttocks (gluteal) tensing
- chewing on clothes, fingers, fingernails, toes, assorted items
- chin touching
- clapping
- clothes pulling, tearing
- cracking knuckles, jaw
- cuticle picking, chewing
- elbow touching behind back
- extending neck
- eye—blinking, rolling, looking toward ceiling, bulging, squinting, winking
- facial contortions, grimacing
- fingers—movements, smelling, pulling, snapping
- flapping arms
- flexing—ankles, wrists, arms, knees, toes, feet
- foot—dragging, shaking, tapping
- freezing movement
- groin thrusting
- gyrating
- hair—brushing out of eyes, tossing, twisting, pulling
- hand fiddling
- head—banging, jerking, shaking, turning, tossing
- hitting self, others
- hopping
- involuntary mimicking of another person's motions (echopraxia)
- jabbing
- jaw—snapping, thrusting, cracking
- jumping

T

- kicking
- kissing self or others
- knee—bending, knocking, extending
- knuckle cracking
- leg—jerking, tensing, extending
- licking
- lifting shoulders
- lips—pursing, pouting, smacking, popping
- mouth—opening, pouting, grimacing, clenching
- neck—twisting, pulling, stretching
- nose—twitching, wrinkling, touching
- obscene/inappropriate gestures (copropraxia)
- obscene writing or drawing (coprographia)
- odd facial expressions
- palm touching
- picking skin, scabs, at lint, lips, cuticles
- pinching
- pulling back pen while writing
- pulling clothes, hair
- pulling out hair (trichotillomania)
- rapid jerking parts of body
- reflex inhibition
- repetitive twisting (dystonic) postures from muscle contractions
- scratching
- shaking head, feet, arms, legs, hands
- shivering
- shoulder—shrugging, lifts, rolls
- skipping
- smelling hands, fingers, objects
- sniffing
- snorting
- somersaulting
- spitting
- squatting
- squinting
- stepping backwards
- stomping
- stooping
- tearing things
- tensing parts of body, muscle groups

- throwing things
- toes—scrunching, flexing
- tongue thrusting
- touching objects, pressure points, self or others (haphemania)
- twirling hair
- twirling in circles
- walking backwards
- walking on toes
- writhing movements

Vocal tics

- air swallowing
- animal sounds (barking, braying, chirping, meowing, mooing, oinking, quacking, etc.)
- barely audible muttering
- belching, burping
- blocking tic (unable to get sound out)
- blowing on fingers, self, objects, others
- blowing sounds
- breathing tics
- calling out
- change in voice tempo, tone, volume, pitch, intonation
- clacking
- clearing throat
- clicking teeth
- clicking tongue
- coughing
- cursing or making socially taboo comments or inappropriate phrases (coprolalia)
- gasping
- groaning
- grunting
- gurgling
- guttural sounds from back of throat
- hiccupping
- hissing
- holding breath
- honking
- humming
- laughing
- making unintelligible noises

- moaning
- muttering
- noisy breathing
- puffing expirations
- repeating words (echolalia), parts of words, phrases, repeating parts of words, one's own words (palilalia)
- screaming
- shouting
- sniffing
- sniffling
- snorting
- spitting
- squeaking
- squealing
- stammering
- stuttering
- sucking sounds
- swallowing air
- talking to oneself
- throat clearing
- vocalizing: "Hey," "Wow," and "tsk" and "pft" noises
- wheezing
- whistling
- yelling
- yelping

The advocacy organization Tourette's Disorder Information lists some symptoms that are not officially recognized but have been reported by the Tourette community: heat sensitivity, light sensitivity (especially flickering light), excessive water drinking, excessive and constant thirst (polydipsia), sleeping difficulties, tactile hypersensitivity (includes itchiness and scratching), and self-injurious behaviors (e.g., poking eye, biting, banging head).

Here is some final advice from Jane Zwilling, Jen's mother: "There are transient tics that children may experience. If your youngster demonstrates tics, you may want to let them know that you notice and ask if they are bothered by it. Chances are the child will say 'no,' so, at that point, it is best to just let it be. The more attention one calls to the tics, the more anxious the child gets and, in fact, the worse the tics become. The less attention paid to them the better. Also, kids with TS are very suggestible because of the misbalance of the chemicals in their brains, so, if you talk about their tics, they do actually tic more. So, educate the important people in their environment, and, unless the child needs help with something that the tic is causing, let it be."

Cause

The cause of TS points to a genetic component because there is such a high incidence in family history with TS patients. If you have TS, according to Dr. Freeman, the chance of one of your children having a tic spectrum disorder is approximately 50 percent for males and 30 percent for females. And even its comorbid disorders have an inheritable connection.

Jean Cottraux, M.D., Ph.D., of the Anxiety Disorder Unit, Hospital Neurologique, in Lyon, France, says, "The most inherited forms [of anxiety] are associated with Tourette disorder."

David E. Comings, M.D., says in his book, *Tourette Syndrome and Human Behaviour*, "Tourette Syndrome is one of the most common genetic conditions affecting humanity and many more carry the trait."

Neurochemistry also plays a big part in that there are abnormalities of dopamine and serotonin in the brain, which is indicated by the positive response to pharmacological intervention.

Diagnosis

For a TS diagnosis, a child must exhibit several different types of involuntary tics, specifically multiple motor tics and at least one vocal tic, for at least one year. The child needs to exhibit the tic for a year in order for this diagnosis because "transient" tics in children are common for short periods of time, occurring in about one in five to one in ten of normal children. The transient tics eventually disappear, and the children get better.

For an official TS diagnosis, a child cannot be tic-free for a period of three months within the twelve-month-required diagnostic period. It is a good idea to keep track of your child's type and frequency of tics.

But even the criteria described above can be problematic. TS is sometimes a particularly tough disorder to diagnose and treat because it is often concurrent with other Alphabet Disorders such as ADHD, APD (auditory processing disorder), and OCD. Some TS children have LDs and sleep and anxiety disorders. Along with those come eating and conduct disorders. TS is one of those Alphabet Disorders that rarely shows up by itself.

Colleen Wang, R.N., medical V.P. of the TSA, says it best: "Tourette Syndrome rarely exists in isolation and is part of a global neurological dysfunction, which includes but is not limited to tics, and dysinhibition. Where does one draw the line? Is 'this' a symptom of 'Tourette Syndrome' or is it part of 'ADHD' or 'OCD' or does it really matter? Tourette Syndrome is … something more akin to 'cross wiring' and the reality being that daily function requires one to deal with what is thrown at one regardless as to what it is called."

The most common path of diagnosis is by starting with the family pediatrician, who will refer the child to a neurologist after observing the child's tics and receiving a history from the parent regarding the duration of the tics along with other relevant information. The good-news/bad-news aspect of this is that almost any doctor can diagnose TS, but, unfortunately, that's because it has become so prevalent.

There isn't one specific diagnostic test for TS, although some doctors use imaging tests like MRIs, CAT scans, EEGs, or blood tests to rule out other conditions that might have symptoms similar to TS.

There are scales, however, that doctors utilize to determine the severity of the disorder—mild, moderate, severe—but these scales rely on subjective input because what one patient might describe as mild, another might feel is severe.

Treatment

There is no cure for TS, but there are several ways to approach the treatment: behavioral therapy, psychological counseling, occupational therapy, and medication. ERPT, a desensitizing approach, habit reversal therapy, and relaxation therapy are all treatments used for TS. None, however, has been conclusively proved to be the ultimate long-term treatment for the disorder. The treatment varies according to how the TS manifests itself in the child.

Medication can be prescribed to treat certain symptoms that negatively impact the child's academic or social life

The pharmacological approach is usually a last-resort approach. In the United States, treating tics with medicine is often off-label, which means that the drug has not yet been approved for children or it has not yet been approved to treat tics by the Food and Drug Administration.

Medicines used to treat tics include clonidine, clozapine, guanfacine, pimozide, risperidone, haloperidol, and botulinum toxin (Botox) for short-term treatment. No medications should be administered to a child without first consulting a doctor.

Although TS is a physical condition, it impacts the child psychologically, so visiting a pediatric psychiatrist or psychologist often helps. Not only is it a way to get some concerns off their chests, the children can learn antistress relaxation techniques and discover ways to deal with anxiety and tics.

Prognosis

The prognosis for TS is good in that many of the tics children suffer from fade, or even disappear, as they grow older. With the proper treatment TS can be, for the most part, kept under control.

Sources and resources

David E. Comings, *Tourette Syndrome and Human Behavior* (Monrovia, CA: Hope Press, 1990).

Tourette's Information Center (www.thetic.info)

Tourette Information Site (www.tourette-syndrome.info)

Tourette Syndrome Association (718-224-2999); (www.tsa-usa.org)

Tourette Syndrome (UK) Association (0845-458-1252; 020-7793-2357); (www.tsa.org.uk)

Tourette Syndrome Foundation of Canada (800-361-3120); (www.tourette.ca)

Tourette Syndrome Information (www.tourettes-disorder.com)

Tourette Syndrome–Now What? (for families of the newly diagnosed) (http://tourettenowwhat.tripod.com)

Tourette Syndrome Online (www.tourette-syndrome.com)

Tourette Syndrome Plus (www.tourettesyndrome.net)

WE MOVE (www.wemove.org)

T

W

WD (Wilson's Disease)

WS (Williams Syndrome)

WD

Wilson's Disease

Terms used in this chapter: NIH (National Institutes of Health); WD (Wilson's disease)

Did you know?

Most people ingest more copper than they need without any problems, but, if a child has the genetic disorder WD, one mushroom might prove fatal.

Named for neurologist Samuel Alexander Kinnier Wilson, M.D., WD, if left undetected and undiagnosed, could lead to serious illness or death due to copper poisoning, which is the disorder's main characteristic.

Children with WD have bodies that retain copper. Their livers, therefore, do not release copper into the bile as it normally would. Copper collects in the liver and eventually starts destroying the organ's tissue, causing copper to be released directly into the bloodstream, making this problem a systemic concern. Copper build-up will harm the kidneys, the urinary system, and the musculoskeletal system; cause brain damage; disrupt the central nervous system; and promote liver failure and eye damage. It can also lead to death.

WD affects approximately one in 30,000 people, and its symptoms usually appear between the ages of 6 and 20 years.

According to the NIH, WD is a rare, inherited disorder that shows up in late childhood or early adolescence as acute hepatitis, liver failure, or progressive chronic liver disease in the form of chronic active hepatitis or cirrhosis of the liver. A third of those with WD will also experience psychiatric symptoms such as an abrupt personality change, bizarre and inappropriate behavior, and depression accompanied by suicidal thoughts, neurosis, or psychosis.

Signs and symptoms

Since onset is often late and since parents are most often carriers, adult as well as children's symptoms are listed:

- abnormal posture
- acute hepatitis
- anemia
- body twisting
- cirrhosis
- clumsiness

- copper excess, especially in eyes, brain, kidney, and liver
- depression
- difficulty swallowing (dysphagia)
- drooling
- fluid build-up in the lining of the abdomen
- heart problems (cardiomyopathy, dysrhythmias)
- high levels of amino acids
- impaired muscle tone
- infertility
- insomnia
- jaundice
- Kayser-Fleischer ring—this is the main diagnostic characteristic of WD. It is a rusty, brown ring around the eye's cornea. It can be observed through an eye exam.
- lack of coordination when attempting voluntary movements (ataxia)
- loss of fine motor skills
- low platelet and white blood cell count
- menstrual irregularities
- migraine headaches
- neuroses
- pancreatitis
- personality changes
- premature arthritis
- premature osteoporosis
- protein, uric acid, and carbohydrates in urine
- psychosis
- repeated miscarriages
- repetitive body movements (dystonia)
- rigid muscles
- seizures
- slowness of movements (bradykinesia)
- slurred speech
- softening of the bones
- sustained muscle contractions
- swelling of liver
- swelling of spleen
- too little parathyroid hormone that helps regulate total body calcium (hypoparathyroidism)
- tremors in the head, arms, hands, and legs
- vomiting blood
- weakening of muscles used for speaking (dysarthria)

It is very important to know that children with WD may not exhibit any signs or symptoms of being ill. But they must be treated, even if it is mild or "nonapparent" WD. Without treatment, they will die.

Cause

WD is an autosomal recessive disease, which is a genetic condition that is found in children who have received two copies—one from each parent—of a non-sex-linked chromosome. Since the parents have only one copy of the gene each, they are carriers and, therefore, do not exhibit the trait because it is recessive. In WD, carriers might have mild abnormalities of copper metabolism, and therefore not reported in family histories. With both parents as carriers, there is a one in four chance of the child's developing the disease. The gene is not sex-linked, meaning it can affect a child of any sex.

The responsible gene, ATP7B, is located on chromosome 13. While most WD cases are inherited, some are caused by spontaneous mutations in the gene.

Diagnosis

Tests are available to measure the copper levels in the blood, urine, and liver: serum ceruloplasmin test, a twenty-four-hour urine copper test, and a liver biopsy are other diagnostic tools. The child will also be tested for the presence of the Kayser-Fleischer ring through an ophthalmologic slit-lamp examination.

In a particular family, if the precise mutation is identified, a genetic diagnosis for other family members is possible by haplotype analysis. This requires a blood sample from both the patient and a relative. The samples are compared to each other. Haplotype testing helps to find symptom-free siblings who have the disease so that they may be treated before they become ill.

More than two hundred different mutations of ATP7B have been identified thus far. Therefore, it has been difficult to devise a simple genetic screening test for WD.

One in one hundred individuals in the general population carries one abnormal copy of the WD gene. All siblings and children of those with WD should be tested for the disorder. Testing is easy and safe, and the treatments are simple and effective. Failure to treat WD, however, can cause severe disabilities and death.

It is crucial to diagnose WD as early as possible, since severe liver damage can occur before there are any signs of the disease. Children with WD can very possibly appear as if they are in good health.

WD is a lifelong disorder, requiring drugs to eliminate copper from the body and arresting the continuation of copper accumulation.

Treatment

A child suspected of having WD or who has been diagnosed with WD should see a WD specialist. WD is a very treatable condition: the disease can be stopped, and the symptoms can improve.

The preferred treatment with no serious side effects is zinc salt, which blocks copper absorption in the stomach. Penicillamine and trientine, which increase urinary excretion of the copper, do have unwanted and serious side effects. Other less-toxic drugs such as tetrathiomolybdate are being researched but are not yet approved for use.

The child will most likely be put on a low-copper diet that involves avoiding mushrooms, nuts, chocolate, dried fruit, organ meats such as liver, soy, dried beans, mineral water, bran breads, shellfish, and other high-copper items.

In rare cases where there is severe liver damage from disease, a liver transplant may be needed.

The Wilson's Disease Association warns that those with WD should never completely stop treatment, stating it "will result in death, sometimes as quickly as within three months. Decreasing dosage of medications also can result in unnecessary disease progression."

Prognosis

WD requires a lifetime of treatment, but as the National Digestive Diseases Information Clearinghouse (NDDIC) reports, "If the disorder is detected early and treated correctly, a person with Wilson's disease can enjoy completely normal health."

Sources and resources

National Digestive Diseases Information Clearinghouse (www.digestive.niddk.nih.gov)
National Institutes of Health (www.nih.gov)
Wilson's Disease Association (www.wilsonsdisease.org)

WS

Williams Syndrome

Terms used in this chapter: ADHD (attention-deficit/hyperactivity disorder); FISH (fluorescence in situ hybridization); LD (learning disability); MR (mental retardation); NIH (National Institutes of Health); NINDS (National Institute of Neurological Disorders and Stroke); WS (Williams syndrome)

Sound familiar?

While Heather Flaharty was pregnant with her son Caleb, he stopped growing in the third trimester. It turned out she had IUGR (intrauterine growth restriction), and the doctors concluded that the umbilical cord was abnormal, one umbilical artery instead of the normal three. Doctors checked Caleb out extensively while still in the womb for any potential abnormalities, and they said he was fine. They induced labor, and on December 12, 1997, Caleb was born. The doctor who delivered Caleb remarked about how small the placenta was. Heather says he seemed surprised as if he had never seen that before.

Caleb, at 4 pounds, 11 ounces, would "scream loud enough to wake up the dead," Heather says. He screamed and cried continually. His whole body would tighten up as if he were in agony. She was told it was colic. "I really, in my heart, knew that it wasn't normal colic," says Heather, who already had an older son. "But I guess young mothers have a tendency to exaggerate, so, the doctor didn't take me seriously." The crying continued for months, sometimes for four or five hours on end.

Caleb made very little eye contact and was not comforted by cuddling. The only thing that would console him was very loud classical music—Mozart would always quiet him down.

As he got older, he was not reaching milestones. After several months, Heather noticed that he was not smiling or laughing. Her oldest son was born smiling. Caleb was not your typical happy baby. "It was very hard to feel a bond with him," Heather says. She felt all alone: "I could not get a baby sitter. Nobody was there to help."

The next milestone Caleb didn't reach was sitting up on his own. He could barely do that until he was about 9 months. When he did finally sit, he started to rock. He'd sit on the couch for hours, just rocking back and forth. By his first birthday, he was starting to smile, and even occasionally laugh. He started walking at 18 months. All this time, the doctor kept saying, "He will catch up. If he doesn't by the time he is 3, then we will start to worry."

"I get so mad thinking back on that nowadays," Heather says.

Caleb, always anxious, was fascinated by any toys that had music and lights. He was very disturbed by loud or out-of-the-ordinary noises and was startled by angry tones of voice or crying. He was fascinated by people's faces. He would grab someone's face and look up their nose or pry open their mouth and look inside. He would pry open their eyelids and look in their ears. "It was so strange," Heather recalls. Caleb became very social—overly social, says his mother. "Caleb would have happily gone home with a stranger and probably never missed me," she says.

At 3, he was still not meeting milestones. The doctor recommended that he be evaluated for speech therapy but was still not worried about Caleb's development. Caleb was very hyper, and visual cues to behave from adults did not affect him. He was very clumsy and would walk straight into anything that was between him and what he wanted. He was not good with spatial relationships. Caleb's teeth were soft and small and he needed anesthesia to have crowns put on. The nurse who monitored him noticed he had a heart murmur. His doctor said he would outgrow it.

When Caleb was enrolled in a typical preschool, his teachers "put up with him" for a month and then recommended he be evaluated. The evaluation indicated he was developmentally delayed by two or three years, so he was referred to a special-needs preschool.

"It was very hard for us to hear," recalls Heather, "even though we knew something wasn't right."

Caleb stayed in preschool until he was 6, during which time he was diagnosed with ADHD and put on medication. He attended a regular kindergarten, which was difficult for him. In first grade, he spent half the day in a special education class and half in a regular class. At this time, he was diagnosed with PDD–NOS (pervasive developmental disorder–not otherwise specified), an autism spectrum disorder, because of his tendency to perseverate or repeat activities as well as his having trouble with transitioning throughout the day. He also had social issues—invading others' personal space and lacking meaningful friendships.

Before second grade, he went to a new pediatrician who seemed very concerned about Caleb's small stature and delays. She referred his parents to an endocrinologist for testing—all came back fine. "I was actually shocked," says Heather. "I expected something to be wrong." The endocrinologist, however, was not satisfied and referred Heather and her husband for genetic counseling.

One day, while channel surfing, Heather watched the Medical Incredible show on the Discovery Health channel and saw a preview for a show about a woman with WS. "I got a very strange feeling," says Heather. "She looked so familiar to me. I almost passed out. She acted just like Caleb. She looked like Caleb. She had the same problems as Caleb. Problems like not being able to do simple math or tie her shoes, but having a mysterious ability for music." (Caleb has a natural ability to harmonize and can name any band or instrument when he hears them. He can play simple songs by ear on the piano and will listen to music for hours. While not every WS child has musical ability, the majority does, and it is a distinctive symptom of WS.) Heather looked the syndrome up on the Internet and found lots of children who looked and acted like Caleb.

"I knew, in my heart, that we finally had our answer."

There was a small doubt, though, because many WS children have severe heart problems as newborns and Caleb only had a murmur. The profile still fit otherwise.

Finally, the genetics appointment came around. Heather told the doctors about the television show, and they agreed. "Caleb showed off his cocktail-party personality and worked his charms on them," she says. They ended up testing him only for WS, and the test came back positive five weeks later. It was a big relief.

Caleb does not have the typical deletion of twenty-eight genes, but a smaller deletion. He was found, however, to have a heart problem after all those years. He has a mild form of aortic regurgitation. It is something to keep an eye on, but it might not have been found until it was too late if he hadn't gotten his diagnosis. Heather attributes the late diagnosis to Caleb's lack of major health problems and lack of awareness of WS on the doctors' part.

"I encourage parents to stand up for their children," says Heather. "If you feel that something is not right with your child, you are probably right. Insist on more testing. Do not give up on your child just because the doctor says, 'Don't worry.' Push for answers. I wish I had done it earlier. There are a lot of good support groups and resources no matter what your child's diagnosis is."

Caleb has WS—Williams syndrome.

Did you know?

WS is an unusual disorder in that it can cause great strengths as much as it can cause great weaknesses.

WS, which was first recognized in 1961 by New Zealand cardiologist J. C. P. Williams, M.D., is a rare genetic disorder distinguished by its specific "pixie-like" facial appearance, which becomes more prominent with age. As the child develops, mild-to-moderate MR or LDs, overfriendliness, and elevated anxiety and empathy are manifested. The disorder, which equally affects males and females, is estimated by the Williams Syndrome Association (WSA) to occur in one in 7,500 births and can be determined at birth. However, many of the symptoms and signs of WS may not be apparent at birth.

Many children with WS exhibit autistic behaviors, including language delays, repetitive behavior (perseverating), gross motor skill problems, hypersensitivity to sounds, and food pickiness. Aside from distinctive physical abnormalities, what differentiates WS kids from autistic children is the high level of sociability these children exhibit. It is also believed that 75 percent of WS children will be diagnosed with some degree of MR.

The sensory issues that affect these children cause many WS kids to be hypersensitive to sound (hyperacusis), with particular frequencies or sound levels becoming painful, or at least uncomfortable, to the child. They also suffer from tactile defensiveness, by being hypersensitive to touch. These sensory conditions often diminish with age.

There are several physical problems that are common to WS children. Cardiovascular disease, caused by the narrowing of arteries, is the most significant medical problem. One of the twenty-five genes that are missing from the 7 chromosome in WS children is the gene that produces elastin, a protein that gives elasticity to blood vessels and other tissues in the body. It is believed that possessing only a single copy of this gene causes blood vessels to narrow.

There are several complications associated with WS that can be life-threatening:

- Blood vessel narrowing can cause heart failure.
- Elevated calcium can lead to calcium deposits in the kidney and other kidney problems.
- There have been rare cases of children with WS having complications, including death, with anesthesia.

These children are confusing to those not familiar with WS because they have abilities that range from MR to giftedness.

Signs and symptoms

- ADHD
- affinity for music
- almond-shaped eyes

- blood vessel narrowing as child gets older
- colic and irritability in infancy
- curvature of the spine
- dental abnormalities
- developmental delay
- distinctive pixie-like facial appearance
- elevated blood calcium levels (hypercalcemia)
- excellent long-term memory
- excellent memory for faces
- excellent vocabulary
- excessively social personality
- extra skin fold of the upper eyelid covering the inner corner of the eye (epicanthic fold)
- far-sightedness
- feeding problems
- flattened nasal bridge
- full lips and open mouth
- hearing loss in late childhood
- heart problems
- high blood pressure as child gets older
- heightened blood calcium levels (hypercalcemia)
- hernias
- initially delayed speech
- inward bend of the pinky (clinodactyly)
- kidney abnormalities
- LDs
- learning-by-hearing strength
- limited joint mobility (joint laxity)
- long midline from upper lip margin to lower nose (philtrum)
- long neck
- low birth weight and gain
- low muscle tone
- mild-to-moderate MR
- muscle rigidity
- narrow face
- narrowing in the aorta
- narrowing of pulmonary arteries
- oval ears
- partial absence of teeth
- poor fine motor skills

- poor suck and swallow abilities when eating
- poor tooth enamel
- puffiness around eyes
- reflux
- seizures
- sensitive hearing (hyperacusis)
- severe gag reflex
- short stature relative to family
- sloping shoulders
- small chin
- small upturned nose
- specific phobias
- sunken chest
- tactile sensitivity and defensiveness
- talkativeness
- unusually compassionate
- visual-spatial disability
- vomiting
- white, lacy, star-like pattern on iris of blue- and green-eyed children
- wide mouth
- widely spaced teeth

Cause

WS occurs when a portion of DNA material on chromosome 7 is randomly missing. Twenty-five genes are missing on the chromosome. It is not necessarily inherited, however, but, according to the NINDS, individuals who have WS have a 50 percent chance of passing it on if they decide to have children.

The NINDS reports the following:

NINDS and the NIH have funded many of the research studies exploring the genetic and neurobiological origins of WS. In the early 1990s, researchers located and identified the genetic mutation responsible for the disorder: the deletion of a small section of chromosome 7 that contains approximately 25 genes. NINDS continues to support WS researchers including, for example, groups that are attempting to link specific genes with the corresponding facial, cognitive, personality, and neurological characteristics of WS.

Diagnosis

Early indications of WS include the child's pixie-like appearance, elevated calcium level in the infant's blood, and observation of a narrowed aorta.

The blood test for the Williams chromosome deletion is called a FISH test. The genetic defect is found in 99 percent of Williams patients. The FISH test is comprised of a blood sample treated with two specific colored markers that give off a "fluorescent" light when exposed to ultraviolet light. The Williams Syndrome Foundation (WSF) explains how WS is then determined:

> One of the markers attaches to each of the two copies of chromosome number seven in a cell. When both copies of chromosome possess the elastin gene, an additional fluorescence of another color is seen attached at another location to each of the two chromosome 7s. But, as is the case in more than 95 percent of the WS children tested, only one copy of chromosome 7, not two, will show the fluorescent spot for the elastin gene. If the FISH test shows the elastin gene to be missing from one copy of chromosome 7, then the individual tested can be diagnosed with WS.

Treatment

There is no single type of treatment for this syndrome. One aspect of WS, however, is its physical nature and that needs constant monitoring. The child's cardiovascular health should always be under medical scrutiny. Seventy-five percent of WS kids have a mild-to-severe heart condition. In regard to the hypercalcemia and the overabundance of blood calcium, supplemental calcium and vitamin D should be avoided.

It is recommended by most WS experts that all treatment be coordinated with a geneticist who is experienced with WS.

There are several tests that are needed for proper ongoing health of WS children:

- echocardiography with Doppler (for showing blood vessel narrowing)
- kidney ultrasound (for potential renal abnormalities)
- periodic blood pressure checks

As with most disorders, early intervention at home and at school that includes teaching self-help skills increases the likelihood of a successful independent or semi-independent life.

Different types of therapy are helpful: Music therapy, physical therapy (particularly for joint stiffness), and speech therapy can help. Even though WS children have strong speech abilities, a speech therapist can help a WS child exploit his or her verbal strengths to help compensate for other deficiencies.

Music therapy is perhaps one of the most important aspects of working with WS children. Often regarded as savants, WS children have a great affinity and a natural talent for music.

Brendan A. Maher, Ph.D., in the November 26, 2001, issue of *The Scientist*, pointed out that "while their [children with WS] attention span for many tasks is fleeting, they will spend hours listening to or making music. Research is scarce, but some evidence shows a high incidence of perfect pitch, and an uncanny sense of rhythm among this group. One boy with Williams syndrome was taught to tap a complicated 7/4-time rhythm with one hand while keeping 4/4-time with the other."

Parents of WS children will notice dental irregularities that are symptomatic of WS: somewhat small, widely spaced teeth, bite (occlusion) deviations, and abnormal tooth appearance and shape. Nowadays these problems can be resolved by cosmetic and orthodontic corrections.

Groin (inguinal) and umbilical hernias are common, and the kidneys are affected both structurally and functionally. WS children commonly have low muscle tone and joint laxity or immobility. As the children get older, they might be prone to stiffness of their joints but can easily be rehabilitated through physical and occupational therapy and build their strength, muscle tone, and joint range of motion.

Prognosis

WS has no cure. The prognosis for individuals with WS varies, and, depending on the severity of the disorder, functionality has a wide range. While some WS adults live independent lives, enjoying successful academic experiences and finishing high school, vocational school, or college, the majority do not live independent of caregivers, often in supervised group homes. The lifespan of individuals with WS depends on their medical status and specific difficulties and complications linked with the disorder, but, because of the heart abnormalities, the life span is usually shortened.

As mentioned earlier, the hypersensitivity diminishes with age.

Sources and resources

Brendan A. Maher, "A Flood in Genomics," *The Scientist*, Nov. 25, 2001, 1.
National Heart, Lung, and Blood Institute (NHLBI) (800-575-WELL [9355]);
    (www.nhlbi.nih.gov)
National Institute of Neurological Disorders and Stroke (www.ninds.nih.gov)
Williams Syndrome Association (248-244-2229); (www.williams-syndrome.org)
Williams Syndrome Foundation (949-824-7259); (www.wsf.org)

XXYS (XXY Syndrome)

XXYS

XXY Syndrome

Terms used in this chapter: APD (auditory processing disorder); IEP (individualized education program); LD (learning disability); XXYS (XXY syndrome)

Sound familiar?

For 33-year-old Illinois IT consultant Christopher Jon Olesch, growing up was not easy; he had many physical and mental challenges. He was tired all the time, but everyone close to him figured it was caused by bad eyesight. When he was 5, he was considered legally blind. As he got older, his vision worsened. Even today, he can't keep up with his vision changes, due mainly to cost—he hasn't seen his eye doctor in four years.

His next biggest struggle was with hearing. He had a constant ringing in his ears that he just couldn't alleviate. He remembers saying when he was younger that he heard the "noise my brain makes" when he plugged his ears.

It's hard to say which of his symptoms was the worst, he says, because "all of them played a role." He has communication difficulties (which he says "are similar to a form of mild autism") that he imagines would have been easier to deal with had they been corrected at a younger age. Suffering from APD, sometimes he doesn't process exactly what others say, so it's difficult for him to have conversations. He has "learned to deal with only understanding 30–50 percent of everything, and then just nodding and agreeing."

As Chris got older, his symptoms worsened still. Doctors kept treating the symptoms rather than trying to figure out the cause.

"Psychologically it was very difficult for me," he recalls. "I was a little confused until about puberty. My parents thought I would turn out gay because, as I got older, I lost all interest sexually."

When Chris reached adulthood, his symptoms continued to worsen. He was unable to exercise because he found it too exhausting. His mother sent him to several psychiatrists because his emotional state see-sawed. The psychiatrists continued to treat the symptoms, which seemed to make things worse. It wasn't until he turned 30 that he went to his doctor and asked for a testosterone test. "When I got the results," he recalls, "I scored so low even my doctor was amazed I was still walking about." His testosterone level was a 41—the average is 450–800.

After he started on a daily regime of testosterone, most of his symptoms subsided. He even began to grow some body hair for the first time.

He's currently struggling with arthritis, degenerative spine problems, and weight issues that vary with the amount of testosterone the doctors supply. He says he was "beginning to feel human again," when he was on a higher dose of testosterone, but it was lowered by half and he regressed. "If I could just find a doctor that understands [my disorder], I think I could get back on track."

In 2004, Chris was diagnosed with gynecomastia or pronounced breast development.

Chris' symptoms now include APD; poor concentration; arthritis in his hips, spine, and knee; occasional loss of feeling in his left leg; extreme migraines; insomnia at night and tiredness all day; and mild narcolepsy. Except for two minor symptoms, which occur in infancy that he doesn't recall, Chris has every symptom listed below in "Signs and symptoms."

Chris, who recently married, says, "I wish there was more awareness in the medical field about [XXYS] and what sort of crap untreated adults have to put up with."

Chris has XXYS—XXY syndrome.

Did you know?

XXYS or KS (Klinefelter's syndrome), named for Harry Klinefelter, M.D., an endocrinologist at Massachusetts General Hospital in Boston, Massachusetts, who first described the disorder in 1942, is a disorder that affects males who have an extra X chromosome in most of their cells. Instead of having the typical male XY chromosomal pattern, they have XXY. The National Institute of Child Health and Human Development (NICHD) reports that about one of every five hundred males has an extra X chromosome, but many don't have any symptoms. Scientists believe the XXY condition is one of the most common chromosome abnormalities in humans.

XXYS affects all phases of typical development: these children have difficulty with expressive language; socially, they tend to be shy and have trouble relating to their peers; physically, they are less muscular and have less facial body hair. This is all due to their deficiency in making testosterone. They also have breast development in puberty, which sometimes disappears in time.

It is important to start treatment as early as possible because, with treatment, including psychological therapy, most XXYS boys lead normal lives.

Signs and symptoms

- academic problems
- auditory processing problems
- breast development (gynecomastia)
- broad hips
- decreased auditory recall
- defiant or rebellious
- delayed speech
- ear infections
- helpful attitude
- increased risk for autoimmune disease such as type I (insulin dependent) diabetes, autoimmune thyroiditis, and lupus erythematosus

- infertility in almost all cases
- LDs
- little facial and body hair
- low energy level
- low self-confidence
- obedient
- overweight
- poor coordination
- poor gross motor skills
- poor memory
- quiet demeanor
- reading problems
- reduced strength
- rounded body type
- sit up, crawl, and walk later than other infants
- small testes
- speech-language deficits, including poor expressive speech
- taller than males in their family and taller than peers, after age 4
- trouble "fitting in" with other boys
- undemanding as baby
- weak bones
- weak muscles
- writing disabilities

Cause

The cause of the syndrome is the extra X chromosome, but the reason that occurs is open to debate. As with most other Alphabet Disorders, no one can really determine a specific cause. While advanced maternal age increases the risk for XXYS, it is not the primary cause as has been believed—50 percent of the time, it has been determined that the extra chromosome comes from the father. XXYS, caused by chromosomal mutations, is not considered an inherited disorder.

Diagnosis

If there is a reason to test because of family history or age of parents, XXYS can now be diagnosed before birth, through amniocentesis (sampling fluid surrounding the fetus) or chorionic villus sampling (CVS), which is conducted in the first trimester, testing cells taken from the placenta. Another test is the karyotype, where a small blood sample is taken, a chromosomal test is conducted, and a genetic map is created.

Treatment

XXYS kids can benefit from many educational modifications and services through an IEP to help their LDs and speech problems. Speech-language therapy and services are most important. These boys are often visual learners, so using visual cues is often the course of therapy. Academic modifications such as providing notes and taking multiple-choice tests (not writing essays or taking open-ended tests) can help XXYS boys succeed academically and, in turn, feel better about themselves not only in an academic setting, but in general. Physical, occupational, and psychological therapies can also greatly benefit the XXYS child. Physical education modifications might also be required.

There are also medical treatments, particularly testosterone replacement therapy (TRT), which usually starts around puberty and can come close to normalizing the symptoms of XXYS. Testosterone can not only help the child attain more masculine features, but it also adds to the general strength and health of the child. Breast reduction surgery is an alternative for those who need it.

Prognosis

The prognosis is good for children with XXYS if there is early detection, intervention, and proper treatment. Symptoms such as speech-language and LDs must be addressed, but it is also very important to have the proper psychological counseling. Some older research has shown high incidences of psychological disturbance for XXYS boys, but those statistics are in question because of the population studies from which they were derived. There are many illnesses that are associated with this disorder including type I diabetes, breast cancer, lupus and non-Hodgkin's lymphoma, COPD (chronic obstructive pulmonary disease), and others, so medical vigilance is very important. Supplementing testosterone can be a life-changing treatment for those with XXYS.

Sources and resources

47XXY (www.47xxy.com)

American Association for Klinefelter Syndrome Information and Support (AAKSIS) (888-466-KSIS [5747]); (www.aaksis.org)

Klinefelter Organisation (www.klinefelter.org.uk)

Klinefelter Syndrome Support Group (www.Klinefeltersyndrome.org)

National Institute of Child Health and Human Development (www.nichd.nih.gov)

Z

ZS (Zellweger Syndrome)

Z

ZS

Zellweger Syndrome

Terms used in this chapter: MR (mental retardation); ZS (Zellweger syndrome)

Did you know?

Named after Hans Zellweger, M.D., a Swiss-American pediatrician, ZS is a rare, congenital disorder that affects infants. This metabolic syndrome affects the body's major organs—brain, kidneys, and liver—because there is a reduction or complete absence of peroxisomes, the cell structures that clear the body of toxic substances in those organs.

ZS is one of four related diseases called PBDs (peroxisome biogenesis disorders), which are included in a group of inherited diseases called leukodystrophies, which damage the brain's white matter and also affect metabolism in the blood and organ tissues. The four PBDs include ZS, the most severe; NALD (neonatal adrenoleukodystrophy); RMCD (rhizomelic chondrodysplasia); and IRD (infantile refsum disease), which is the mildest of the group.

Because the toxins are unable to be broken down, iron and copper begin to build up in the blood and tissue, causing the severe problems associated with this syndrome.

Present at birth, ZS is estimated to occur in one out of 50,000 to 100,000 births, affecting males and females equally. ZS is an autosomal recessive defect, which means the defective gene was passed on by both parents and that each future child has a 25 percent chance of being born with the syndrome.

Signs and symptoms

- asymmetrical ears
- bone defects in hand, legs, and feet
- calcification of the kneecaps (patella)
- cataracts
- cysts in kidneys and brain
- deformed ear lobes
- dilation of renal pelvis and obstruction of urine flow (hydronephrosis)
- distinctive facial deformities
- enlarged liver
- excess neck skin folds
- extra crease or fold in eyelids (epicanthic fold)
- flat-looking face

- gastrointestinal bleeding
- glaucoma
- hearing problems
- heart defects
- high forehead
- high levels of iron and copper in blood
- inability to move
- inability to suck or swallow
- jaundice
- lack of muscle tone (hypotonia)
- large anterior soft spot (fontanelle)
- low and broad nasal bridge
- MR
- narrow ribcage
- prenatal growth failure
- reduced or absent reflexes
- respiratory distress
- retinal degeneration
- seizures
- shallow ridges beneath the eyebrow
- small lower jaw (micrognathia)
- underdeveloped brain
- underdeveloped eyebrow ridges
- vision problems, including blindness

Cause

The metabolic and neurological abnormalities that cause ZS's symptoms occur during fetal development, due to mutations in the PXR1 gene, which has been mapped to chromosome 12. ZS and its sister disorders are caused by genetic defects in brain development and the formation of myelin, the white brain matter found in the cerebral cortex, which coats and insulates nerves, aiding in the conduction of data between the brain and other parts of the body. The syndrome is characterized by the child's inability to break down fatty acids into simple compounds.

Diagnosis

Usually it is the distinctive shape of the head and face that provides a clue to this disorder. Since ZS causes the build-up of very-long-chain fatty acids (VLCFAs), a test for VLCFA can be performed to confirm the ZS diagnosis, along with other genetic testing.

Treatment

There is no one particular course of treatment for children with this disorder. Because the genetic damage occurred during the fetal stage, it is too late to prevent the many problems associated with the disorder, so most of the treatments involve dealing with easing ZS's symptoms.

ZS children are susceptible to life-threatening respiratory problems, so there should be constant vigilance to prevent pneumonia and other respiratory distress.

Other dysfunctions such as feeding problems, liver dysfunction (through bile acid treatments), and seizures (through antiseizure medication) can also be addressed. There are also children with ZS who live long enough to benefit from occupational, speech, and physical therapies.

Prognosis

ZS has no cure. There is not a very good prognosis for ZS—with its survival rate of a year and usually not beyond six months, due to the main symptoms of gastrointestinal bleeding, liver failure, or respiratory distress. There are some children, however, who have lived well beyond the usual six-month period.

Sources and resources

United Leukodystrophy Foundation (800-728-5483); (www.ulf.org)
Zellweger Baby Support Network (www.zbsn.org)

Resources

General resources

A

Academic Alliance Foundation/Healthcare for Africa (703-294-6551); (www.academicalliancefoundation.org)

Academy of Cognitive Therapy (ACT) (610-664-1273); (www.academyofct.org)

Advocates for Children's Health Affected by Mercury Poisoning (A-CHAMP) (www.a-champ.org)

Alexander Graham Bell Association for the Deaf (www.agbell.org)

Alliance for Technology Access (707-778-3011); (www.ataccess.org)

Alphabet Disorders Association (www.alphabetdisorders.com)

American Academy of Audiology (800-AAA-2336); (www.audiology.com)

American Academy of Child and Adolescent Psychiatry (AACAP) (202-966-7300); (www.aacap.org)

American Association for Pediatric Ophthalmology and Strabismus (www.aapos.org)

American Association of People with Disabilities (800-840-8844); (www.aapd-dc.gov)

American Council of the Blind (www.acb.org)

American Foundation for the Blind (www.afb.org/afb)

American Lung Association (800-548-8252; 800-LUNGUSA); (www.lungusa.org)

American Pregnancy Association (972-550-0140); (www.americanpregnancy.org)

American Psychiatric Association (APA) (888-357-7924); (www.psych.org)

American Speech-Language-Hearing Association (800-638-8255); (www.asha.org)

Americans with Disabilities Act Information and Technical Assistance (www.ada.gov)

APD-UK (www.apduk.gov)

Aphasia Hope Foundation (www.aphasiahope.org)

The Arc (national organization on mental retardation) (301-565-3842; 800-433-5255); (www.thearc.org)

The Association for People with Severe Handicaps (TASH) (www.tash.org)

Australian Association of Special Education (AASE) (www.aase.edu.au)

C

Centers for Disease Control and Prevention (CDC) (404-498-1515; 800-311-3435); (www.cdc.gov)

Child & Adolescent Health Measurement Initiative (www.cahmi.org)

Children's Defense Fund (www.childrensdefense.org)

Children's Eye Foundation (817-891-1144); (www.childrenseyefoundation.org)

Children's Hospital Boston (617-355-6000); (www.childrenshospital.org)
Chromosome Disorder Outreach, Inc. (561-395-4252); (www.chromodisorder.org)
Council for Exceptional Children (www.cec.sped.org)
Andrew Cuddy, *The Special Education Battlefield: A Guide to the Due Process Hearing and Other Tools of Effective Advocacy* (Ithaca, NY: Ithaca Press, 2007).

D

Data Resource Center for Child & Adolescent Health (www.childhealthdata.org)
Depression and Bipolar Support Alliance (800-826-3632); (www.dbsalliance.org)

E

Early Intervention Program: A Parent's Guide for Children with Special Needs—New York State Department of Health (www.health.state.ny.us/nysdoh/eip/index.htm)
Easter Seals (312-726-6200; 800-221-6827); (www.easterseals.com)
Educational Audiology Association (EAA); (800-460-7322); (www.edaud.org)
Epilepsy Foundation (800-332-100); (www.epilepsyfoundation.org)

F

Family Village (www.familyvillage.wisc.edu)
Family Voices (506-872-4774); (www.familyvoices.org)
Federation for Children with Special Needs (617-236-7210); (www.fcsn.org)
Fetal Alcohol Spectrum Disorders (www.fasdcenter.samhsa.gov)

G

The Genetic Alliance (www.geneticalliance.org)
Genetics Home Reference (www.ghr.nlm.nih.gov)
Grassroots Environmental Education (516-883-0887); (www.grassrootsinfo.org)

H

Helen Keller International (212-532-0544; 877-535-5374); (www.hki.org)

I

Independent Panel for Special Education Advice (IPSEA)/UK (www.ipsea.org.uk)
Individuals with Disabilities Education Act (IDEA) Homepage (www.ada.gov)
International Birth Defects Information Systems (www.ibis-birthdefects.org)
Internet Mental Health (www.mentalhealth.com)
Internet Special Education Resources (ISER) (www.iser.com)

J

Johns Hopkins Medicine (www.hopkinsmedicine.org)

K

Kindergarten Interventions and Diagnostic Services (KIDS), Inc. (940-497-5437; 800-594-4649); (www.kidsinc.com)

L

Learning Disabilities Association of America (412-341-1515); (www.ldaamerica.org)

M

March of Dimes Foundation (888-663-4637); (www.marchofdimes.com)

Maternal and Child Health Information Resource Center (MCHIRC) (www.mchb.hrsa.gov/mchirc/chusa)

Mayo Clinic (480-301-8000); (www.mayoclinic.com)

Med Help International (www.medhelp.org)

Mental Health Resources (www.mentalhealth.about.com)

Muscular Dystrophy Association (www.mda.org)

N

NASEN (National Association for Special Educational Needs)/U.K. (www.nasen.org.uk)

National Alliance on Mental Illness (NAMI) (800-950-6264); (www.nami.org)

National Aphasia Association (www.aphasia.org)

National Association for Parents of Children with Visual Impairments (NAPVI) (www.spedex.com/napvi)

National Association for the Visually Handicapped (www.navh.org)

National Association of Cognitive-Behavioral Therapists (NACBT) (www.nacbt.org)

National Association of the Deaf (www.nad.org)

National Braille Press (www.nbp.org)

National Center for Biotechnology Information (www.ncbi.nlm.nih.gov)

National Center for Environmental Health (www.cdc.gov/nceh)

National Center for Gender Issues and ADHD (www.ncgiadd.org)

National Center for Learning Disabilities (212-545-7510; 888-575-7373); (www.ld.org)

National Center on Birth Defects and Developmental Disabilities (NCBDDD) (www.cdc.gov/ncbddd)

National Clearinghouse on Post-secondary Education for Individuals with Disabilities (Heath Resource Center) (www.heath.gwu.edu)

National Dissemination Center for Children with Disabilities (NICHCY) U.S. Dept. of Education, Office of Special Education Programs (800-695-0285); (www.nichcy.org)

National Heart, Lung, and Blood Institute (NHLBI) (301-592-8573);
    (www.nhlbi.nih.gov)
National Information Centre for Metabolic Diseases (Children Living with Inherited
    Metabolic Diseases/CLIMB) (www.climb.org.uk)
National Institute of Arthritis and Musculoskeletal and Skin Diseases (NIAMS)
    (301-495-4484; 877-226-4267); (www.niams.nih.gov)
National Institute of Child Health and Human Development (NICHD)
    (800-370-2943); (www.nichd.nih.gov)
National Institute of Environmental Health Sciences (NIEHS) (www.niehs.nih.gov)
National Institute of Mental Health (NIMH) (301-443-4513; 866-615-6464);
    (www.nimh.nih.gov)
National Institute of Neurological Disorders and Stroke (NINDS) (800-352-9424);
    (www.ninds.nih.gov)
National Institute on Deafness and Other Communication Disorders (NIDCD)
    (800-241-1044); (www.nidcd.nih.gov)
National Institutes of Health (301-496-4000; 301-402-9612); (www.nih.gov)
National Kidney Foundation (212-889-2210; 800-622-9010); (www.kidney.org)
National Mental Health Association (NMHA) (703-684-7722; 800-969-6642)
    (www.nmha.org)
National Organization for Rare Disorders (NORD) (203-744-0100; 800-999-6673);
    (www.rarediseases.org)
National Society of Genetic Counselors (312-321-6834); (www.nsgc.org)
Nemours Foundation (www.nemours.org)
New Horizons Un-Limited (414-299-0124); (www.new-horizons.org)
NYU Child Study Center (www. aboutourkids.org)

O

Optometrists Network (www.strabismus.org)

P

Pediatric Neurology.com (www.pediatricneurology.com)

R

Resources for Children with Special Needs, Inc. (www.resourcesnyc.org)

S

Scottish Rite Foundation/RiteCare Childhood Language Program (for children with
    communication disorders) (202-232-3579); (www.scottishrite.org)
Society for Deaf Children (866-895-4206; 800-942-2732); (www.deafchildren.org)
Special Educational Needs Legal Services (www.senlegal.co.uk)

Stanford University School of Medicine (http://med.stanford.edu)

Substance Abuse and Mental Health Services Administration (www.mentalhealth.samhsa.gov)

T

The Association for People with Severe Handicaps (TASH) (www.tash.org)

U

United Cerebral Palsy (800-872-5827; 202-776-0406); (www.ucp.org)

United Nations International Children's Emergency Fund (UNICEF) (www.unicef.org)

U.S. Department of Education (www.ed.gov)

U.S. Food and Drug Administration (FDA) (888-463-6332); (www.fda.gov)

U.S. Office of Special Education and Rehabilitative Services (OSERS) (202-245-7468); (www.ed.gov/about/offices/list/osers/index.html)

W

WE MOVE (movement disorders) (www.wemove.org)

World Craniofacial Foundation (972-566-6669; 800-533-3315); (www.worldcf.org)

World Health Organization (WHO) (www.who.int)

Y

YOUR DAY AWAY (www.yourdayaway.com) Organization for parents and guardians of children with special needs

Specialty resources

Autism

Action for Autism/India (www.Autism-India.org)

Alphabet Disorders Association (www.alphabetdisorders.com)

American Speech-Language-Hearing Association (ASHA) (800-638-8255); (www.asha.org)

Autism Africa (www.autismafrica.com)

Autism Canada Foundation (519-695-5858); (www.autismCanada.org)

Autism Europe (www.autismeurope.org)

Autism Independent UK (www.autismuk.com)

Autism Info Australia (www.autisminfo.org.au)

Autism International Foundation (www.autisminternationalfoundation.org)

Autism Key (www.autismkey.com)

Autism National Committee (AUTCOM) (www.autcom.org)

Autism Network International (ANI) (http://ani.autistics.org)

Autism–PDD Support Network (www.autism-pdd.net)

Autism Research Institute (ARI) (619-281-7165); (www.autism/index.com.asp)

Autism Resources (www.Autism-Resources.com)

Autism Society Canada (613-789-8943; 866-476-8440);
    (www.autismsocietycanada.ca)

Autism Society of America (301-657-0881; 800-328-8476); (www.autism-society.org)

Autism South Africa (www.autismsouthafrica.org)

Autism Speaks (212-252-8584); (www.autismspeaks.org)

Autism Spectrum Australia (ASPECT) (www.aspect.org.au)

Autism United (516-933-4050); (www.autismunited.org)

CDC Act Early Report (www.cdc.gov/actearly)

Center for Autism and Related Disabilities (University of Central Florida)
    (www.ucf-card.org)

First Signs (www.firstsigns.org)

Future horizons (www.Fhautism.com)

Lebanese Autism Society (www.autismlebanon.org)

MAAP Services for Autism, Asperger's, and PDD (219-662-1311);
    (www.maapservices.org)

National Autistic Society/U.K. (www.nas.org.uk)

National Institute on Deafness and Other Communication Disorders Information
    Clearinghouse (800-241-1044); (www.nidcd.nih.gov)

O.A.S.I.S. Online Asperger Syndrome Information and Support
    (www.udel.edu/bkirby/asperger)

Spectrum Magazine (www.spectrumpublications.com)

Eating disorders

Academy for Eating Disorders (AED) (847-498-4274); (www.aedweb.org)

Alliance for Eating Disorders Awareness (www.eatingdisorderinfo.org)

American Dietetic Association (www.eatright.org)

Anorexia Nervosa and Related Eating Disorders, Inc. (www.anred.com)

Asociacion Civil de Lucha Contra Desordenes Alimentarios (en español)
    (www.alda.org)

AWARE Foundation (www.awarefoundation.org)

Center for the Study of Anorexia and Bulimia (212-333-3444);
    (www.icpnyc.org/CenterForStudy.nxg)

Dads and Daughters (www.dadsanddaughters.org)

The Dressing Room Project (828-318-4438); (www.thedressingroomproject.org)

Eating Disorder Referral and Information Center (www.edreferral.com)

Eating Disorder Research Program, University of Minnesota (612-627-4494);
    (www.med.umn.edu/psychiatry/research/eatingdisorders/home)

The Eating Disorders Action Group/Halifax, NS (902-443-9944); (www.edag.ca)

Eating Disorders Anonymous (www.eatingdisordersanonymous.org)

Eating Disorders Association, Ireland (www.bodywhys.ie)

Eating Disorders Association (UK) (www.b-eat.co.uk)

Eating Disorders Association of WA (Western Australia)
  (www.healthyplace.com/Communities/eating_Disorders)

Eating Disorders Coalition (www.eatingdisorderscoalition.org)

The Elisa Project (214-369-5222); (www.theelisaproject.org)

Healing Connections, Inc. (www.healingconnections.org)

Jessie's Wish (804-378-3032); (www.jessieswish.org)

International Association of Eating Disorders Professionals (IAEDP) (www.iaedp.com)

Marino Therapy Centre, Dublin (marinotherapycentre@gmail.com)

National Association of Anorexia Nervosa and Associated Disorders (ANAD)
  (847-831-3438); (www.anad.org)

National Eating Disorders Association (NEDA) (800-931-2237);
  (www.nationaleatingdisorders.org)

National Eating Disorders Screening Program (NEDSP)
  (www.mentalhealthscreening.org)

Overeaters Anonymous (www.overeatersanonymous.org)

Somerset and Wessex Eating Disorders Association (www.swedauk.org)

Something Fishy (www.something-fishy.org)

Weight-control Information Network (877-946-4627); (www.win.niddk.nih.gov)

WINS (We Insist on Natural Shapes) (800-600-WINS)

Learning disabilities

British Dyslexia Association (0118 966 2677); (www.bdadyslexia.org.uk)

Canadian Dyslexia Association (613-722-2699); (www.dyslexiaassociation.ca)

Dyscalculia Centre (www.dyscalculia.me.uk)

dyscalculiaforum.com (www.dyscalculiaforum.com)

Dyscalculia.org (www.dyscalculia.org)

Dyslexia Teacher (www.dyslexia-teacher.com)

International Dyslexia Association (410-296-0232; 800-ABCD-123);
  (www.interdys.org)

Learning Disabilities Association of America (412-341-1515); (www.ldaamerica.org)

Learning Disabilities Worldwide (www.ldworldwide.org)

National Center for Learning Disabilities (888-575-7373); (www.ld.org)

National Joint Committee on Learning Disabilities (www.ldonline.org)

The Nemours Foundation (www.nemours.org)

NLD Online (831-624-3542); (www.nldline.com)

Nonverbal Learning Disorders Association (860-658-5522); (www.nlda.org)

Recording for the Blind & Dyslexic (Audio Services) (212-557-5720);
  (www.rfbd.org/New_York.htm)

Schwab Foundation for Learning (800-230-0988); (www.schwablearning.org)

Index